MW01286425

Books by Paul Brodeur

Fiction

The Sick Fox
The Stunt Man
Downstream

Nonfiction

Asbestos and Enzymes
Expendable Americans
The Zapping of America

The
Zapping
of America

Paul Brodeur

W · W · Norton & Company · Inc ·

New York

The
Zapping
of America

Microwaves, Their Deadly Risk, and the Cover-Up

First Edition

Grateful acknowledgment is made for permission to quote from the following: EMP
Radiation & Protective Techniques, by L. W. Picketts et al. (1976), reprinted by
permission of John Wiley & Sons, Inc.

Library of Congress Cataloging in Publication Data

Brodeur, Paul.
    The zapping of America.

    "Part of this book appeared originally as a series of articles in *The New Yorker.*"
    Includes index.
    1. Microwaves—Hygienic aspects—United States.
2. Microwaves—Environmental aspects—United States.
3. Microwaves—Physiological effect.   I.   Title.
RA569.3.B76   612'.01448'1   77–12787

                    ISBN 0-393-06427-1

            1 2 3 4 5 6 7 8 9 0

TO
Adrienne
AND
Stephen

Part of this book appeared originally as a series of articles in *The New Yorker*, in slightly different form.

Contents

	Acknowledgments	xiii
1	From Radio to Radar	1
2	Early Warning	16
3	The Cover-Up Begins	32
4	The Human Factor	42
5	The Cataract Connection	54
6	Some Illumination	72
7	An Unhealthful Post	95
8	Exaggerated Reactions	107
9	Project Pandora Revisited	116
10	The Cancer Connection	125
11	The Genetic Time Bomb	132
12	Irretrievably Messed Up	153
13	An Aggressive Study	164
14	Well Aware of the Hazards	179
15	The Tip of the Iceberg	188

16 | Some Intense Exposures   198
17 | Some Poor TV Reception   212
18 | The "Golf Ball"   219
19 | The Money Trail   230
20 | Some Further Unraveling   250
21 | A New Game of Gap   265
22 | Seafarer   280
23 | Some Loose Ends   286
24 | The Mind-Control Connection   293
25 | The Zapping of America   302
     Epilogue   319
     References   327
     Index   333

ACKNOWLEDGMENTS

The author wishes to express his appreciation to William Shawn, the editor of *The New Yorker,* who provided him with the idea for this project; to Charles Patrick Crow, of *The New Yorker,* who edited the part of the book that appeared in the magazine; to Edwin Barber, of W. W. Norton, who edited the book; to Anne Mortimer-Maddox, who helped with the research; to Barton Reppert, of the Associated Press, who first investigated the Moscow Embassy Affair; and to the hundred or so concerned people within and without the government, who came forward with the information, assistance, and advice which made the rest of this book possible.

The
Zapping
of America

1

From Radio
to Radar

Back in 1891, when electric lights were first installed in the White House, President and Mrs. Benjamin Harrison, like many other Americans, were reluctant to turn them on or off for fear of getting shocks. In fact, they always had someone else do it for them. Presidential anxiety about electric switches disappeared during the second term of Grover Cleveland, presumably because flipping them produced no demonstrably adverse effects upon members of the presidential staff, and by 1900—after a decade of scientific discoveries that included X-rays, radio waves, radioactivity, and the electron—no one in the White House, from President McKinley on down, had the slightest qualm about operating one of Thomas Alva Edison's incandescent lamps. By then, Edison was being rivaled for position of wizzard of the age by the Italian electrical engineer and entrepreneur Guglielmo Marconi, the inventor of long-distance wireless telegraphy and the pioneer in its use for ship-to-shore communication, who had already sent messages across the English Channel and would cap a series of spectacular accomplishments by announcing, in December

1901, that the letter "s" had been transmitted in Morse code from Poldhu, Cornwall, to St. John's, Newfoundland.

Wireless telegraphy—the use of electromagnetic waves to transmit telegraph signals through space—had first been proposed in 1892 by Sir William Crookes, an English publisher and experimenter, and had first been demonstrated in 1894, initially over a distance of a hundred yards, and then over a distance of half a mile, by the English physicist Sir Oliver Joseph Lodge. In 1895, Wilhelm Conrad Roentgen, a German physicist at the University of Würzburg, discovered X-rays (a discovery that is often said to mark the beginning of modern physics), and these two breakthroughs constituted the first harnessing of electromagnetic radiation—radiant energy in the form of invisible waves moving through space or matter. The existence of electromagnetic radiation had been predicted in 1864 by James Clerk Maxwell, the director of the Cavendish Laboratory, at Cambridge University. Maxwell had concluded that electromagnetic radiation consisted of electric and magnetic fields moving together, that such radiation could be produced by electric charges in motion, and that they traveled in much the same manner as water waves. He also concluded that they traveled at the speed of light, and that light was therefore a visible form of electromagnetic radiation, which differed from other forms only in wavelength—the distance between corresponding points of two consecutive waves—and in frequency of vibration, expressed as the number of waves that pass a given point in a second.

Maxwell's brilliant postulations were not accepted by the scientific community until 1888, when a German physicist named Heinrich Rudolph Hertz produced and detected the first man-made electromagnetic radiation by sending a powerful electric charge across a spark gap and thereby causing a smaller spark—evidence of the presence of an electric field—to jump across a second gap some distance away. In addition to proving that Maxwell was right, Hertz's experiments inspired a long line of inventors and engineers, beginning with Marconi, to devise equipment for generating and receiving electromagnetic radiation in the radio-frequency range, and to use such waves for telecommunication. (Another outstanding pioneer of wireless telegraphy was the German physicist Ferdinand Braun, who shared the Nobel Prize for physics with Marconi in 1909.) In the early days, the ingenuity of the inventors and engineers often outstripped that of the theoreticians, who were forced to play catch-up. Long-range radio transmission, for example, was considered manifestly impossible by the scientific community, because of the earth's curvature and the fact that electromagnetic waves could travel only in straight lines. Marconi's remarkable achievement of 1901, therefore, cried out for explanation. It came in 1902, when Oliver Heaviside, an English mathematician, and Arthur Edwin Kennelly, an American electrical engineer at Harvard University, independently postulated the existence of the ionosphere: a region of electrons and electrically charged particles in the upper atmosphere —between 30 and 250 miles above the earth—which by reflecting radio waves back to earth extends the range of their transmission far beyond the mere line of sight.

By 1907, thanks to the discovery by an American inventor, Lee De Forest, of a radio-frequency-wave detector that proved to be far more sensitive than the crystals then in general use, and to its subsequent refinement as a generator of radio-frequency waves as well as an amplifier of speech, the transmission of actual speech through space had become a possibility. By 1915, thanks to the further refinement of De Forest's invention, radiotelephony had become a reality, and the electronic age was at hand. In April of that year, spoken words were transmitted from Montauk Point, on Long Island, to a receiver on top of the du Pont Building, in Wilmington, Delaware, a distance of 214 miles; in May, successful transmission was made from Montauk to a receiver on St. Simons Island, off the coast of Georgia, a distance of 800 miles; and during the summer a transmitter in Arlington, Virginia, broadcast speech that was heard and understood, albeit heavily burdened with static, in California, in Panama, in Paris, and as far away as Honolulu, a distance of 4,900 miles. In the early 1920s, commercial broadcasting was initiated—the first station was KDKA, in Pittsburgh, which began transmitting in November 1920—and, fascinated by it as by few technological developments since, thousands of people began assembling their own receivers at home. By this time, the term "wireless telegraphy" had become obsolete. In England, the new phenomenon was called wireless; in the United States and elsewhere, it was known as radio.

For more than a decade after the first transoceanic transmission of speech, static was the great obstacle to the rapid development of radio. At first, it was thought that either some method of minimizing static would have to be devised or the levels of transmitted power would have to be raised—an expensive proposition—until the radio signal prevailed. Since early in the century, it had been believed that radio waves of long wavelength and low frequency—waves stretching for several miles and oscillating at from thirty to sixty thousand cycles a second—were best suited to transmission over long distances; that waves of shorter length and higher frequency, such as those about 650 yards long and vibrating in the neighborhood of five hundred thousand cycles a second, were best suited to shorter distances; and that radio-wave propagation would become progressively poorer as the frequencies became higher. In spite of the fact that these shorter waves had been used extensively and successfully for long-distance ship-to-shore telegraphy, such theories still prevailed in the 1920s. As a result, when the Bell System people began to develop a transatlantic radiotelephone program, they planned to transmit at the long-wave frequency of sixty thousand cycles. Because the ionosphere turned out to consist of several layers, however, and because it was found to fluctuate widely from day to night, from summer to winter, and during the eleven-year sunspot cycle, the outlook for long-wave transmission became less and less favorable, and in 1927, even as Bell inaugurated a public telephone service to London, it was realized, belatedly, that good reception could be obtained only during the low-static winter months.

Hoping to salvage their program, the proponents of long-wave transmission planned the construction of twelve gigantic antennas, covering fifty square miles of land, in Maine. It was a project that became an instant casualty of the stock-market crash of 1929. Meanwhile, ever the pioneer, Marconi had developed small, highly directional shortwave antennas that concentrated low levels of transmitted energy into narrow beams, and—together with amateur radio operators, who had been granted government permission to transmit in the shortwave band, because it was thought to be useless for long-distance transmission, but who were actually sending messages across the Atlantic as early as 1921—had undertaken to demonstrate that frequencies extending beyond one and a half million cycles a second were far more efficient for transoceanic radio than the sixty-thousand-cycle frequency employed by Bell.

By 1925, Marconi had been able to receive shortwave signals sent from Cornwall to the Caribbean island of St. Vincent—a distance of

2,300 miles—using a carrier frequency of three million cycles a second; by 1927, the Marconi Company had set up shortwave telegraph links between Britain and Canada, India, Australia, and South Africa; and in that year a shortwave telephone on the British liner *Carinthia* established contact with London from the middle of the Pacific. Not surprisingly, the long-wave diehards in the Bell System soon capitulated, the controversy involving long waves and shortwaves came to an end, and in 1930 the company's radiotelephone service to London was being transmitted over three shortwave channels. This marked an important turning point in the history of telecommunications, for the entire trend since then has been toward the development of equipment capable of generating higher and higher frequency (and therefore shorter and shorter) radio waves, whose capacity for carrying messages has proved to be greater and greater.

For a while, the radio-frequency frontier stood at waves that were about ten yards long and oscillated at about 30 megacycles—that is, thirty million cycles—a second. By 1933, however, French and English engineers had set up a radio-communications system across the Strait of Dover using waves a little over seventeen centimeters, or about seven inches, long, whose frequency was what then seemed an incredible 1,750 megacycles a second. They called this system Microray Wireless. The term proved to be prophetic, for within a few years all the ultrahigh, superhigh, and extremely high frequencies—those frequencies lying just below the infrared region of the electromagnetic spectrum and ranging in wavelength from about a hundred centimeters, or forty inches, down to a millimeter, or about a twenty-fifth of an inch—came to be known as microwaves.

Since microwaves are reflected by electrical conductors such as metal and by obstacles such as raindrops, and since they can be focused into intense, compact, and highly directional beams by antennas and conveniently carried by waveguides, they soon found application in radar. Radar aims microwaves at a target in short bursts, or pulses, picks up the microwaves reflected by the target, and measures the distance to the target on the basis of the elapsed time between outgoing and returning pulses, which move, like all electromagnetic radiations, with the speed of light. During the Battle of Britain, the English land-based radar system, using microwaves of about fifty centimeters, was able to detect German bombers and measure how far away they were with great accuracy. (In 1942, this same radar system facilitated an important scientific discovery by picking up an intense form of interference that was initially thought to be enemy jamming but that further investigation proved to be caused by radio waves emanating from the sun.)

It was soon apparent, however, that microwaves of much shorter length and higher frequency would be necessary for radar equipment light and compact enough to be carried in planes, thus enabling them to drop bombs with accuracy through overcast, and to be installed on naval ships, which needed similar radar for detecting aircraft, for gunfire control, and for night fighting. Such radar rapidly became available, owing to improvements made by the British in the pulsed magnetron—a device capable of generating microwaves that were only ten centimeters in length and vibrated at a frequency of three thousand megacycles. This range became known as the S-band. Consequently, the Allies were able to bomb German cities through fog and clouds, and the American Navy was given a decisive edge over the Japanese fleet in the Pacific.

As the war progressed, the military kept asking for radar with more accuracy and better definition, and so the search for higher and higher microwave frequencies continued. S-band radar was soon followed by X-band, then by K-band, and when V-E Day arrived a K/2-band radar was under development, using microwaves of less than a centimeter in length and with a frequency of forty-eight thousand megacycles. By that time, the Bell Telephone people had also developed a highly successful microwave radio-relay telephone system for the Army. As a result, long-distance telephone transmission by wire line soon became obsolete. A microwave radiotelephone system using line-of-sight relay towers was opened between Boston and New York in November 1947—the same year in which large-scale television broadcasting, also transmitted on microwave frequencies, got under way. By 1951, a coast-to-coast radiotelephone system had been established; it consisted of 107 hops, each about thirty miles long, and it used the tops of buildings, the peaks of mountains, and two-hundred-foot towers on the plains of the Midwest. By 1960, more than a third of Bell's intercity telephone communication was being provided by microwave relay.

Since the end of the war, the growth of sources generating microwaves and other radio-frequency waves has been phenomenal.

During the past thirty years, the number of radio-frequency transmitting devices authorized by the Federal Communications Commission—a figure that does not include military devices or transmitters—has risen from 50,000 to more than 7,000,000. The first microwave-telephone relay tower was built on Asnebumskit Mountain, near Worcester, Massachusetts, in 1946; today, nearly 250,000 microwave-telephone and television-signal relay towers—each with several microwave-generating sources—are strung across the United States. Other microwave relay towers provide links for motorist-aid call boxes along highways, and private microwave links have been set up to transmit data from computers in one city to computers in another. In 1945, there were only 6 television stations in the country; today, there are almost 1,000 all of them transmitting at either very high or ultrahigh frequencies, and they are received by 121,000,000 television sets. At the end of the war, there were 930 radio stations; today, there are nearly 8,000 AM and FM stations. In addition, there are about 15,000,000 Citizen's Band radio transmitters broadcasting on shortwave frequencies into homes and vehicles throughout the nation.

Besides the tremendous increase in the use of microwaves for radio and television broadcasting, and for line-of-sight telephone and television relay systems, hundreds of immensely powerful microwave transmitters—some with antennas that scatter microwaves from the upper layers of the troposphere, 7 to 10 miles above the earth—have been installed in the United States and overseas during the past twelve years to serve as links for civilian and military satellite-communications systems. During 1976, two powerful microwave broadcasting satellites were placed in orbit in a fixed position relative to earth, 22,300 miles above the equator, where, using extremely high frequencies in the billions-of-cycles-per-second range in order to penetrate the ionosphere, they are relaying telephone conversations, television and radio broadcasts, and printed material to antennas at receiving stations across the nation. Similar broadcast satellites are providing microwave-communications links with ships at sea and offshore oil rigs. Radar navigational systems have been established in almost all airports, and are found on virtually all commercial vessels, as well as on thousands of pleasure craft. Radar surveillance systems are being installed in harbors around the country. Police radar operates on microwave frequencies, as do many burglar-alarm systems, shoplifting-detection devices, and automatic garage-door openers.

Because of security classification, no one knows the full extent of the proliferation of microwaves by the Army, the Navy, and the Air Force, in this era of electronic warfare, but it is unquestionably enormous. From the swarm of communications and surveillance satellites that look down on earth from outer space; through the vast network of high-power tracking and scanning radars that are strung across the Arctic and much of the rest of the world; through guidance systems for the armada of nuclear missiles and antimissile missiles that girdles the globe; through radar and radar-jamming equipment that has been installed on hundreds of warships and thousands of aircraft; down to tiny range finders for tank gunnery, and hand-held radiation detectors for foot soldiers, the military has developed an almost insatiable maw for microwave and other electromagnetic devices, employing them in virtually every installation and conveyance it commands. Even more highly classified are the microwave eavesdropping operations of the National Security Agency—a twenty-thousand-man organization with headquarters at Fort Meade, in Maryland—whose special mission to listen in on and protect domestic communications, to intercept foreign messages, and to break foreign codes has been made easier by the fact that microwave transmissions are far simpler to intercept than messages carried on wire lines, and has been made more difficult by the fact that the Russians have been listening in for several years on long-distance telephone calls in the United States with microwave antennas set up on the roofs of their embassy in Washington and their consular offices in several other cities across the nation. Equally secret, though employing electromagnetic radiation of a different sort, are the Department of Defense's electromagnetic pulse (EMP) projects, multimillion-dollar programs designed to simulate the immense surges of radiant energy accompanying nuclear explosions. EMP could have a jamming effect on the electronic and computer systems of the Navy's warships, of strategic bombers, and of the thousand-odd Minuteman intercontinental ballistic missiles that have been installed in underground silos in the American Midwest and West by the Air Force. And most secret of all are the directed-energy weapons programs being developed by the Defense Nuclear Agency, the Navy, and the Air Force, which will employ high-power microwave beams, laser beams, and charged-particle beams to render enemy missiles inoperative either by disrupting their electronic guidance systems, or by destroying their nuclear warheads.

Other uses for microwaves have evolved from the long-held knowledge that human and animal tissues, like other substances that absorb radio-frequency waves, are heated by them. Indeed, physicians have been treating patients with long-wave diathermy for almost a century and with shortwave diathermy for more than forty years. As of 1972, there were about fifteen thousand microwave-diathermy machines in use in the United States; today, their number is believed to have increased significantly, and it is estimated that two million Americans are treated annually with microwave radiation by nonphysicians for such ailments as arthritis, bursitis, muscle soreness, sprains, and congested sinuses. Since 1926, radio-frequency currents have been used by surgeons to make incisions in tissues such as the brain, the prostate, and the liver, in order to effect simultaneous cauterization and control bleeding.

The fact that microwaves heat tissue has also formed the basis of a multimillion-dollar microwave-oven industry, which had its inception back in 1945, when the Raytheon Company, of Waltham, Massachusetts, filed a patent proposing that microwaves be used to cook food. Today, microwave ovens are among the best-selling appliances in the nation, with several million of them in use in homes, restaurants, and institutions across the land, and with annual sales approaching nine hundred thousand. In the food industry, microwaves have been used to dry potato chips and pasta; to roast soybeans, coffee beans, sunflower seeds, and peanuts; to proof and fry doughnuts; to precook bacon; to temper various meats; and even to facilitate the shucking of oysters. Elsewhere in industry, microwave ovens and furnaces are used to dry yarn, paints, ceramics, paper, leather, wood, tobacco, cellulose and pulp, textiles, pencils, match heads, and wet books, and also to cure chemicals, rubber, resins, nylon, rayon, and urethane. In addition, microwaves are being tested for use in agriculture—the radiation being applied directly to the soil in order to kill weed seeds, weeds, and harmful soil-borne insects.

If the present use of microwaves seems diverse, the possibilities for their future application appear limitless. Communications engineers predict that by 1980 broadcast satellites will be able to handle seventy thousand or more conversations at once, almost as many as could be

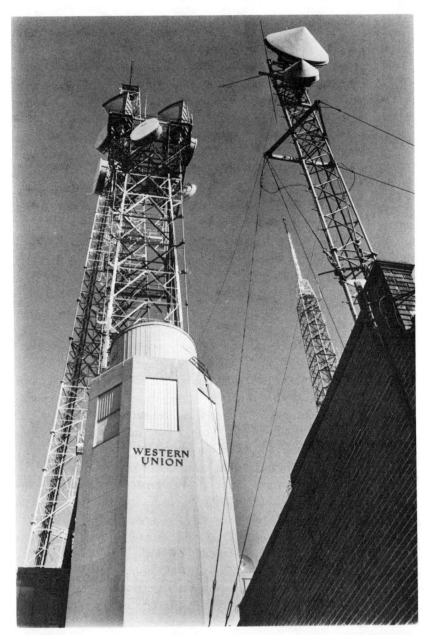

A radio-frequency and microwave transmitting complex in northwest Washington, D.C. The tower at far left contains a TV transmitter, an FM radio transmitter, and numerous two-way radio systems. The second tower from the left is part of a Western Union microwave junction station that acts as a distribution point for the Washington area. The third tower from the left is a standby TV transmitter. The tower and antennas on the far right belong to the Washington Gas Light Company.

PHOTO BY ROBIN TOOKER

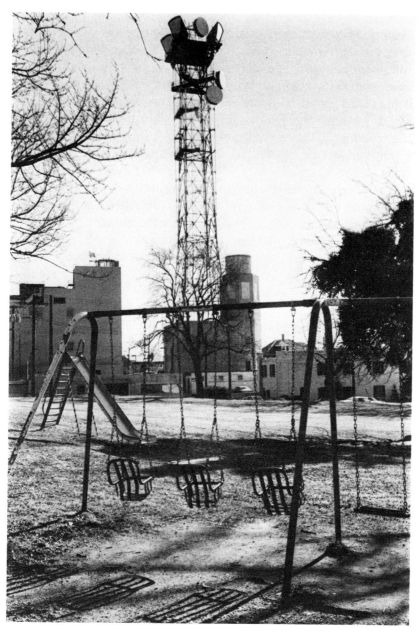

Another view of the Western Union junction station. PHOTO BY ROBIN TOOKER

handled by large cables or microwave links on the ground. Microwave broadcasting satellites will one day be transmitting directly from space to rooftop antennas on earth. The development of cheap solid-state devices for generating microwaves will result in dozens of new products, including pocket telephones. Microwave radiation is being tested for use in medicine as a diagnostic tool and for warming blood, for retarding tumors, for healing skin wounds, for studying the functions of the brain, for monitoring respiration, and for thawing frozen animal organs. A newly developed system for keeping track of the whereabouts of trucks and other commercial vehicles will require each vehicle to carry a transmitter that will broadcast continuous microwave signals to receivers installed along highways, which, in turn, will relay the signals to a surveillance center. Electronic license plates will send out microwave signals if a vehicle breaks down or runs out of gas, or is stolen. Another projected use for microwaves is a radar-augmented braking system for automobiles. (It will prevent highway accidents by beaming microwave radiation ahead of a vehicle and utilizing the reflection from other vehicles to activate brakes automatically if collision is imminent.) Still another scheme that is being seriously considered here and in Europe calls for the use of microwave furnaces to change liquid nuclear waste materials to solid form for easier and safer disposal. And perhaps the most grandiose of all envisions the orbiting of satellite power stations consisting of gigantic arrays of solar cells, which will capture the sun's energy, convert it into microwaves, and beam the microwaves to a vast receiver complex here on earth, where they will be converted into electric current.

Far out as much of this may seem, a good deal of it was first conceived of years ago by Nikola Tesla, a brilliant and eccentric electrical engineer and visionary, who was born in Croatia in 1856, and emigrated to the United States in 1884. Tesla's many inventions included the famous Tesla transformer and the induction motor, which helped to make his high-voltage alternating electrical systems practical. In 1893, he predicted the advent of radio broadcasting, referring to it as "the transmission of intelligible signals without the use of wires." In the same year, his alternating-current system supplied all the lighting and power for the Chicago World's Fair, and Tesla himself capped a demonstration of his recent inventions by allowing one million volts of high-frequency alternating current to pass through his body. In 1895, Tesla's alternating-current system was used to generate hydroelectric power at Niagara Falls, which is considered to be one of the most significant feats in engineering history.

Between 1897 and 1905, Tesla worked on a system for the wireless transmission of power, and in 1899, while living in Colorado Springs, he lit two hundred incandescent lamps with electrical current transmitted through the earth over a distance of 26 miles. While in Colorado, he also used a giant oscillator to produce hundred-foot-long lightning strokes. In 1898, Tesla demonstrated a remote-control guidance system for ships at the first annual Electrical Exhibition in Madison Square Garden; in 1900, he predicted in an article in *Century Magazine* that radio waves would one day be used to detect moving objects, such as ships at sea; in 1915, he predicted the development of radio-controlled missiles similar to the V-1 and V-2 rockets used by the Germans in World War II; and in 1934, on the occasion of his seventy-eighth birthday, he announced the invention of a death ray capable of destroying enemy airplanes at a distance of 250 miles. The last idea proved to be an eerie harbinger of the military's projected use of electromagnetic radiation as an antirocket weapon that will render incoming enemy missiles inoperative by disrupting their electronic circuitry or destroying their warheads. It was also prophetic of the recent disclosure that the Soviet Union and the United States have developed hunter-killer satellites armed with laser beams which can search out and destroy each other's reconnaissance satellites in the vast reaches of space.

Past and future grand schemes aside, it is small wonder that as a result of their multiple and miscellaneous applications microwave and other radio-frequency radiations have already become widespread in the environment. Just how widespread is not known. Congestion of microwave communications channels, however, is already a serious problem in a number of cities, including New York, and in some urban areas the radio background created by microwaves and other high-frequency radio waves is estimated to be from one hundred to two hundred million times as great as the natural radio-frequency background provided by the sun. Many environmentalists claim that the cities of the nation are being saturated with microwaves. Some of them call it electronic smog. The government has also expressed concern about the situation. In December 1971, the

Electromagnetic Radiation Management Advisory Council—a nine-member group that was established in December 1968 by the President's Office of Telecommunications Policy—issued a report entitled "Program for Control of Electromagnetic Pollution of the Environment," which dealt with the possible biological hazards of microwaves and other radio-frequency energy. In its assessment of the problem, the council stated, "The electromagnetic radiations emanating from radar, television, communications systems, microwave ovens, industrial heat-treatment systems, medical diathermy units, and many other sources permeate the modern environment, both civilian and military." The report went on, "This type of man-made radiation exposure has no counterpart in man's evolutionary background; it was relatively negligible prior to World War II." After describing the growth of electromagnetic-radiation sources that had taken place since 1940, the report continued, "Power levels in and around American cities, airports, military installations and tracking centers, ships and pleasure craft, industry and homes may already be biologically significant."

One paragraph later, the report said, "Unless adequate monitoring and control based on a fundamental understanding of biological effects are instituted in the near future, in the decades ahead, man may enter an era of energy pollution of the environment comparable to the chemical pollution of today." After stating that "research in the field of long-term, low-level effects of electromagnetic radiation on living systems has been near a standstill in this country," and after estimating that "the population at risk is not really known; it may be special groups; it may well be the entire population," the report warned that "the consequences of undervaluing or misjudging the biological effects of long-term, low-level exposure could become a critical problem for the public health, especially if genetic effects are involved." It went on to recommend that a five-year microwave-research program, starting in 1972 and costing $63,400,000 —an increase of nearly $60,000,000 over what had previously been allocated for microwave research—be undertaken to determine the long-term effects of low-level microwave radiation on human beings.

If the new studies should indicate the existence of a health hazard from such exposure, the population at risk may well be every man, woman, and child in the land. In the meantime, the problem remains one of the most baffling and controversial medical questions ever posed, involving several different scientific disciplines, the largest communications and entertainment industries in the world, and, in the view of the Department of Defense, the national security. According to the council's report, one of the major problems in evaluating "the possible biological effects of long-term, low-level irradiation of living systems by microwave and other radio-frequency radiations resides in the paucity of information concerning the basic mechanisms of interaction between the electromagnetic field and the living system." What the report never states outright, however—perhaps because its authors assumed that everyone already knew it—is that human beings are considered to be transparent to long-wave radio waves and absorbent to shortwave radio frequencies and to microwaves, just as they are considered to be transparent and absorbent to such other forms of electromagnetic radiation as X-rays and sunlight. This phenomenon was stated succinctly in 1926 by the Soviet naturalist Vladimir Ivanovich Vernadskii, who wrote, "We are surrounded and penetrated, at all times and in all places, by eternally changing, combining, and opposing radiations of different wavelengths." When Vernadskii wrote those lines, he was referring to electromagnetic radiation emanating from the sun and the stars. He had no way of knowing that within fifty years his observation would apply as well to radiation generated here on earth by his fellow-man. Nor, of course, could he have guessed that radiation beamed by his compatriots into the American Embassy in Moscow would create an international cause célèbre.

2

Early Warning

The first biological experiments with electromagnetic energy were conducted by Luigi Galvani, an eighteenth-century obstetrician and surgeon, who lived in Bologna. Galvani is best known for his discoveries concerning the chemical effects of electric current, which led to the coining of the term "galvanism" and to the invention of the battery by his colleague and rival Alessandro Volta, and thus paved the way for the age of electric power. As a medical doctor, Galvani was interested mainly in anatomy and physiology, and this interest led him to perform numerous experiments with electricity on animals. Chief among these was his observation, around 1786, that the leg muscle of a frog placed at some distance from the spark of an electrostatic machine—a device for generating sparks—would twitch if touched by a scalpel when the machine was turned on. Experiments in the remote stimulation of nerves with electricity were not conducted again for more than a hundred years—possibly because they appeared to have little practical value—although in the meantime electric current was used for treating headaches and fatigue in human beings.

Then, in 1890, the prodigious Tesla performed some experiments showing that tissues became heated when subjected to high-frequency electric current of radio wavelength. Tesla pointed out possible medical uses of this phenomenon, but he soon became interested in wireless telegraphy, and credit for pioneering in the field of electrotherapy went to Jacques Arsène d'Arsonval, a French physician and physicist and director of the laboratory of biological physics at the Collège de France, who, independently and at about the same time, demonstrated that high-frequency electric currents penetrated deeply into the body and elevated the temperature of living tissue. D'Arsonval conducted many experiments to determine the biological effects of high-frequency electric current, recording both physiological and behavioral reactions in test animals, and proving that currents of two hundred thousand cycles a second diminished the activity and strength of diphtheria toxin. He also used high-frequency current to treat disorders of the skin and mucous membranes in human beings. D'Arsonval called his new method of treatment diathermy, which means "heating through," and he predicted that it would someday become a valuable tool of medicine. In the beginning, he was looked upon as something of a dreamer by his fellow-doctors, but by 1900 diathermy machines were being used to stimulate blood flow and to treat a wide variety of aches and pains.

By then, too, the X-rays that had been discovered five years earlier by Roentgen (who had noticed that whenever high-voltage electrical current passed through a gas-discharge tube some barium platinocyanide lying nearby began to glow) were rapidly becoming invaluable tools of medicine. Because of their photographic effect, their extraordinary power to penetrate, and their ability to cause certain substances to fluoresce, X-rays were being used to diagnose bone fractures and in fluoroscopy—a form of radiophotography invented by Edison in 1896 which enabled physicians to view the innards of patients over an extended period. Since X-ray tubes were considered a great novelty, they were employed not only by doctors and dentists but also by engineers, laboratory workers, teachers, students, and other laymen, who experimented with them almost at random. The results were sometimes surprising and often painful.

Within six months of the discovery of X-rays, people working with them found that large doses of radiation could cause reddening and blistering of the skin, and that even small repeated doses could produce serious skin lesions. This characteristic of X-rays proved to be a double-edged sword. On the one hand, it led directly to radiation therapy—the use of X-rays to destroy cancerous tissue and prolong life—and, on the other hand, it showed that X-rays could themselves produce cancer, and painful death, as in the case of Clarence Dally, a young assistant to Edison, whom Edison had frequently irradiated while he was perfecting the phosphorescent screen of his fluoroscope machine, and who died of the effects a few years later. In spite of such experiences, ignorance of the adverse biological effects of X-rays— particularly their long-term, cumulative effect—persisted for decades, and was complicated by the apparent compulsion of an eminently practical and empirical-minded age to put every new discovery to use. For example, when it was found, shortly after 1900, that X-rays had the effect of alleviating pain, they were employed in the treatment of arthritis, bursitis, and shingles, and for many years they were used to treat tonsillitis, adenoids, acne, and ringworm in children. As for the physicians involved, few of them bothered to protect either themselves or their patients from anything other than skin burns. Indeed, it was common practice for doctors to test how well their fluoroscopes were working by placing their hands in the X-ray beam. As a result, many doctors developed cancer of the skin.

Meanwhile, in 1900 the German physicist Max Planck had proposed a law for electromagnetic radiation—the quantum theory— which marked the beginning of an arduous effort by scientists to unravel the mysteries of how radiation interacts with matter. Planck set forth the hypothesis that radiation did not necessarily exist as continuous waves but could also take the form of particles, or quanta, of energy. He postulated that the energy emitted by matter —energy in the form of either light or other electromagnetic radiation—was directly related to its frequency, and that the higher the frequency the greater the energy contained in each quantum. In 1905, Planck's theory was given further definition by Albert Einstein's special theory of relativity, which explained how the propagation of electromagnetic radiation, consisting of quanta that contained varying amounts of energy, was compatible with the fact that all radiation traveled at the speed of light. By 1916, Einstein had formulated some fundamental equations describing the exchange of energy that took place when radiation and matter interacted, and during the early 1920s concrete evidence of the particle nature of electromagnetic radiation came with the discovery that collisions between quanta—

or photons, as they were soon to be called—of radiant energy and the electrons in particles of matter accounted for a great many of the physically observable effects of radiation.

Physicists studying the properties of the various electromagnetic radiations customarily arranged them according to frequency and wavelength in what has come to be known as the electromagnetic (or radiant-energy) spectrum. At the long-wave, low-frequency end of this spectrum are radio waves—the longest of which stretch for thousands of miles and vibrate at about ten cycles per second (or hertz, as they are now called). At the other end of the spectrum are gamma rays—extremely high-frequency radiation emitted by radioactive substances such as radium, uranium, and artificially radioactive isotopes and during atomic and thermonuclear explosions as a consequence of disintegrations of atomic nuclei. The wavelength of gamma rays—well-nigh infinitesimal—is measured in terms of angstroms (one angstrom is one-tenth of a millimicron, which is a billionth of a meter), and the frequency of these rays is registered in millions of trillions of hertz. In between radio waves and gamma rays, in ascending order of frequency, are microwaves, infrared radiation, visible light, ultraviolet radiation, and X-rays.

Since the energy contained in a given photon was known to be proportional to its frequency, physicists who continued to study the interaction of the various radiations with matter became aware that X-rays and gamma rays, because of their exceedingly high frequencies, were capable of changing the internal structure of atoms and molecules, and that this capacity was directly related to their tremendous photon energy and their enormous penetrating power. As a result, the electromagnetic spectrum was divided into two categories —ionizing radiation and non-ionizing radiation. The first category covered X-rays and gamma rays, which have sufficient energy to dislodge orbital electrons from atoms, creating electrically charged, highly unstable, and chemically reactive atoms, called ions, which, because they inevitably damaged the cells of living tissues, were capable of disrupting life processes and of causing genetic mutations. The second category covered all the lower-frequency radiations.

Because the language of physics was new, constantly changing, and markedly different from that of biology, the physicists and medical scientists of half a century ago were rarely able to communicate with one another. Awareness of the biological consequences of ioniz-

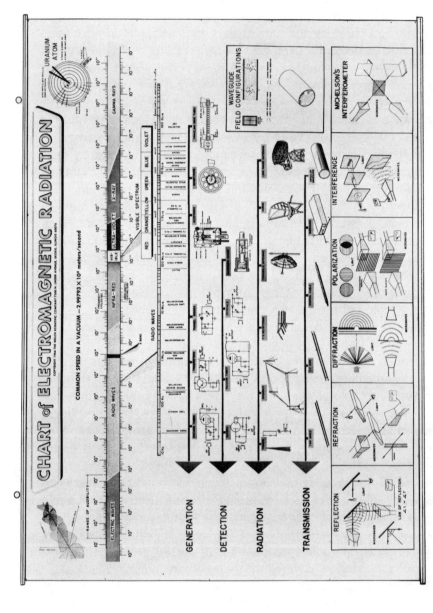

Chart of Electromagnetic Radiation Spectrum. COURTESY OF SARGENT-WELCH SCIENTIFIC COMPANY

ing radiation continued to depend for a long time upon the appearance and observation of disease and damage in human beings. As early as 1916, the incidence of skin cancer on the hands of radiologists was such that the British Roentgen Society recommended safety measures for X-ray use, and by 1922 the American Roentgen Ray Society had established a radiation-protection committee. In 1925, the year in which cancer of the jawbone was found in women who had been in the habit of licking paintbrushes to obtain a fine point as they made watch dials luminous with applications of radium, delegates to the First International Congress of Radiology, in London, recommended a safe level of exposure to X-rays at one-tenth the amount necessary to cause skin burn—a standard that has since been drastically reduced. In 1928, delegates to the Second International Congress, in Stockholm, adopted a standard unit of measurement for X-rays, and called it the roentgen. However, this was merely a preliminary to formulating a system of dosimetry applicable to X-rays, for the roentgen—a unit devised by physicists—provided a measure of the amount of energy delivered (and the degree of ionization produced) in a cubic centimeter of air, and not of the amount of energy absorbed by tissue, which, of course, determines the degree of ionization produced in human beings. In spite of this, the roentgen was mistakenly used as a unit of absorbed energy for many years. Not until 1953, in fact, was this measurement correctly defined, by a unit called the rad—an acronym for "radiation absorbed dose"—which measures the X-ray energy that is absorbed per gram of tissue.

In the meantime, radiation standards were more or less voluntary, and were aimed solely at protecting doctors and radiologists, who, assuming that diagnostic X-rays were harmless, proceeded to give pelvic X-rays to pregnant women—a practice that resulted in a significant increase of leukemia and other types of cancer among the children of these women—and who also treated cases of infertility in women by irradiating their ovaries with X-rays. As for the radiologists, during the early 1950s the incidence of leukemia among them was found to be a thousand percent higher than that of all other physicians combined. By then, of course, concern over the biological effects of ionizing radiation had been aroused by the tremendous amount of radiation sickness, as well as by the increase of leukemia and genetic damage, among the citizens of Hiroshima and Nagasaki who survived the atomic holocaust of 1945. Today, aware that X-ray damage is cumulative, and that any exposure, however slight, to ionizing radiation entails some degree of risk, medical authorities are virtually unanimous in the opinion that no unnecessary X-ray examination should ever be carried out.

During the sixty-odd years it took for medical scientists to comprehend the potent biological hazards associated with X-rays and other ionizing radiation, the extensive region of the electromagnetic spectrum occupied by radio-frequency energy was regarded in this country and almost everywhere else as having little or no biological significance. To begin with, this belief was simply a result of the fact that adverse health effects similar to those engendered by X-rays were not observed in people treated with diathermy or otherwise exposed to radio-frequency waves. And once the phenomenon of ionization was identified the idea was reinforced by the additional belief that the photon energies of radio waves and microwaves—tiny compared with those of X-rays and other ionizing radiation—were not sufficient to dislodge electrons from atoms. As for the heating effect of radio-frequency energy, this was explained by the fact that ions and electrically polarized molecules of water in tissue invariably attempt to orient themselves with a rapidly oscillating electric field, which results in molecular collisions that produce friction, and thus a general rise in temperature.

Since no immediate harmful effects from the heating of tissues by radio-frequency waves were observed in human beings, there was no apparent cause for alarm. During the 1920s, the development of generators capable of producing shorter and shorter radio waves for telecommunication also made it possible to use shorter and shorter waves in diathermy, and by the 1930s shortwave therapy was much in vogue. As early as 1924, however, Dr. Joseph Williams Schereschewsky, a specialist in occupational disease employed by the Public Health Service, where he eventually became medical director, and the founder of the Cancer Research Center at the Harvard Medical School, began a series of extensive experiments to determine the biological effects of shortwave radiation in mice and other test animals. Dr. Schereschewsky soon discovered that the effects of exposure to certain wavelengths were markedly different from those of exposure to other frequencies. He found, for example, that high doses of radiation at frequencies ranging from eighteen million to sixty-six million cycles a second were especially lethal to mice, which died from being overheated, but that frequencies of ninety million to a hundred million cycles per second could be used to cure tumors in the animals without causing any significant rise in their body temperature. (He would no doubt have been amused to learn not only that half a century later scientists would rediscover this finding, but that the National Cancer Institute would initiate a major program to investigate the possible use of radio-frequency and microwave heating in the treatment of cancer.) For his part, Dr. Schereschewsky ascribed these curative effects to heating of the tumor cells, which, he concluded, was produced in an entirely different manner from the heating induced by ordinary long-wave diathermy.

Over the next few years, considerable investigation of the effects of shortwave radiation was undertaken by other researchers, especially in Europe, and in the thirties a lively controversy broke out between scientists who claimed that shortwaves had special, nonthermal biological effects, including metabolic changes in tissue, and scientists who insisted that no specific action other than heating had been adequately demonstrated. The argument was not resolved to anyone's satisfaction, and in this country it was temporarily laid to rest in 1935 by a report to the Council on Physical Therapy of the American Medical Association, which concluded that "the burden of proof still lies on those who claim any biologic action of these currents other than heat." By then, diathermy machines capable of generating electric currents at frequencies of up to ten million cycles a second were in widespread use, and shortwave therapy was being employed not only by general practitioners to treat muscular inflammation, sinus trouble, lung infections, and gynecological disorders but also by some ophthalmologists to treat uveitis, which is inflammation of the inner eye. Since there were no published reports of any adverse effects of such clinical practices, there was still no concern in medical circles that any problem existed. Indeed, the only problem associated with shortwave diathermy in those days was that, because the machines were inadequately shielded and were being operated on communications channels, they were disrupting overseas shortwave-telephone circuits.

During the next decade, few experimental studies of the health effects of radio-frequency energy were undertaken in the United States. Not only were there no apparent hazards associated with its use but during the war the sheer military importance of radio and radar far outweighed any other considerations. In the absence of scientific work, however, a whole folklore, based on a mixture of intuition, observation, and apprehension, grew up around the biological effects of shortwaves and microwaves, expressing itself in the form of black humor, scuttlebutt, and quasi-medical practices. As early as the late 1930s, engineers from the Bell Telephone Laboratories' shortwave-radio research station, in Deal, New Jersey, were kidded at annual beer busts by colleagues from other divisions of the company, who sang songs parodying the work of the Deal engineers on the basis of rumors that it was rendering them sterile. During the early part of the war, stories about the sterilizing effects of radar beams spread like wildfire, especially in the Navy, where enterprising radarmen were known to charge a fee for giving microwave "treatments" to shipmates going ashore on liberty. At the same time, many sailors in the fleet believed that radar could cause their hair to fall out. By the spring of 1942, faced with a crescendo of rumors and inquiries about radar, the Navy undertook a medical study of forty-five civilians who had been working with experimental radar at the Naval Research Laboratory, in Washington, D.C. This study, which included periodic physical examinations and blood tests, found no sign of sterility, unusual baldness, or any other adverse biological phenomena in these men. Indeed, the only thing to turn up was that some of them complained of headaches, eye pain, and a flushed feeling in the face whenever they were exposed to microwaves emanating from radar antennas. Such symptoms were considered interesting but subjective, and when the results of the study were published, in the *U.S. Naval Medical Bulletin* for July 1943, the conclusion was drawn that there was "no clinical evidence of damage to these personnel." Careful note was also taken that, compared with the standard diathermy machines of the day, the power output of the radar being tested at the Naval Research Laboratory was not only low but inefficient.

The fact that no clinical changes were observed in the Navy's study may well have been due to the short duration of exposure on the part of the civilian employees, and to the relatively low power output of the radar being used early in the war. In 1940, the pulsed magnetron developed by the British was capable of delivering an average power of only ten watts into an antenna; by the end of the war, however, in order to extend the range of radar, the power output of the magnetron, which Raytheon was turning out at the rate of two thousand a day, had been increased more than a hundredfold, and radar technicians were sometimes known to pass idle moments using microwave beams to make eggs explode or to toast marshmallows. Such phenomena soon provided electrical engineers and inventors with inspiration. For example, the idea of using microwaves for cooking occurred to Dr. Percy Spencer, of Raytheon, one day in 1945, when, after feeling the warmth of a microwave emanation on his hand, he used the beam to pop some popcorn. These phenomena also gave pause to the handful of medical scientists who were then interested in the possible biological consequences of microwaves. These researchers were aware that the body compensates for a general rise in temperature through perspiration, and for localized heating through a marked increase in blood flow. They were also aware that, because circulating blood acts as a coolant, muscle tissue, which is well equipped with blood vessels, can withstand localized heating far more readily than tissue with poor blood circulation, such as the eyes and the testes. Since they had long known that thermal cataracts could develop in the eyes of glassblowers, steel puddlers, and other workers exposed to the heat of infrared radiation, they found themselves wondering whether the eyes of people who were occupationally or accidentally exposed to the heating effects of microwaves might not be similarly affected. Accordingly, during the 1940s a number of investigators began to conduct experiments on the eyes of test animals, using large doses of high-power microwave radiation, on the assumption that this was necessary for the production of sufficient heat to induce the formation of cataracts.

The power, or intensity of the beam, of microwaves and other electromagnetic radiation is customarily expressed in terms of power density, which is the amount of energy that flows each second through a square measure of space. Like the roentgen, power density is not a unit of absorbed energy, and it is usually stated in terms of milliwatts per square centimeter; for example, the power density of the sun's energy detectable on the surface of the earth at the equator is about 100 milliwatts per square cer..imeter. The investigators who performed the early microwave experiments on test animals, however, exposed the eyes of rabbits and dogs to power densities of up to 3,000 milliwatts per square centimeter. They found that ten-minute exposures to such radiation could produce thermal cataracts, for what they were doing amounted to cooking the eyeball, which, like the transparent white of an egg in a frying pan or in a pot of boiling water, becomes irreversibly opaque when it is subjected to sufficient heat. In addition to producing thermal cataracts with high doses of microwaves, the early experimenters were able to produce lesions in the brains of rabbits and severe testicular damage in rats and dogs without causing the animals any apparent discomfort. However, since these effects and the power densities at which they occurred could not be correlated with any known exposures of human beings, they created little stir in either medical or military circles. As a result, few precautions were taken by people working with radar, in spite of the fact that by the late 1940s standard high-power radar beams were capable of igniting steel wool at a distance of 100 feet.

Then, on October 11, 1951, a microwave technician employed by the Sandia Corporation—a company engaged in the development of missile-guidance systems for the Army, at Sandia Base, near Albuquerque, New Mexico—came to Dr. Frederic G. Hirsch, the company's medical director, complaining of a sudden blurring of vision. Dr. Hirsch diagnosed his patient as suffering from bilateral cataracts with acute inflammation of the retina. His report of the case noted that for the previous eleven months the man had been operating an experimental microwave generator connected to a horn antenna that dissipated microwave radiation into a room. It also took note of the fact that the operator had made a regular practice of putting his hand into the antenna to determine from the heating effect whether the equipment was generating energy. When he did so it was necessary for him to look into the antenna to place his hand properly. At the time, Dr. Hirsch estimated that the intensity of the radiation to which the man had been subjected was about 100 milliwatts per square centimeter. In the conclusion of his report he recommended that the case be used "as a means of recalling the attention of ophthalmologists, industrial physicians, and microwave operators to the potentialities of microwave radiations in order that the use of this form of energy will be accompanied by appropriate respect and precautions."

In 1970, after an interval of nearly twenty years, Dr. Hirsch, who had by then become assistant research director of the Lovelace Foundation for Medical Education and Research, in Albuquerque—an outfit that specializes in biomedical and environmental studies for the armed forces and various government agencies—reevaluated his findings, claiming that the magnitude of his patient's exposure to microwaves had been far greater than the original estimate, which had rested on data that were subject to military restrictions. As might be expected, however, his initial report attracted widespread attention when it was published, in the American Medical Association's *Archives of Industrial Hygiene and Occupational Medicine* for December 1952. Concern was expressed in some quarters that, in addition to the eye and the testes, other areas of the body with relatively poor blood circulation, such as the cavities of the gastrointestinal tract, the gall bladder, and the urinary tract, might prove vulnerable to microwave damage. As a result, many new studies of the effects of microwaves on test animals were initiated, and over the next few years numerous attempts were made by various organizations to determine levels of exposure that were hazardous and levels that were safe. Because inadequate data existed concerning the quantity of microwave energy that must be absorbed to produce adverse biological effects, however, these efforts amounted to little more than guesswork. In April 1953, scientists and doctors attending a symposium at the Naval Medical Research Institute found themselves in agreement with Hirsch's suggestion that power densities of 100 milliwatts per square centimeter were damaging; in November of that year, Bell Telephone Laboratories engineers estimated a safe level of exposure to be one-tenth of a milliwatt per square centimeter— one-thousandth of the hazardous level suggested by Hirsch's findings —and in June of the following year the General Electric Company, apparently convinced that its employees could withstand ten times as much microwave radiation as Bell's, established a supposedly safe level of one milliwatt per square centimeter.

In part, the confusion and uncertainty over what constituted a safe level of exposure to microwaves stemmed from a complex set of variables that made it impossible to duplicate the conditions of typical human exposure in experimental animal studies, and that made it extremely difficult to extrapolate to man the biological effects observed in those studies. How, for example, could the results of microwave irradiation of the eyes of test animals, whose heads were of necessity held in place, be accurately correlated with the exposure of, say, a radar technician, especially when it was known that even small variations in the distance from the eye of an animal to the source of the microwave energy could produce marked differences in the severity and the extent of the opacities produced? But the situation was complicated far more seriously by the fact that microwaves were an indispensable component of missile-guidance systems and of radar, and were thus necessary to virtually every offensive and defensive strategy being devised by military men, who during the 1950s were wholly caught up in the contemplation of nuclear warfare and of ways to keep the balance of terror tipped in favor of the United States. With so much at stake, the reaction of the military to the prospect that microwaves might pose a biological hazard turned out to be ambivalent. In fact, more than five years passed between the publication of Dr. Hirsch's original findings and any attempt by a branch of the armed forces to establish even a tentative hazardous level of microwave radiation.

Meanwhile, in September 1955, at the Mayo Clinic, in Rochester, Minnesota, representatives of the medical profession, the armed forces, various academic institutions, and industry, hoping to arrive at some interim solution to the problem, held a symposium on the physiological and pathological effects of microwaves. Many of the data presented at this meeting dealt with the power densities and exposure times required to produce cataracts in the eyes of test animals. There were also studies concerning the production of hyperthermia—the medical term for abnormally high fever—which included a paper delivered by scientists from the Naval Medical Research Institute reporting the death of dogs that had been exposed for thirty minutes to microwave radiation with a power density of only forty milliwatts per square centimeter.

As with the development of cataracts, however, hyperthermia in animals provided few clues to the amount of microwave radiation that could be absorbed and tolerated by the human body. For one thing, the rate of absorption of microwaves and their conversion to heat in various animal species depended upon such widely varying factors as the thickness and texture of the animal's fur and skin; the ratio of the surface area being irradiated to the animal's total body size; and the total body size in relation to the wavelength or frequency of the radiation to which the animal was being subjected. For another thing, although it was thought that a human being's ability to perspire allowed him to withstand much higher doses of microwaves than could be tolerated by fur-bearing animals, the absorption of microwave radiation by the human body also depended upon the frequency (and, therefore, the penetrating power) of the radiation, and on the thickness and resistance of the skin, fat, and muscle through which the radiation was passing. Moreover, since the physiological effects of microwave absorption could, in turn, be affected by temperature, humidity, and wind velocity—factors influencing the heat loss of all animals—it was apparent to scientists attending the Mayo meeting that they would face a dilemma of extraordinary proportions if they attempted to establish a safe level of human exposure on the basis of animal studies alone.

As it happened, a way out of this dilemma was proposed by Herman P. Schwan, a professor of electrical engineering in the Department of Biomedical Electronic Engineering of the University of Pennsylvania's Moore School of Electrical Engineering, in Philadelphia. He suggested that a maximum safe level of exposure for human beings could be set at ten milliwatts per square centimeter. Professor Schwan had first proposed this level to the Navy in 1953, having arrived at it on theoretical grounds: he based it on the fact that energy derived from the metabolism of food is normally dissipated by the surface of the human body, when at rest, at the rate of about five milliwatts per square centimeter, and on the assumption that an additional heat load of this size could be applied by external forces such as microwave irradiation without causing a significant rise in the body's temperature. Since there were no studies to indicate that a power density of ten milliwatts could cause hyperthermia in animals, and since there were animal studies showing that ten milliwatts could be applied directly to the eye and tolerated for long periods without the production of cataracts, Professor Schwan's proposal seemed eminently sensible to the scientists attending the Mayo meeting.

Moreover, the proposal appeared to be corroborated by a clinical study, presented at the meeting, that reported no serious biological changes in radar workers exposed to power densities of up to thirteen milliwatts at the Lockheed Aircraft Corporation in Burbank, California. This study was conducted by Dr. Charles I. Barron, medical director of the California division of Lockheed, who, in describing his reasons for undertaking it, stated that animal studies reporting adverse effects from exposure to microwaves had "all too often found their way into lay publications and newspapers," and added, "Unfortunately, the publication of this information within the past several years coincided with the development of our most powerful airborne radar transmitters, and considerable apprehension and misunderstanding has arisen among engineering and radar test personnel." Starting in the spring of 1954, Dr. Barron examined 226 men being regularly exposed to microwave fields with power densities of up to thirteen milliwatts per square centimeter, as well as 88 control subjects, who were prohibited from entering zones where the power density exceeded one and six-tenths of a milliwatt. Upon comparing the results of these examinations, Barron discovered that there were significant changes in the white-blood-cell counts of the men in the two groups. There was a marked decrease in polymorphonuclear cells and a disproportionate increase in monocytes and eosinophils in the men who were more heavily exposed to radiation. (All of these are leucocyte white-blood cells.) Barron described his findings as "paradoxical and difficult to interpret." Later, he ascribed them to a laboratory error.

As for a high incidence of eye pathology among the men in the more heavily exposed group, he reported that all but one case had been determined to be unrelated to radar exposure. Dr. Barron's report noted in passing that twenty-five percent of the radar workers experienced heating effects when they were exposed to radar of X-band frequencies; that men exposed to S-band frequencies complained of buzzing vibrations, pulsations, and tickling sensations about the head and ears; and that there were also occasional complaints of fatigue, headache, and aching eyeballs. The fact that these complaints were similar to complaints voiced more than ten years earlier by radar workers at the Naval Research Laboratory was not mentioned by Dr. Barron, who was aware of the Navy study, and either went unnoticed or was considered unimportant by other scientists attending the Mayo meeting. They were apparently more interested in Dr. Barron's conclusion that there was "no indication of increased significant pathology" among workers exposed to microwave power densities of up to thirteen milliwatts per square centimeter. In any case, after the Mayo meeting, the ten-milliwatt level that Professor Schwan had based solely on thermal considerations came to be regarded as providing a safe maximum level of continuous whole-body exposure to microwave radiation, and during 1957 and 1958, it was adopted as a tentative standard by the Army, the Navy, the Air Force, the Bell Telephone Laboratories, and the General Electric Company.

3

The Cover-Up
Begins

By the late 1950s, virtually all the investigations into the biological effects of microwaves were being either conducted or financed by the Department of Defense, which had assigned the Air Force the responsibility of developing a program of coordinated research in the three branches of the armed services. This program, known as the Tri-Service Program, was in operation from 1957 until 1961. Its essential objective, as later described in testimony given at a Senate hearing by a high-ranking Air Force officer, was "to acquire, through laboratory experimentation, a basis for validating protective criteria to insure a safe radiation environment for personnel at the least possible cost to military operations." Most of the research reported in the program's four annual conferences was undertaken with the preconceived idea that all microwave effects were thermal in nature. Therefore, the task, as seen by the Tri-Services Program, was to acquire data validating the ten-milliwatt level that had already been adopted by the military as a theoretically safe level of continuous whole-body exposure to microwaves. Consequently, the vast majority of the animal experiments performed under the auspices of the Tri-Service Program used microwave exposures of more than 100 milliwatts per square centimeter, and few studies of any kind were undertaken to determine whether low-level or nonthermal effects might exist, even though this possibility had been suggested from the outset by Professor Schwan, who had also stated his opinion that no one should undergo whole-body exposure even to 10 milliwatts for more than an hour.

There were, of course, some exceptions to the general trend. One was a study conducted by scientists at the Naval Medical Research Institute, who reported that testicular damage resulting in temporary sterility could occur in test animals exposed to power densities of only five milliwatts per square centimeter. Another was an animal study conducted by Russell L. Carpenter, a professor of zoology at Tufts University, in Medford, Massachusetts, whose findings not only suggested that pulsed microwaves, such as those used in radar, might have a nonthermal effect in producing cataracts, but also raised the possibility that cataracts might occur through the cumulative effect of repeated exposures to low-level microwave radiation. However, the military sponsors of the Tri-Service Program did not regard the results of these studies as raising any doubt about the validity of the arbitrary ten-milliwatt level that had been adopted. Nor, for that matter, did they so regard the findings of experimental studies by other scientists suggesting the existence of nonthermal effects upon the endocrine systems of male rats; upon the normal development of chick embryos; upon the antigenic reactivity of human gamma globulin; and upon the electrical potentials of nerve fibers of the central nervous system.

As for nonthermal, or low-level, effects upon human beings, since this aspect of the problem had been discounted to begin with, it was virtually ignored during the entire Tri-Service Program. On one occasion, though, it was treated as a joke. That happened during the third annual conference, in Berkeley, California, in 1959, when the plant physician of the Sperry Gyroscope Company, of Great Neck, New York—a division of the Sperry Rand Corporation—described the mental distress and loss of morale that had occurred in a radar plant during World War II after nineteen workers in a row became the fathers of girls. According to the physician, rumors began flying around the plant that a man exposed to the emanations of radar could father female children only, and these rumors were dispelled only when the senior engineer of the microwave division "came through for the company and with flying colors produced a 'bouncing' baby boy." After telling this story to illustrate "how the human mind may distort the true facts in this 'mysterious' realm of radar," the plant physician warned his colleagues that "the innate desire to spread rumors and the fear of anything relatively new and unexplored can still be a major problem in this field." He did not venture any reason for the consecutive births of the nineteen girls, however. As it happened, his company had taken great care to screen outdoor radar units at installations in the New York metropolitan area, and in other densely populated places, with wire mesh designed to reflect and disperse microwave radiation, and he offered no explanation for this, either.

By the time of the fourth and final Tri-Service conference, which was held in New York, in August 1960, it was apparent that the military-industrial complex had developed almost complete immunity to any information that might place the ten-milliwatt level in question. By then, it was known that the power of the microwave-radiating equipment, which had risen within the previous twenty years from average outputs of ten watts to almost a million watts, would soon be increased tremendously in order to meet the demands of the space age. And it was realized that the antennas of such equipment, even when they were pointed skyward, could easily leak radiation in amounts that might prove hazardous to human beings. Indeed, it was no secret that the power density of leakage from radar at some of the Ballistic Missile Early Warning System sites greatly exceeded the ten-milliwatt level, and that the Navy's fleet commanders were vigorously opposing any enforcement of the level, because average microwave exposures on the flight decks of aircraft carriers were far greater and could not be lowered without drastic curtailment of operations. It had even come to light that the Navy was extremely concerned about the danger that stray radio or radar waves might cause the premature firing of missiles or trigger the explosion of their nuclear warheads.

In spite of such revelations, the ten-milliwatt standard was affirmed as being both safe and practical. During the final Tri-Service conference, its chairman, Colonel George M. Knauf, of the Air Force, declared that "this level has proven to be an operationally feasible one"; that "our research has not demonstrated a need to modify this level"; and that "there is virtually no disagreement in this country on this level as insuring a safe working environment." Colonel Knauf went on to announce that the ten-milliwatt level not only had been adopted by the fourteen member nations of Supreme Head-quarters Allied Powers Europe and the North Atlantic Treaty Orga-nization but also had been endorsed by the Soviet delegation to the Third International Congress on Medical Electronics, which had been held in London a few weeks earlier. According to Colonel Knauf, who had just returned from London, members of the Soviet delegation had told him that the results of their microwave studies generally concurred with those conducted under the auspices of the Tri-Service Program. To the accompaniment of such assurances, the Tri-Service era came to an end. The idea that the only hazard posed by microwave radiation was thermal remained firmly entrenched in the minds of most American investigators; continued research into the biological effects of microwaves faltered for want of additional funding; and an air of complacency concerning the problem settled over the country for nearly a decade.

It seems likely that during Colonel Knauf's conversation with the Russian scientists in London something was lost in translation, for soon afterward it became known that the official Soviet standard for a safe level of occupational exposure to microwave radiation for an entire working day was not ten milliwatts per square centimeter but, rather, one-thousandth of that amount, or ten microwatts. At first, this information was discounted as a Soviet attempt to embarrass the United States, which had been setting up radar warning systems around the world. Over the next few years, however, it became apparent that the Russians had based their standard primarily on the effects of low-level microwave radiation on the central nervous sys-tem, which they had observed in the course of many large-scale, long-term clinical investigations of workers exposed to microwaves and also from experimental animal studies. Indeed, it turned out that the Russians had recognized unusual effects of radio-frequency en-ergy on the human central nervous system as early as 1933 and had been studying the problem ever since.

During World War II, Soviet scientists had taken complaints of headache, eye pain, and fatigue on the part of Russian radar workers seriously enough to conduct full-scale investigations of them, whereas in the United States similar complaints had been dismissed as "subjective symptoms." During the 1950s, extensive clinical studies of thousands of people exposed to microwave radiation were conducted by the Institutes of Labor Hygiene and Occupational Diseases of the Academy of Medical Sciences in Moscow and Leningrad, by the Gorky Institute, and by the State Institute of Physiotherapy, whereas in the United States only one such study—that of the 226 radar workers at Lockheed—was undertaken. Accordingly, by the late fifties Soviet scientists had amassed a vast amount of information concerning the neurological and physiological effects of low-intensity microwave radiation on human beings, whereas their American counterparts, largely because of the bias and constraint hampering the Tri-Service Program, had for the most part contented themselves with demonstrating the heating effects of high-level microwaves on fur-bearing test animals.

Soviet investigators found that in addition to headache, eye pain, and weariness, workers undergoing prolonged exposure to microwaves complained of stabbing pains in the heart, dizziness, irritability, emotional instability, depression, diminished intellectual capacity, partial loss of memory, loss of hair, hypochondria, and loss of appetite. As for functional changes in the central nervous system, the Soviet investigators discovered that exposure to microwave radiation of low intensity could cause alterations in the normal rhythm of brain waves recorded in electroencephalogram patterns, and that radiation of high intensity could provoke hallucinations and other perceptual changes. During electrocardiographic examinations of microwave workers, they noted numerous changes in cardiovascular functions, including bradycardia—slowing of the heart rate. They also noted changes in blood pressure. These discoveries caused some of them to recommend that people with cardiovascular abnormalities be excluded from work involving exposure to radio-frequency energy. The investigators found changes in the protein composition of the blood of Soviet microwave workers, and shifts in white-blood-cell counts similar to those that had been observed in the blood of the Lockheed workers but dismissed as uninterpretable. In addition to ocular pain, eye strain, and eyelid tremor, they found that some workers exposed to low-intensity microwave radiation had little perception of the color blue and had difficulty in seeing white objects, and that other workers had developed cataracts after exposure to higher power densities. The Soviet investigators also turned up a great number of endocrine responses to radio-frequency radiation, including increased thyroid activity, slight enlargement of the thyroid gland, sterility, and decreased lactation in nursing mothers. Moreover, they claimed to have found that an unusually high number of female children were being fathered by microwave workers.

Just how serious Russian scientists considered the effects of microwave radiation to be, and how radically different their outlook was from that of their American counterparts, can be seen in a report called "The Effects of Radar on the Human Body," which was published in July 1962 by the U.S. Army Ordnance Missile Command's liaison office at the Bell Telephone Laboratories, in Whippany, New Jersey, where part of the Nike-Zeus antiballistic missile defense system was developed. The Army report was based on a translation of a book entitled *The Biologic Action of Ultrahigh Frequencies,* written by Professor A. A. Levitas and Dr. Zinaida V. Gordon, of the Institute of Labor Hygiene and Occupational Diseases of the USSR Academy of Medical Sciences, and published in Moscow, in 1960. "We might assert that prolonged and systematic irradiation even by weak and comparatively long-wave fields cannot pass without leaving a trace on humans since it is artificial," the Russian authors declared in their preface. "As for powerful high-frequency fields, there is incontrovertible evidence confirming the necessity of taking the most serious measures of protection."

The fact that the Russians had already acted upon such evidence was apparent in the "Safety Regulations for Personnel in the Presence of Microwave Generators," which had been approved by the Chief of State Sanitary Inspector of the USSR back in November 1958. According to the Army report, these regulations not only stipulated that no worker should be exposed to more than ten microwatts per square centimeter during an entire working day, but laid down strict guidelines for work practices which were (and still are) unheard of in microwave plants and installations in the United States. For example, the Russian regulations did not allow microwave generators in areas where other work was being performed, and required that the antennas of these generators be directed so as to avoid irradiating the people who were operating or servicing them. (By contrast, workers in many American radar factories had long been

allowed to walk right through the main beams of microwave generators.) Russian safety regulations also required that "the radiation
intensity must be measured systematically no less than every two
months, in areas where microwave generators are tuned, tested, and
operated as well as in neighboring areas and adjoining rooms"; that
"measurements should be taken while the generators are operating
at maximum emission power"; and that "in the case of experimental
and research work, the radiation intensity must be checked after each
change in the working conditions, after changing equipment to operate on another power or frequency, after a change in the arrangement
or construction of test equipment, or when other conditions affecting
the radiation are changed." Needless to say, such precautions in
radar facilities in the United States were virtually nonexistent.

There was other evidence of contrast in the Levitas-Gordon book.
For example, after taking note of Dr. Barron's determination that
the eye pathology among the Lockheed workers was unrelated to
radar exposure, the Russians had this to say:

> In an examination we conducted of the eyes of 370 persons working
> with microwave generators, we found that some of them were com-
> plaining of lacrimation, pain, and fatigue of the eyes at the end of the
> working day. In these cases, irritation of the mucosa of the eyelids and
> eyeball was frequently noted. An investigation of the deep refractory
> media of the eye disclosed changes in the crystalline lens in most of
> the people.

The Soviet scientists went on to point out that progression of such
changes was noted in the eyes of people who had been exposed to
microwave radiation with an intensity of several milliwatts per
square centimeter, and that "This has led us to believe that under
definite conditions, microwave radiation can cause the formation of
cataracts." Small wonder that the Soviet safety regulations of 1958
required microwave workers to wear protective goggles whenever
they were exposed to a radiation level of one milliwatt per square
centimeter. By contrast, of course, the United States standard allowed microwave workers to be exposed day in and day out to ten
times this amount of radiation with no provision whatsoever for
protective goggles or, for that matter, for any other preventive measures.

Incredible as it may seem, when news of the Soviet findings

reached the United States, it did not cause uneasiness or provide impetus for new research into the biological effects of microwaves, but, instead, was generally greeted with skepticism by the scientific and medical community and with suspicion by the military-industrial complex. There were many reasons for these reactions. To begin with, there had always been profound traditional differences in scientific approach between American and Soviet biologists. The Soviet biologists had been greatly influenced by the theories of the Nobel Prize–winning physiologist Ivan Petrovich Pavlov concerning the fundamental controlling role of the central nervous system in the entire human organism. As a result, they tended to look for microwave effects in the modification of nervous-system function. American scientists, by contrast, had always tended to be skeptical of behavioral data and to trust only those effects which could be observed, quantified, and then duplicated in experimental studies. As a result, they tended to regard as hearsay Soviet conclusions that appeared to be based largely on examinations of workers who had been exposed to microwave radiation. Another reason for rejecting the Soviet findings was that translations of the Russian experiments were often grossly inaccurate. Still another was that many of the reports of the experiments lacked the kind of detailed information on how they were conducted which American investigators considered necessary in order to evaluate and duplicate them. Above all, however, was the fact that, having assumed to begin with that the only possible biological effect of microwaves was the heating of tissue, American biologists were still hopelessly mired in the tradition and orthodoxy of the thermal theory.

As for the military, since microwaves were indispensable to virtually all the nation's offensive and defensive weapons systems, any objective evaluation of microwave hazards on its part was bound to be, as it had been for nearly fifteen years, a casualty of the Cold War. That is to say, for reasons they perceived to be of national security military people felt obliged to protect the ten-milliwatt level at all costs and to ignore, deny, or, if worst came to worst, suppress any information about adverse effects of low-intensity microwave radiation. In 1962, however, a bizarre discovery at the United States Embassy in Moscow threw the Department of Defense and the various agencies of the intelligence community into confusion over the possible neurological and behavioral effects of microwaves. At that time, security experts who were conducting an electronic sweep of the embassy to detect hidden listening devices found that the Russians were beaming low-intensity microwave radiation into it from a building across the street. (Searches of the embassy had been going on periodically since 1952, when security people discovered that the carved wooden Great Seal of the United States, which the Russians had presented to Ambassador Averell Harriman at the end of the Second World War, had been bugged; indeed, it was this same eagle that Ambassador Henry Cabot Lodge had displayed before the Security Council of the United Nations on May 26, 1960, on the occasion of his famous speech concerning Soviet perfidy.)

At first, it was believed that the microwaves being beamed into the embassy had something to do with the normal eavesdropping operations that virtually all nations conduct against one another. It was soon realized, however, that the Russians were using multiple frequencies and widely fluctuating microwave beams with highly irregular patterns, which did not appear to be applicable to intelligence gathering. As time went on, the motive for the Soviet microwave bombardment of the embassy became the subject of intense scrutiny by various American intelligence agencies, including the Central Intelligence Agency, whose officials had become belatedly aware of the vast amount of research that the Russians had conducted on the effects of microwaves upon human behavior. For the usual security reasons, this scrutiny was carried on with the utmost secrecy, and cloaked in the usual euphemisms. The microwave beams being directed at the embassy were referred to as the Moscow Signal; the investigation of them was dubbed Project Pandora; and information about it was parceled out on a strict "need to know" basis, which, as it turned out, excluded most of the State Department employees at the embassy who were being irradiated. CIA agents interviewed scientists who they knew were involved in microwave research, asking them such questions as whether it was reasonable to believe that microwaves beamed at human beings from a distance could affect the brain and alter behavior.

In the autumn of 1965, the Institute for Defense Analyses—a think tank that does work for the Department of Defense—convened a special task force to assess the problem, and studies were undertaken to duplicate some of the Russian experiments showing that microwaves affected the central nervous system of test animals. In addition, the Advanced Research Projects Agency (ARPA)—a highly secret organization within the Department of Defense, which was engaged in developing a wide variety of electromagnetic weaponry, including electronic sensors and other devices that were designed to detect enemy movement on the Ho Chi Minh Trail and elsewhere in Vietnam—set up a special laboratory at the Walter Reed Army Institute of Research, in Washington, D.C., where, over a number of years, experiments were conducted in which rhesus monkeys were irradiated with microwaves at power densities and frequencies similar to those of the Moscow Signal. Although the results of these experiments were called inconclusive, they remained unknown until quite recently, for the Department of Defense classified them as secret. However, similar studies undertaken since have clearly demonstrated that microwaves can exert a profound effect upon the central nervous system and the behavior of rhesus monkeys and other primates.

4

The Human Factor

At the summit meeting in Glassboro, New Jersey, in June 1967, President Lyndon Johnson asked Premier Alexei N. Kosygin to call a halt to the irradiation of the embassy in Moscow. As it happened, during the same month the first of several bills providing that electronic products be designed and manufactured so as not to emit radiation endangering the public health and safety was introduced in Congress. The proposed legislation came about as a result of public disclosure by the General Electric Company that it was recalling ninety thousand color television sets whose shunt-regulator tubes were found to be emitting X-rays in excessive amounts. Initially, therefore, Congress was concerned with the hazard of ionizing radiation given off by TV sets, by medical X-ray machines, and by artificial radioactive materials used in industry. However, by the time the Senate Commerce Committee got around to holding hearings on the problem, in May 1968, the measures had been expanded to include non-ionizing radiation as well.

As might be expected, none of the testimony presented at the hearings gave the senators any inkling that the Defense Department and the CIA were gravely concerned about the possibility that low-intensity microwave radiation could affect human behavior. On the contrary, the Defense Department sent over two high-ranking officials from its Defense Research and Engineering branch, plus a high-ranking medical officer from each branch of the armed forces, to assure the senators that military-sponsored research into the biological effects of microwaves had been adequate, that the ten-milliwatt level was safe, and that nobody in the Army, the Navy, or the Air Force was being exposed to hazardous amounts of microwave radiation. (Apparently, no one in the Defense Department had given much thought to the voluminous Soviet literature on the low-level effects of microwaves, or, for that matter, to a medical bulletin issued by the Air Force in December 1965 which, under the heading "Unexplained Response of Man to Radar," stated that "epigastric distress and/or nausea may occasionally occur at as low as five to ten milliwatts per square centimeter.")

As for the Soviet findings, the only witness in five days of hearings to address this subject directly was Professor Charles Susskind, of the Department of Electrical Engineering of the University of California at Berkeley, who told the committee that American investigators had scarcely bothered to look for nonthermal effects of microwaves. After observing, "We cannot very well dismiss a whole body of scientific literature just because it is Russian," Professor Susskind urged that the Soviet experiments be duplicated in order that they might be corroborated or disproved. He also said, "Although ionizing radiation seems to loom larger as a hazard, it would not surprise me in the least if non-ionizing radiation were ultimately to prove a bigger and more vexing problem."

As it turns out, Professor Susskind had very good reason for thinking so. Back in 1961 he had performed an experiment for the Air Force which still calls for further investigation. Susskind and a colleague, Susan Prausnitz, exposed 200 male mice to radiation in the X-Band frequency range, which was generated by an Air Force radar transmitter. The mice were irradiated at a power density of 100 milliwatts per square centimeter for four and a half minutes a day, over a period of fifty-nine weeks. The longevity of the mice did not appear to be affected by these conditions. However, when the researchers performed autopsies on irradiated animals that had died during the course of the experiment, and compared them with autopsies performed on control animals that had not been exposed to microwaves, they discovered testicular degeneration in forty percent of the dead irradiated mice, and in only eight percent of the control animals. Even more alarming, they found cancer of the white blood cells—both lymphatic leucosis and lymphatic leukemia—in fully thirty-five percent of the irradiated mice, as compared with ten percent of the controls.

While most of the testimony given at the Commerce Committee hearings supported the ten-milliwatt level, some testimony cast doubt upon it and reflected the confusion and uncertainty surrounding the whole problem. Perhaps the most surprising source of such testimony was Professor Schwan, who not only had proposed the ten-milliwatt level to begin with but also had been chairman of the Sectional Committee on Radiofrequency Radiation of the American Standards Association—a private organization largely funded by industry and the government, and now called the American National Standards Institute. In 1966 this organization had recommended that the ten-milliwatt level be adopted as an official standard. Professor Schwan told the committee that much more research would be needed to determine whether long-term exposure to low-intensity microwave radiation was harmful; whether a level of exposure that was safe for adults would turn out to be safe for children; whether microwaves could interact with tissue on a molecular or microscopic level; and whether microwaves could cause genetic damage or impairment of nervous-system function.

Professor Schwan went on to point out that investigators who tried to acquire information about microwave injuries were encountering difficulties from employers, and he deplored a tendency on the part of the military and industry "to dismiss the possibilities of microwave-induced damage in order to avoid legal and compensation problems." After defending the ten-milliwatt standard as "the best we can formulate on the basis of presently available knowledge," he admitted that it had been "crudely set" and "badly needs refinement." According to Professor Schwan, the ten-milliwatt level had not been formulated with any regard to frequency, yet there was "good scientific reason to believe that the standard ought to be frequency related, since the lower-frequency radiation penetrates much deeper in the body and can heat it more effectively than higher frequencies." He also pointed out that the standard "becomes practically meaningless in the presence of complex field configurations"—highly irregular and unpredictable wave intensities that often occur in close proximity to microwave-generating equipment—and so it could not be safely applied to microwave ovens. About the specific hazards of the ovens, Professor Schwan had this to say: "If microwave ovens should become very popular, which may be quite possible, and if there occurs a leak in a microwave oven and if a housewife happens to be standing in front of that leak accidentally, then she could be hit by a severe dose of microwaves. And if the oven is placed so that the radiation hits her face, she may be blinded."

This statement by Professor Schwan had a considerable impact on the Senate Commerce Committee, for surveys of microwave ovens made in two states and the District of Columbia had shown that even when their doors were shut, anywhere from a sixth to a quarter of them leaked radiation in excess of the ten-milliwatt level. (This level had been adopted as a voluntary performance standard by all microwave-oven manufacturers.) Of thirty ovens delivered to the Walter Reed Army Medical Center, twenty-four had to be rejected because they were leaking radiation up to twenty milliwatts per square centimeter. Indeed, the Senate hearings marked the beginning of a long and bitter controversy over the safety of microwave ovens, which still continues. In a statement submitted for the record, the Raytheon Company—then the nation's largest manufacturer of domestic and commercial microwave ovens—assured the committee that microwave leakage from its ovens was substantially less than ten milliwatts per square centimeter, and that, in any case, unlike X-rays, microwaves did not have a cumulative effect. On the other hand, Professor Carpenter, of Tufts University, wrote the committee, "We have clearly demonstrated a cumulative harmful effect of microwave radiation on the eye, so that single exposures to radiation which are not of themselves harmful may become truly hazardous if they are repeated sufficiently often."

Faced with testimony that was inconclusive, incomplete, and often contradictory, Congress, not surprisingly, threw up its hands over the enormously complex and long-neglected problem of exposure to microwave radiation and passed the Radiation Control for Health and Safety Act of 1968. Basically, the act authorized the Secretary of Health, Education, and Welfare to establish a broad program to coordinate, conduct, and support research on radiation hazards, and to develop and administer performance standards that would minimize unnecessary emissions of X-rays and other radiation from electronic products. However, it contained no provision whatever for the development and promulgation of standards governing the actual exposure of not only consumers but the general population to microwaves and other non-ionizing radiation. Nor did it give anyone any statutory authority to develop emission standards for electronic equipment under the control of the federal government, though the government was then (as it is now) far and away the largest single user of microwave devices in the United States. The extent to which Congress's hands were tied in this regard was clearly stated in a letter sent on June 5, 1968, to Senator Warren G. Magnuson, chairman of the Commerce Committee, by the acting general counsel for the Department of Defense:

> It is understood, however, that the development of product standards to protect the public health will not necessarily preclude the use of devices, e.g., radars, communications transmitters, etc., which are designed to intentionally emit large quantities of radiation. The use of such devices is often essential to meet requirements of the national defense. It is anticipated that in developing standards, the Department of Health, Education, and Welfare will give consideration to the use and purpose of these devices and will consult with other federal agencies on the development of standards which could have such an effect on these devices. Moreover, if standards are developed that do have an effect on the operation of devices essential to the national defense it is understood that this will be a matter subject to exemption under section 360 (A) (b).

After the 1968 act was passed, the Environmental Control Administration's Bureau of Radiological Health was given responsibility for administering its provisions, and dutifully set out to establish performance standards for television sets, microwave ovens, certain kinds of electron tubes used in schoolrooms, and diagnostic X-ray equipment. The work was necessary, of course, but it hardly began to deal with the real dimensions of the microwave problem. This had been described for the Commerce Committee by James G. Terrill, Jr., director of the National Center for Radiological Health, who had testified at the outset of the hearings that as a result of the widespread use of microwave generators for military purposes, radio navigation, tracking, communications, food ovens, and various industrial processes, the entire population of the United States was subject to some microwave exposure, and that the number of persons exposed to excessive levels of microwave radiation was unknown. Indeed, the Radiation Control for Health and Safety Act, with its narrow focus and its many limitations, amounted to little more than a license for continuing the vast proliferation of microwave devices that, having gone on unabated since World War II, had brought about this very situation.

One of the most significant contributions of the Bureau of Radiological Health in carrying out the provisions of the 1968 act was to propose a three-day symposium on the Biological Effects and Health Implications of Microwave Radiation. Sponsored by the Medical College of Virginia, the symposium was held in Richmond in September 1969, and it marked the first time since the final Tri-Service conference, in 1960, that leading microwave scientists had gathered to discuss their work. As might be expected, there was plenty to catch up on. In the nine-year interval the notion that the only serious hazard posed by microwave radiation was thermal had been seriously challenged both here and abroad. The need for additional research had become apparent.

Practically everyone who attended the Richmond symposium agreed in principle that studies should be undertaken to determine whether microwave damage could occur at the cellular or molecular level; whether the biological effects of microwaves were cumulative; whether microwaves could influence the central nervous system and alter the behavior of human beings; and whether they could cause genetic damage.

In some ways, therefore, the symposium marked a long-overdue turning point in the general attitude of American scientists toward microwave research. In other ways, however, it marked a drawing up of battle lines between scientists who tended to discount the possibility of nonthermal, or low-level, effects—in some cases, apparently, because their research was being financed by the military or by the microwave industry—and scientists who, no matter who was financing their work, believed that the possibility of such effects should be thoroughly investigated. To a great extent, the symposium also reflected a continuation of the ambivalence and uncertainty that had always characterized the efforts of scientists to come to grips with the biological problems posed by radio-frequency energy. This ambivalence was nowhere more apparent than in the attitudes expressed toward the Soviet literature on microwave effects—attitudes that ranged from outright dismissal of the Soviet findings, through doubts about the methodology employed to arrive at them, to a plea by one scientist who, after reminding his listeners that Soviet work on the low-level effects of X-rays and other ionizing radiation had first been ridiculed and then acknowledged as accurate by American investigators, urged them to "accept your Russian colleagues as co-equal scientists of integrity" and to use the Russian findings as a lead in conducting further research.

Although no Soviet scientists were able to accept an invitation to the Richmond symposium, Dr. Karel Marha, director of the department of high frequency of the Institute of Industrial Hygiene and Occupational Diseases in Prague, was on hand to describe research that had been undertaken in Czechoslovakia. According to Dr. Marha, investigators from his department had visited some 200 workplaces—including factories where microwave devices were manufactured, radio and television stations, and radar centers—and had found a wide variety of neurological problems among the people who were employed in them. "Typical symptoms are pains in the head and eyes and fatigue connected with overall weakness, dizziness, and vertigo when standing for a long period," Dr. Marha told the symposium. "Sleep at night is restive and superficial, and there is sleepiness during the day. Exposed individuals are subject to changing moods; they often become irritated to the point of becoming intolerable. Hypochondriac reactions are manifested along with feelings of fear. Sometimes those affected feel nervous tension, or, on the contrary, mental depression connected with inhibition of intellectual functions—mainly decreased memory. The afflicted workers complain of a feeling of strain in the skin of the head and forehead; their hair falls out; they complain of pains in the muscles and in the heart region connected with irregular heart beating and breathlessness."

According to Dr. Marha, Czechoslovak investigators had found that some of these effects could be induced at power densities as low as one-tenth of a milliwatt per square centimeter—a hundred times less than the American standard. He went on to explain that because the effects of repeated irradiation were thought to be cumulative, and because large variations had been found in the sensitivities of different people, the Czechoslovak standard for exposure to microwaves incorporated a safety factor of ten, and was thus similar to the standard that was in force in the Soviet Union. Pregnant women were specifically prohibited from working in areas where these levels were exceeded.

As it turned out, the reason for this drastic prohibition was described at some length in a book entitled *Electromagnetic Field and the Life Environment,* which Dr. Marha and two of his colleagues had recently written. In the section dealing with the biological effects of radio-frequency energy, Dr. Marha pointed out that morphological alterations caused by microwave radiation could result in "changes of the reproductive cycle, in a decrease in the number of offspring, in the sterility of the offspring, or in an increase in the number of females born." Dr. Marha went on to observe that "no decrease in fertility was noted in persons working in rf [radio-frequency] fields, but as far as the number of children born is concerned, girls distinctly predominate." After stating that irradiation of pregnant women and female animals apparently increases the percentage of miscarriages, Dr. Marha described a case of birth defect which occurred after a mother was treated with shortwave diathermy at the beginning of her pregnancy. He then wrote as follows: "Other authors have also reported that the rf field definitely impairs embryogenesis in both humans and animals, particularly in the beginning stages. The development of the fetus is retarded, congenital defects appear, and the life expectancy of the infant is reduced."

It is not known how many of the scientists who attended the Richmond symposium read Dr. Marha's book when it was translated into English and published in 1971 by the San Francisco Press. It is known, however, that after delivering his paper at the symposium, he was subjected to some tough questioning, especially by Dr. Lawrence Sher, of the University of Pennsylvania. Dr. Marha handled himself with aplomb. For example, when Dr. Sher told him that "we are subject to many possible insults from our environment," and asked him how he could justify limiting microwave radiation to intensities that precluded the smallest possible effect by a safety factor of ten, Dr. Marha gave a reply that epitomized the profound difference in thinking and approach between scientists in the countries of Eastern Europe and those in the United States. "Our standard is not only to prevent damage but to avoid discomfort in people."

In emphasizing the human factor, Dr. Marha put his finger on a strange deficiency in the microwave research that had been carried on in this country. For more than twenty years, countless dogs, cats, rabbits, rats, and other test animals had been irradiated (or zapped, as some American scientists are fond of saying) with microwaves of various frequencies and power densities in order to induce cataracts, sterility, or sleep, or to produce fever, brain damage, or death. All this experimental work had, of course, been performed with the idea of determining a safe level of exposure for human beings. Yet, curiously, except for a study limited to the ophthalmological effects of microwaves, no broad survey had ever been undertaken in the United States to determine the health experience of radar workers and other people who had been exposed to microwaves over long periods. In short, during the whole of these two decades—a time in which there had been an incredible drive to exploit the commercial and military importance and uses of microwaves—the actual biological effects of microwaves on human beings had been virtually ignored by all but a few of the researchers who were investigating the problem.

As it happened, the Richmond symposium was attended by several scientists who had chosen not to ignore the effects of microwaves upon human beings. One of them was Dr. Allan H. Frey, a biophysicist working for Randomline, a research firm in Huntingdon Valley, Pennsylvania, who had done some pioneer research in the effects of microwaves upon the nervous system. Frey's interest in microwaves had begun in 1961. At the time, he was working in the General Electric Company's Advanced Electronics Center, at Cornell University, and he also held a contract from the Office of Naval Research to investigate the effects of radio-frequency energy on the nervous system and on behavior. By chance one day, he met a technician from General Electric's radar test facility in Syracuse, who told Frey that he could hear radar. Frey knew that people were supposed to be able to hear only acoustical energy, but instead of rejecting the man's contention out of hand he arranged to visit the test facility.

"The fellow worked near a radar dome," Frey has since recalled. "And when I walked around there and climbed up to stand at the edge of the pulsating beam, I could hear it, too. I could hear the radar going *zip-zip-zip.*"

During subsequent field tests, Frey determined that human beings could indeed hear pulsed microwaves at frequencies ranging from 300 to 3,000 megahertz—the portion of the radio-frequency spectrum at which electromagnetic energy passes into and through the head, and which includes the frequencies used for radar, television, shortwave radio, microwave ovens, and microwave communications-relay towers. He also found that, depending upon the width of the pulse and its rate of repetition, radio-frequency sound was perceived as buzzing, ticking, hissing, or knocking; that it could be induced several hundred feet from an antenna the instant the antenna's transmitter was turned on; that it could occur at average power densities far below the ten-milliwatt level; that it could be perceived by people who were blindfolded and people who were deaf; and that it always seemed to come from within or a short distance behind the head.

When Frey published these findings, in the early 1960s, in *Aerospace Medicine* and in the *Journal of Applied Physiology,* he was laughed at by most of the people who were investigating the biological effects of microwaves:

> It was as if none of them was prepared to accept or even listen to what I had hit upon. But I knew that my data were correct and that I was right. There was no question about it. Incidentally, I wasn't the first person to report the perception of sound in a radar field. Just after the Second World War ended, some engineers who were developing radar for the Airborne Instruments Lab wrote up a one-page report on the phenomenon and brought it to the attention of an expert on hearing. The expert proceeded to assure them that it was impossible to hear radar. He told them the whole thing was probably just a question of teeth rattling, and to forget about it. So they did. Ironically, somebody in the company's promotion department got hold of the paper and ran it in an advertisement—a believe-it-or-not, look-how-wonderful-radar-is kind of thing. After I published my findings, I got some pretty strange letters. One of them came from a fellow in Chicago. He wrote that my article made him so relieved he hardly knew how to express himself. It seems he had been entertaining grave

doubts about himself for years—ever since 1943, in fact, when he was in the Air Force and, while strolling along the perimeter of his base one day, distinctly heard the radar antenna. When he told the base medical people about it, they hospitalized him for psychiatric examination. Finally, after a series of exhaustive tests, they told him that his skull must be some kind of resonating cavity, and let him go. I've often wondered how many other stories there are like that.

Undaunted by the initial reaction to his findings, Frey set out to try to determine how microwaves could produce the sensation of sound. He soon demonstrated through human and animal studies that the sound of radar could not be conveyed to the ear by any mechanical vibration of the teeth, eardrums, skin, bone, or muscle. Since he knew that the microwave frequencies that induced the perception of sound could penetrate into the brain, he decided to explore the possibility (already under investigation by Soviet scientists) that electromagnetic waves might be able to excite the nerve tissue of the brain directly. To investigate this possibility, he implanted electrodes in the brains of cats and began to record their brain waves as light traces on an oscilloscope. He then irradiated the heads of the cats with pulsed microwaves at average power densities as low as thirty microwatts per square centimeter—a level of intensity nearly 350 times less than the ten-milliwatt standard. When he did so, there was unmistakable and incontrovertible evidence on the oscilloscope that the brain—including the hypothalamic area, where emotions are believed to originate—shows a strong reaction to stimulation by microwave energy.

In addition to studying the effects of microwaves on the nervous system, Frey performed experiments on the hearts of frogs. During these experiments, he found that when he synchronized pulsed microwave energy with the heartbeat cycle he could not only alter the rhythm of the heartbeat but cause the heart to stop beating altogether. By the time of the Richmond symposium, in 1969, all this work had been published, and Frey was finally beginning to win the respect of his colleagues. This did not deter him from admonishing them about the narrowness and rigidity of their thinking and their approach to microwave research. Frey urged his fellow-scientists to forget mathematical calculations that supposedly proved microwaves could not affect nerves and to recognize that very little was known about the workings of the nervous system, and even less about the possible interaction of radio-frequency energy with neural function. Commenting on the headache phenomenon described by Dr. Marha, he said his own work had convinced him that it was a real effect, and one that should be further explored. "I have not done so with humans because I think there is an ethical question," Frey continued. He then made a statement that no other American microwave researcher had ever made in public. "I have seen too much," he said. "I very carefully avoid exposure myself, and I have for quite some time now. I do not feel that I can take people into these fields and expose them and in all honesty indicate to them that they are going into something safe."

5

The Cataract
Connection

One of the most controversial figures to emerge from the tangle
of controversy surrounding the biological effects of microwaves over
the last decade has been Dr. Milton M. Zaret, an ophthalmologist
practicing in Scarsdale, New York, and a clinical associate professor
of ophthalmology at the New York University–Bellevue Medical
Center. Dr. Zaret's involvement with microwaves began in 1959,
when he was asked to conduct a survey to determine the occurrence
of lens defects and cataract formation in the eyes of radar technicians
and microwave workers employed in the armed forces and in the
defense industry. Cataracts were known to occur in the eyes of
workers exposed to infrared radiation, and had been produced in the
eyes of animals exposed to microwave radiation; in addition, there
was by then a documented case in which microwave radiation had
been determined to be the cause of cataract formation in a microwave
worker. Carried out as a joint effort by the medical center's depart-
ments of ophthalmology and industrial medicine, the survey was
financed by the Air Force, and was undertaken as part of the Tri-

Service Program. It marked the start of a long voyage of discovery for Zaret, who eventually came to believe that microwave radiation and other radio-frequency waves posed a far greater health hazard than anyone had ever suspected.

Between the spring of 1960 and the spring of 1963, Zaret examined the eyes of a selected population of nearly sixteen hundred workers who were employed at sixteen military and civilian installations throughout the United States and in Greenland, including Army, Navy, and Air Force bases, missile-tracking facilities, radar-research-and-development laboratories, and factories in which radar systems were being assembled. To insure that Zaret's findings would be made on a wholly objective basis, there were some workers who had been exposed to microwaves and some, as control subjects, who had no history of exposure; and Zaret proceeded to examine them all without knowing who had been exposed and who had not. In every case, an ophthalmological history of the patient was obtained to determine whether there was any hereditary predisposition to cataract formation; the patient's eyes were tested for visual acuity; the lenses of his eyes were examined with a slit lamp, which is a type of microscope that beams light into the eye and makes it possible to scrutinize the lens in minute detail; and three-dimensional photographs of each lens were taken. When the survey was completed, no cataracts were found, but there was a slight excess of minor defects in the lenses of the group exposed to microwaves. Since Zaret knew from clinical experience that such imperfections were not the precursors of cataracts but merely an indication of the normal effect of aging upon the lens, he concluded that they did not serve as an indicator of cumulative exposure to microwaves and were of no clinical significance in determining whether or not microwave workers were at special risk of developing cataracts. Moreover, he noted that since it was impossible to establish with any accuracy the microwave levels to which the workers had been exposed, no conclusions could be drawn from the survey about the safety of the ten-milliwatt level. For these reasons, he stated in his final report that a proposed follow-up survey of lens imperfections in these patients would serve no useful purpose, and he recommended that it not be undertaken.

Although the results of the three-year survey were inconclusive, Zaret had made some unusual observations in the course of it that in time profoundly altered his own thinking about how microwaves could affect the eyes.

> Right off the bat, I saw something very strange. In April of 1960, while I was conducting a pilot study of forty-odd radar workers up at Griffiss Air Force Base, in Rome, New York, I examined a young man in his early twenties who had a cataract on the posterior portion of the lens as well as areas of opacity on the posterior capsule. Now, the capsule is a transparent elastic membrane about ten microns—or one twenty-five-hundredth of an inch—thick which surrounds the lens the way a cellophane wrapper surrounds a piece of candy, and only in extremely rare circumstances do cataractous changes occur in it. The only capsular cataracts I had ever come across had occurred in glassblowers and other workers exposed to the intense heat of infrared radiation, and those cataracts, as might be expected, had developed on the anterior, or front, portion of the capsule. In fact, I had never seen a cataract on the posterior capsule of an otherwise healthy eye before, and I didn't know what to make of it. Since the young man was a juvenile diabetic, however, and since diabetes is known to be a causative factor in the formation of cataracts, there were no conclusions to be drawn from the case. I made a note to reexamine him, but unfortunately he died in the meantime. He was found unconscious at the foot of a microwave relay tower, and he died in what was diagnosed as a diabetic-related uremic coma.

Zaret went on to say that he had made another unusual observation in the summer of 1961, while examining a group of civilian radar workers at the Ballistic Missile Early Warning System installation in Thule, Greenland:

> Two men showed up with pronounced swelling of the lens. Such swelling usually occurs within two weeks of some acute injury or trauma to the eye, so I went to the health-and-safety people at the base and asked them what each of these men had been doing recently. Sure enough, there was an accident report on file for them. It turned out not only that they worked together but that ten days before, while they were working on some microwave generators that had supposedly been shut down, sparks began flying from their screwdrivers. This meant that their tools were acting as receiving antennas, and that they themselves were being irradiated with microwaves. The very nature of their injuries indicated that they had been exposed to power densities that must have greatly exceeded ten milliwatts per square centimeter.

The incredible thing to me was that neither of them could remember feeling anything. Up till then, everyone had always assumed that an amount of microwave radiation sufficient to cause acute injury such as swelling of the lens would also produce the sensation of heat, which microwaves are known to produce in tissue, and that this sensation of heat would be especially felt by the eye, which is exquisitely sensitive to pain. Indeed, part of the mythology long accepted by microwave workers was that you couldn't be hurt by a microwave beam, because you would always be able to feel heat and get out of the way. Yet these two workers insisted that they hadn't felt a thing. It was an ominous finding indeed, for it meant that microwaves could act insidiously to cause serious injury.

As it happened, at about this time several large electronics and communications companies that were taking part in the survey of lens imperfections began sending to Zaret for private consultation employees who had already been diagnosed by other ophthalmologists as having cataracts:

> I saw half a dozen such cases in 1961 and 1962. These patients were sent to me because there was a question as to whether they had been injured by microwave radiation. Of course, every one of them was a potential legal case, and it is to the credit of the companies that they continued to send those cases, for I made it clear to begin with that I would disclose my findings to each patient, and I requested that I be permitted to perform follow-up examinations of them in the future. As things turned out, what I found ultimately changed my whole thinking about microwave cataractogenesis, for slit-lamp examination revealed not only that all six of these patients had developing cataracts but also that the cataracts were forming on the posterior capsular surface. This was a totally unexpected finding—the possibility of such damage had not even been included in the parameters of the survey I was conducting for the Air Force. Naturally, I began looking for similar abnormalities in the people who had been selected for the official survey, and I soon began to find them. In one group of forty-odd radar trouble-shooters from a large electronics company, I found that fully one-third of them had roughening and thickening of the posterior capsular surface—a kind of pre-cataractous scarring that I later came to realize was an early sign of microwave injury.

When Zaret wrote his final report for the Air Force survey, in March 1963, he knew that the criteria upon which the study had been

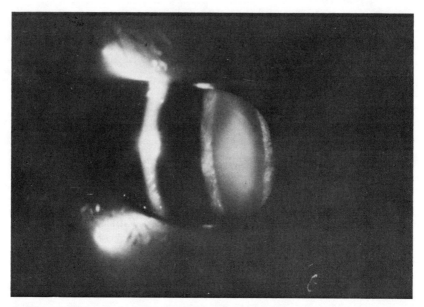

A slit-lamp photograph of a fully developed cataract in a radar worker, showing opacification in both the anterior and posterior capsule of the lens. PHOTO BY MILTON ZARET

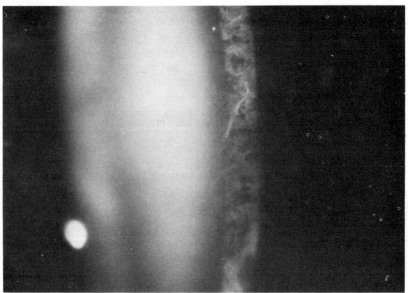

A higher magnification in which the lighter areas clearly show that the posterior capsule has become clouded with cataractous changes. PHOTO BY MILTON ZARET

based—the occurrence of imperfections within the lens—were not a valid method of assessing the ophthalmological hazard posed by microwaves. Within a year, however, thanks largely to the cases he had seen in private consultation, he believed that he had found a way to make this assessment:

> I knew by then that the typical microwave cataract tends to involve the posterior surface of the lens, whereas the typical infrared or heat cataract involves the front surface. This occurs for two reasons: first, because microwave radiation penetrates deeply and heats the whole eye; second, because the iris, with its greater blood circulation, keeps the front portion of the eye cooler than the rear portion. With infrared radiation, on the other hand, absorption occurs maximally at the surface so the temperature is higher at the front surface of the lens than at the rear surface. For these reasons, I suspected not only that microwave injury leading to cataract formation tended to occur first at the posterior capsule but also that posterior capsular cataract was a marker disease for exposure to microwaves. Therefore, I was prepared to make a presumptive diagnosis of microwave cataracts as a clinical entity on the basis that posterior capsular opacification could serve as the special signature of microwave injury. This, in turn, enabled me to start looking for pre-cataractous changes in workers who were being exposed to microwave radiation, and to recommend preventive measures where indicated.

In October 1964, Dr. Zaret published his findings on three cases of posterior capsular cataracts. The data appeared in the final report of a year-long study he had conducted for the Air Force in order to arrive at a new methodology for assessing the cataractogenic effects of microwave radiation. However, the Air Force was apparently unimpressed by the information, for in the same report it announced the termination of its microwave-eye-study program and of any follow-up research. "By this time, I was beginning to wonder about the military's attitude toward the problem of microwave exposure," Zaret said.

> Here I had spent three years examining nearly sixteen hundred microwave workers, and except for one case that didn't count, because diabetes was involved, I hadn't come across a single cataract. Then, right in the middle of my survey, some of the very firms that were taking part in it began sending me patients on the side—patients who had been diagnosed as having cataracts. Why weren't such patients

included in the official survey? Why did they all come from private companies? Why had I not seen any cataracts among military person-nel? Had I been examining a true cross-section of people exposed to microwave radiation? Or was something funny going on in the selec-tion process, because of worries over public disclosure and possible legal problems?

Zaret soon had other reasons to consider the possibility that expo-sure to microwaves was being viewed in a nonmedical manner:

> By this time, I had been approached on a number of occasions by the Central Intelligence Agency. The contacts were innocuous to begin with. At first, the CIA people wanted to know about research I had performed on the ophthalmological effects of microwave and laser radiation. They also wanted me to analyze some of the foreign and American literature on the subject of radiation for them. In 1964, however, they started asking me about the possible behavioral effects of microwaves. They wanted to know, for example, whether I thought that electromagnetic radiation beamed at the brain from a distance could affect the way a person might act. I said that from what I had read primarily in Soviet literature on the subject it seemed conceivable. During 1964 and 1965, I had a number of visits from a medical doctor who worked for the agency. He wanted to know if a device that took pictures at night with an invisible laser beam instead of a conventional flashbulb was safe to use. When I exposed the eye of a rabbit to the beam, I found that it produced an immediate retinal hemorrhage, so I told him that in my opinion the device was not safe. He also wanted answers to a number of theoretical questions. For instance, would a laser beam directed at a listening device planted on a windowsill be liable to injure anyone inside the room that was being bugged? And could microwaves be used to facilitate brainwashing or to break down prisoners under interrogation?

Early in 1965, Dr. Zaret was informed by his CIA contact that the Russians had been irradiating the American Embassy in Moscow with microwaves. "The CIA people seemed puzzled and confused by this development," Zaret recalled.

> Later that year, they invited me to attend a special meeting on the subject at the Institute for Defense Analyses, in Arlington, Virginia, where I met a number of people from the Defense Department's Advanced Research Projects Agency, who were also working on the problem. There appeared to be considerable anxiety in the minds of

some of these people over whether the Moscow Signal, as it was called, was a serious attempt to actually alter the behavior of our personnel at the embassy. This anxiety no doubt resulted from the fact that the signal, which was described in detailed technical terms at the meeting, was not considered to be suitable either for electronic eavesdropping or for jamming electronic listening devices. It was being generated at multiple frequencies and widely fluctuating patterns, and at power densities that never exceeded four milliwatts per square centimeter. Since the Russians considered radiation at this level to be unsafe, and since we had only very limited data on the question, I advised the Department of Defense people to irradiate monkeys with a signal of the same frequency and power density, in order to determine what the signal's behavioral and biological effects upon human beings might be. I told them that in my opinion our government ought to demand that the Russians stop irradiating the embassy at once. I also told them that thorough medical examinations of the embassy staff members should be performed, and that these people should be informed of what had been done to them. Subsequently, some associates and I conducted research for the Advanced Research Projects Agency by replicating a few selected Soviet and Eastern European behavioral experiments on rats and rabbits. We performed this research with the help and assistance of Professors Saul W. Rosenthal and Leo Birenbaum, who are from the Department of Electrical Engineering and Electrophysics of the Polytechnic Institute of New York. In some cases, we were able to confirm the Soviet and Eastern European results and in others we were not. I remember that on one occasion we not only succeeded in replicating a Czechoslovak study of behavioral effects in rats but also observed some unique convulsions in these animals prior to death. When I relayed that information to Washington, I received a telegram from the agency ordering me not to pursue the investigation any further. Later, I was given to understand that, as part of a highly classified operation called Project Pandora, tests to determine the effects of the Moscow Signal were conducted at the Walter Reed Army Institute of Research, in Washington, D.C., and that some deficiencies in the animals' ability to function and to perform tasks were observed. However, I was never told officially of the results of any of these studies.

Meanwhile, Zaret had continued to spend most of his time investigating the effects of microwave radiation upon the eye. In 1963, he had set up his own research foundation to facilitate these efforts, and in 1964, after the Air Force terminated its eye-study program, he

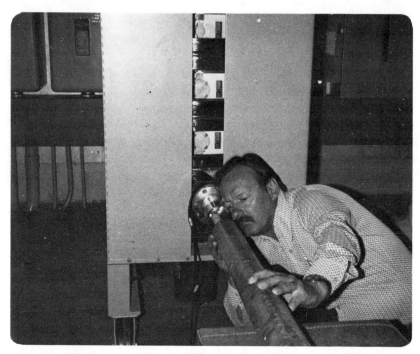

A broadcast technician demonstrating the practice of aligning two sections of a TV transmitter following replacement of a defective klystron tube. During this procedure the remainder of the transmitter is still operating to permit broadcasting to continue. This worker developed a rapidly maturing cataract in the right eye following one such procedure. PHOTO BY BERNARD DANEK

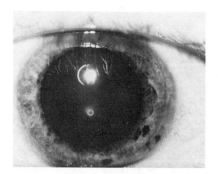

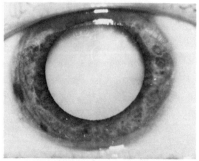

The left eye of the same man showing a relatively normal lens. Ordinarily, cataracts develop simultaneously in both eyes. The fact that this man developed a cataract in his right eye is strong evidence that it was caused by microwave radiation. PHOTO BY MILTON ZARET

The right eye of the broadcast technician in the photograph above showing a fully developed cataract. PHOTO BY MILTON ZARET

undertook for the Army a study of military and civilian personnel who had been exposed to microwaves, in order to look for early signs predictive of eye injury. He also continued to examine patients who were referred to him by industry for private consultation. At that time, only five documented cases of human microwave cataracts were known to exist. Over the next five years, however, Zaret found thirty-nine more cases of incipient or clinically significant microwave cataracts:

> All thirty-nine cases occurred in men who worked for the armed services, the National Aeronautics and Space Administration, and in the electronics industry. Most of the men were engaged in the research and development or the testing and maintenance of high-power radar systems. They averaged about forty years of age, which meant that they were far too young for naturally occurring cataracts, and none of them were known to have any hereditary or pathological predisposition toward the disease. Most important of all, slit-lamp examination showed that each of these thirty-nine men had cataracts of the posterior capsular surface.

By the end of the decade, Zaret had collected and published data on a total of forty-two cases of microwave cataracts, and he also claimed to have found nearly two hundred cases of roughening and thickening of the posterior capsular surface, which he considered to be early evidence of cataract development. He had also lost the contract with the Army for the prospective study:

> The Army decided not to renew the contract in 1968, shortly after I reported posterior capsular changes in seven civilian employees at the Signal Corps base at Fort Monmouth, New Jersey. The chief of Ophthalmology Service at the Walter Reed General Hospital, Colonel Budd Appleton, told me there was no such thing as a microwave cataract. He claimed the only thing one could say was that a patient had a developing cataract due to normal aging. One trouble with this theory was that in many of the forty-two cases I had reported, a cataract had formed in only one eye, whereas senile cataracts usually develop bilaterally. Of course, the military people were anxious about my findings for a number of reasons. First of all, if I turned out to be correct, and if it became widely recognized and accepted that microwaves could cause a specific and recognizable type of cataract, the armed forces were liable to incur some huge medical-legal problems, especially with civilian employees who had been exposed to radar.

Second, and even more important, an enormous part of the nation's weapons-development program for the next decade, including the antiballistic-missile systems, was predicated on the assumption that the ten-milliwatt level was safe. If this standard turned out to be unsafe and had to be lowered, the cost of relocating radar and missile sites and of redesigning equipment would amount to billions of dollars. With so much at stake in the ten-milliwatt standard, the military could scarcely afford to accept any findings that cast doubt on the theory that cataract formation was thermal in origin. But, you see, like the two technicians in Thule, none of my forty-two patients had any recollection whatsoever of experiencing heat or pain in their eyes. This meant that cataracts could be produced by exposure to microwave levels that did not produce acute burn, which, in turn, raised the possibility that cataracts might form in the eyes of people who were chronically exposed to low levels of microwave radiation over long periods—for example, radar technicians or unsuspecting people using microwave ovens that leak.

From this point on, Zaret found himself engaged in a running battle with the military over whether microwaves were responsible for the development of cataracts in the eyes of men who had been exposed to radar. The situation was exacerbated by the fact that a number of ex-servicemen who had worked as maintenance technicians on radar picket planes during the fifties and sixties and had lost their sight as a result of cataract formation had filed disability claims with the Veterans Administration and had also initiated lawsuits against the manufacturers of the equipment they had used. Since there was no conclusive proof of what level of microwave radiation constituted a hazard to the human eye, the military, viewing such claims, together with Zaret's findings, as a threat to the ten-milliwatt level, proceeded to gather statistics and opinions to counter them. Ophthalmologists working for the Army and the Air Force conducted eye surveys showing that lens imperfections and cataracts were not occurring any more frequently in personnel exposed to radar than in personnel who had no exposure. Furthermore, they were unanimous in the opinion that cataracts occurring in the eyes of former radar technicians were no different from those occurring in the eyes of people who had no exposure to radar. They concluded, therefore, that the probability of cataracts being caused by microwave radiation was low unless a specific instance of severe exposure could be documented and correlated with subsequent cataract development, and that the ten-milliwatt level was safe. Since Zaret stood alone in his contention that exposure to microwaves could cause unique changes in the posterior capsule, proof of a specific microwave cataract was considered lacking, and, with one exception, the disability claims of the former radar technicians were disallowed by the Veterans Administration.

As it turned out, the exception was one of Zaret's early patients —a man named Arthur Kay, who had served as a radar trouble-shooter on Navy radar picket planes during the Korean war, and who later developed a cataract. Kay's original claim for disability had been turned down by the VA in 1969. However, with Zaret's help he was subsequently able to furnish information to refute the Navy's contention that he had not been exposed to microwaves, and in 1972, after a VA appeal hearing at which Zaret appeared as his principal witness, Kay won his case. Kay's cause was also aided by Dr. Shields Warren, professor emeritus of pathology at the Harvard Medical School, who had been brought in as an independent consultant by the Board of Veterans Appeals, and who gave the opinion that Kay's cataracts had indeed been caused by microwave radiation.

As for the Navy's contention that Kay and other crew members of radar picket planes had not been exposed to microwaves, its falseness was revealed by the Navy at its nineteenth annual Occupational Health Workshop, which was held in Charleston, South Carolina, in September 1976. At that time, the officer in charge of the Radiation Health Branch of the Navy Environmental Health Center, in Cincinnati, stated that he and some assistants had recently measured the power density of microwave radiation emanating from the radar-antenna dome ten feet aft of the flight-crew ladder on the belly of an old P-2 Lockheed Neptune radar picket plane, and, finding it to be between 300 and 500 milliwatts per square centimeter from a distance of ten yards, they guessed that it would be about 600 milliwatts per square centimeter up close. He further stated that anyone climbing the flight-crew ladder leading into the aircraft could have been exposed to these high intensities.

Since the Kay case, compensation for work-related cataracts has been awarded to five former radar technicians by the VA, and to two air traffic controllers by the Department of Labor. Back in 1971, however, the Navy, which had evidently come to the conclusion that it had embarked on a collision course with Zaret, decided not to renew a contract it had awarded him to study the delayed effects of chronic microwave exposure on primates under conditions simulating human exposure. When Zaret asked for an impartial hearing on the matter, the Navy convened a five-man ad-hoc committee, which, after holding a meeting at the New York City headquarters of the Rand Corporation, upheld the decision to terminate Zaret's contract. The members of this committee included:

• William A. Mills, director of the Environmental Protection Agency's Twinbrook Research Laboratory, in Rockville, Maryland;

• Dr. David D. Donaldson, an ophthalmologist at the Massachusetts Eye and Ear Infirmary, who, as a member of the military's Joint Services Committee on Microwave Ocular Effects, had examined the eyes of former Air Force radar workers;

• Professor Sol M. Michaelson, a doctor of veterinary medicine at the Department of Radiation Biology and Biophysics of the University of Rochester's School of Medicine and Dentistry, who was a leading consultant on microwave radiation to the Association of Home Appliance Manufacturers;

• John M. Osepchuk, a consulting scientist with the Raytheon Company, the world's leading manufacturer of microwave ovens;

• Samuel Koslov, who was then a research scientist with the Rand Corporation and a member of the federal Electromagnetic Radiation Management Advisory Council, who had previously participated in Project Pandora as an official in the Department of Defense, and who has since become Special Assistant for Research to the Assistant Secretary of the Navy.

The fact that representatives of the microwave-oven industry had agreed with the military in opposing Zaret was not surprising, for two reasons. In the first place, Raytheon and other microwave-oven manufacturers also made (and still make) radar and missile-guidance systems. Second, the microwave-oven industry was in the midst of an enormous expansion that would be jeopardized if Zaret's theories about the low-level cumulative effects of microwaves proved to be correct. After the passage of the Radiation Control for Health and Safety Act of 1968, the manufacturers of microwave ovens had undertaken to make technical improvements in their products to keep them from leaking radiation in excess of the ten-milliwatt level, which had been voluntarily adopted by the Association of Home

Appliance Manufacturers. However, in 1969 a four-state survey of microwave ovens by the Environmental Control Administration's Bureau of Radiological Health showed that a third of them failed to meet this limit, and in 1970 a government-industry survey of nearly five thousand ovens revealed that ten percent were exceeding the voluntary standard. The survey indicated that faulty door seals and faulty safety interlocks—devices that are supposed to turn the oven off when the door is opened—were the chief causes of leakage, and that improper servicing and maintenance as well as normal wear and tear were also factors.

No one knew just how many microwave ovens were in use in this country, but estimates for 1969 ranged anywhere from one hundred thousand to two hundred thousand. The Bureau of Radiological Health was sufficiently concerned to recommend that until ovens could be tested for leakage consumers ought to remain at least an arm's length away from them while they were in operation, and that children should not be allowed to watch food cooking through the oven doors. The microwave-oven manufacturers claimed that their products were not leaking radiation at levels that had been proved harmful; that a person being irradiated with unsafe levels of microwave radiation would always be able to feel heat in time to move out of danger; and that the biological effects of microwaves were not cumulative. Nevertheless, when the Bureau of Radiological Health people got around to promulgating a performance standard for microwave ovens, in October 1970, they decreed that as of October 6, 1971, no oven prior to sale should leak radiation exceeding one milliwatt per square centimeter at a distance of five centimeters from its surface, and that no oven after purchase should leak more than five milliwatts over the same distance.

No one knows on what scientific basis, if any, the bureau determined that a five-milliwatt emission standard for microwave ovens would be safe for consumers, let alone how it expected any housewife to ascertain the amount of radiation leaking from a particular oven. It is known, however, that during 1969 and 1970 the bureau carefully studied and documented a case attributing the formation of what it called "typical microwave-radiation cataracts" to levels of exposure that cast doubt upon the safety of the new standard. The case involved a thirty-eight-year-old radiation-safety officer from New Mexico. Between June and December 1968 he had undergone a series of twelve fifteen-minute microwave-diathermy treatments for painfully sprained neck muscles. The diathermy machine with which the patient was treated generated microwave radiation at a frequency of 2,440 megahertz, which also happens to be within the operating-frequency band of the vast majority of microwave ovens that are manufactured and used in the United States. During the winter of 1969, vision in the patient's right eye became hazy; in May, vision in his left eye began to deteriorate; and in July he was diagnosed as having bilateral posterior subcapsular cataracts. This diagnosis was subsequently confirmed by Dr. Donaldson, of the Massachusetts Eye and Ear Infirmary, and by Professor Russell L. Carpenter, a zoologist who had recently retired from the Department of Biology of Tufts University and had become a consultant to the bureau's Northeastern Radiological Health Laboratory, in Winchester, Massachusetts.

After extensive investigation, Donaldson and Carpenter ruled out the possibility that their patient's cataracts could have been caused by diabetes, senility, chronic uveitis, or exposure to cortisone steroids or X-rays. Carpenter then set out to reconstruct the radiation pattern and power levels of the microwave field to which the patient had been exposed—something it had rarely been possible to ascertain with any real accuracy in the case of radar technicians, who usually worked with equipment generating microwaves of different wavelengths and power densities. With the cooperation of the patient and the physician who had given the diathermy treatments, Carpenter duplicated the conditions of therapy as nearly as he could, and was able to determine that the patient's right eye had been exposed to approximately thirty-three milliwatts per square centimeter and his left eye to only about two milliwatts per square centimeter. This was an astonishing finding, and, not surprisingly, the case received prominent mention in the bureau's 1969 annual report to Congress. When Carpenter described it at the fifth annual symposium of the International Microwave Power Institute, which was held in Scheveningen, in the Netherlands, on October 7, 1970, he stated that it provided a "unique example of bilateral cataracts resulting from low-level microwave radiation." Strangely, Carpenter's statement came one day after the bureau announced the promulgation of its five-milliwatt emission standard for microwave ovens. Equally strange is the fact that neither he nor Donaldson ever saw fit to submit their findings for official publication. The case never became part of the medical literature, and it has been virtually forgotten. Indeed, both Carpenter and Donaldson have since written that they knew of no case of cataracts that could be definitely attributed to microwave radiation.

During 1971 and 1972, the controversy over the biological effects of microwaves, which had previously been carried on in scientific and military circles, received considerable public attention, thanks to a series of articles written by columnists Jack Anderson and Les Whitten which appeared in newspapers from one end of the country to the other. Anderson and Whitten began by describing the plight of a group of retired Air Force radar technicians who had developed cataracts after serving as crewmen on Lockheed Constellation EC-121 spy planes, and by questioning the claim of the Air Force that the levels of microwave radiation to which these men had been exposed presented no hazard to their eyes. They went on to say that in 1969 the Air Force had transferred the physician in charge of radiobiology at its Aerospace Medical Division after he had stated publicly that microwave radiation presented a serious hazard to the eyes of servicemen exposed to radar and other microwave devices and that thorough investigations should be made of a whole series of biological effects in order to reevaluate the ten-milliwatt level.

Anderson and Whitten took the Navy to task for terminating its financial support of Zaret's study of the chronic effects of microwaves upon monkeys, and suggested that Zaret's preliminary report that some monkeys had died after being exposed to relatively low levels of radiation might have had something to do with it. (Zaret had informed the Navy in February 1970 that one monkey had died after being irradiated for several hours with only twenty milliwatts per square centimeter, and that "the finding has extremely serious implications.") In subsequent columns, Anderson and Whitten expressed doubts about the safety of microwave ovens, and in May 1972 they broke the ten-year-old story of how the Russians had beamed microwave radiation into the American Embassy in Moscow in the early sixties. In their account of the Moscow incident, Anderson and Whitten revealed that the whole affair had been kept secret from employees at the embassy; that the CIA had speculated that the Russians might be trying to brainwash American diplomats; and that scientists working for the Advanced Research Projects Agency had attempted to come to grips with the mystery by irradiating monkeys and other test animals in a secret study called Project Pandora, whose results were said to have been inconclusive.

As might be expected, Anderson and Whitten came under heavy attack from representatives of both the military and industry, who maintained that many of their assertions concerning the hazards of radar and microwave ovens were either inaccurate or unnecessarily alarming. Curiously, no one in the military or in industry attempted to refute their claim that the Russians had tried to alter the minds and behavior of American Embassy personnel in Moscow with microwave radiation, and in August the Russians themselves lent credence to the claim by voicing a suspicion, during the chess matches in Reykjavik, Iceland, that aides of Bobby Fischer were irradiating Boris Spassky with electronic devices in an effort to cause the Russian master to lose his championship. Be that as it may, back in December 1971 the nine members of the Electromagnetic Radiation Management Advisory Council—the group that had been established three years earlier by the President's Office of Telecommunications Policy—had released a little-publicized report assessing the possible biological hazards of microwaves and other radio-frequency energy in terms that made Anderson's and Whitten's revelations seem fragmentary, if not tame, by comparison. Among other things, the council's report pointed out that microwave radiation was permeating the modern environment; that such man-made radiation had no counterpart in man's evolutionary background; that existing levels of radio-frequency energy might already be biologically significant; and that the consequences of undervaluing or misjudging the biological effects of long-term, low-level exposure could become a critical public-health problem—especially if genetic effects were involved.

Having hinted at the unthinkable in its overall evaluation of the problem, the council proceeded to recommend ways of solving it which promised to continue a business-as-usual approach to the situation. In its "Program for Control of Electromagnetic Pollution of the Environment," which was adopted by the government, the council did not propose a single measure for controlling microwave radiation. Instead, it called for a coordinated five-year, multi-agency, $63-million-dollar research effort to determine whether microwave radiation posed a hazard to health. Moreover, the council delegated primary responsibility for determining the effects of long-term low-level microwave radiation to the Department of Defense, which for twenty-five years had been denying that any such hazards might exist and casting a pall of obfuscation over the entire question, a tactic reminiscent of the metallic chaff dropped from airplanes during the Second World War to create false echoes and blur the enemy's radar.

6

Some Illumination

The publicity generated by the microwave controversy in 1971 and 1972 was bound to have political repercussions, and on March 8, 1973, the Senate's Committee on Commerce opened three days of hearings to determine how the Radiation Control for Health and Safety Act of 1968 (Public Law 90–602) had functioned since its passage. The committee's presiding officer, Senator John V. Tunney of California, spoke first: "Unfortunately, preliminary work by the committee has raised some disturbing questions about radiation safety in this country, and calls into question whether Public Law 90–602 has in fact resulted in big enough steps being taken to insure that long-term and far-reaching radiation damage will be avoided." Senator Tunney went on to say that a major source of concern to the committee was the increasing proliferation of devices emitting microwaves into the environment; that industry would soon be selling two hundred thousand microwave ovens a year; and that "only yesterday the Consumers Union recommended against the purchase of any microwave oven, primarily because of the unknown biological effects of microwaves." Tunney was referring to an announcement that Consumers Union had obviously issued to coincide with the opening of the hearings, and that was being carried in newspapers across the country. In its announcement, Consumers Union stated that it had found measurable radiation leakage in fifteen leading microwave-oven models; that it considered the government's five-milliwatt emission standard inadequate, because there were no data on what quantity of low-level radiation could cause human injury; that although the leakage it had detected was within the five-milliwatt level, a tug on the door of one model and a paper towel caught in the door of another caused leakage far in excess of the government standard; and that it felt the burden of proof was therefore on microwave-oven manufacturers to show that their products were safe.

The first witness at the hearings was John C. Villforth, director of the Bureau of Radiological Health, who praised the government's microwave-research program and defended the five-milliwatt emission standard for microwave ovens, saying, "Although reliable human data [are] not yet available, we do have animal experiments and epidemiological studies to give us confidence that the limit that we have set is reasonable." Villforth subsequently referred questions about the testing of microwave ovens to Dr. Robert L. Elder, deputy director of the bureau and a former director of its Division of Electronic Products, who also defended the five-milliwatt level as valid in terms of the available biological information. Senator Tunney then asked Dr. Elder, "If low-level effects are unknown, why not err on the side of safety—particularly when research that has been done on low-level exposure by the Russians and other researchers in this country, such as Dr. Milton Zaret, demonstrates that it could be injurious to health?" Elder said he believed that in setting up its testing procedures the bureau had erred on the side of safety to begin with. Something he did not mention was that less than a year before, as a member of the American National Standards Institute's subcommittee on radio-frequency hazards, he had recommended that the microwave-protection guide be lowered to one milliwatt per square centimeter.

On the following day, Dr. Clay T. Whitehead, director of the Office of Telecommunications Policy, told the committee that his office was attempting to coordinate studies in the research program recommended by the Electromagnetic Radiation Management Advisory Council, which were being carried out by the Department of Defense together with a dozen different agencies and subagencies. When Senator Tunney asked him if he was satisfied that adequate protection was being given to consumers, and particularly to house-wives using microwave ovens, Dr. Whitehead replied that although he was not an expert in the field, he was convinced that "the stan-dards that we have now are appropriate to the kinds of hazards that we can document through scientific study." Senator Tunney then recalled that in a press release announcing the government's research program Dr. Whitehead had stated that the potential impact of microwave radiation on human beings was unknown, and that the probable effects of long-term exposure to low levels of radiation were not adequately understood. "If this is true," Senator Tunney asked Dr. Whitehead, "wouldn't you agree with the Consumers Union that it would be unwise to expose yourself to any unneeded radiation until more is known?"

"No one should expose himself to any unneeded radiation," Dr. Whitehead replied. "The problem is that so much of the radiation that people are exposed to—microwave ovens, television transmit-ters, and what have you—are all devices that are doing very useful things that people want to do and want done for them. I think the important thing to recognize is that there is no evidence that there is a hazard from low-level energy radiations. It's just that there is some uncertainty in the scientific knowledge, and that we can't rest on our laurels."

The next witness to appear before the committee was Dr. Zaret, who stated at the outset that in his opinion there was a "clear, present, and ever-increasing danger" to the entire population of the United States from exposure to the non-ionizing portion of the elec-tromagnetic spectrum. "The dangers cannot be overstated," Zaret said, "because most non-ionizing radiational injuries occur covertly, usually do not become manifest until after latent periods of years, and when they do become manifest, the effects are seldom recog-nized." Zaret went on to characterize the ten-milliwatt level recom-mended by the American National Standards Institute's subcommit-tee on radio-frequency hazards—an organization from which he had recently resigned—as being patently unsafe, and to blame the De-partment of Defense for leading the country astray by minimizing the true extent of the microwave-radiation hazard. Zaret was partic-ularly critical of the ethics and the safety of a study being conducted at the Naval Aerospace Medical Research Laboratory, in Pensacola, Florida, in which human volunteers were being exposed to radio waves in the extremely-low-frequency portion, or ELF, of the electromagnetic spectrum. This study had been undertaken to assess the possible biological hazards of Project Sanguine, an ambitious scheme —later renamed Project Seafarer—that would bury a gigantic, three-to-four-thousand-square-mile underground radio-antenna system three to six feet below ground in the Upper Peninsula of Michigan, in order to permeate the entire biosphere with extremely-low-frequency radio waves, and thus enable the Navy to communicate with deeply submerged nuclear submarines. Zaret's reservations about the study were subsequently confirmed in part by the fact that blood-serum triglyceride levels rose to abnormally high levels in nine out of ten volunteers following one day of exposure to an extremely-low-frequency magnetic field, and also by the fact that in another study of eleven men exposed to the field there was a significant decline in their ability to perform simple addition. (These results were not made public by the Navy for more than two years, but the Navy ended the human volunteer study, and is now conducting an extensive study of the chronic exposure of monkeys to extremely-low-frequency electromagnetic fields.) Zaret's reservations about Project Seafarer as a whole have also been confirmed in part by the revelation that Soviet and Spanish workers in high-voltage switchyards, who have been occupationally exposed to electric and magnetic fields at extremely low frequencies similar to those employed in Project Seafarer, have experienced instability in pulse and blood pressure, slowed heartbeat, anemia, tremors in the arms and legs, and diminished sexual vigor.* Zaret has since hypothesized that extremely-low-frequency electric fields from sources such as high-voltage power

---

*In this connection, a fierce battle is being waged by environmentalists who are opposed to the New York State Public Service Commission's plans to link nuclear power plants in upstate New York with a network of 765,000-volt power lines. According to Dr. Andrew Marino, a biophysicist at the Veterans Administration Hospital in Syracuse, the sixty-hertz electric fields emanating from these high-voltage power lines can be detected up to a mile away, and since he has observed stunting of growth in mice and alterations in the blood chemistry of rats that were exposed to electric fields of 15,000 volts per meter, which is approximately the strength of the electric field found directly beneath the high-voltage power lines, he believes that the long-term biological effects of electric fields on human beings should be thoroughly investigated before the network of 765,000-volt power lines is installed. It is interesting to note that when beehives are placed directly under the wires of high-tension power lines, the electric field prevents the bees from increasing in number and storing excess honey.

lines might prove to be a partial causative factor in sudden-infant-death syndrome. As for the residents of the Upper Peninsula, they have expressed their reservations about Project Seafarer, which has already cost the nation's taxpayers about a hundred million dollars, by voting against it in special referenda held during the Michigan primary elections in the spring of 1976. Political opposition on the part of the inhabitants of northern Wisconsin and Texas had previously defeated efforts by the Navy to locate the project in those areas.

At the conclusion of his testimony in the 1973 hearings, Zaret told the committee that he had recently observed typical microwave-radiation cataracts in the eyes of a housewife whose only known exposure to microwaves had come from the use of a microwave oven that leaked. "The sun is our strongest natural source of microwaves," Zaret continued. "The microwave-oven-leakage standard set by the Bureau of Radiological Health is approximately one billion times higher than the total, entire microwave spectrum given off by the sun. It is appalling for these ovens to be permitted to leak at all, let alone for the oven advertisements to encourage our children to have fun by learning to cook with them."

Zaret was followed to the witness table by John Osepchuk, of Raytheon, who was accompanied by Professor Michaelson, of the University of Rochester. After announcing that he and Michaelson were appearing on behalf of the Association of Home Appliance Manufacturers, Osepchuk said that he wished to place the controversy over the safety of microwave ovens in perspective by quoting Dr. James A. Van Allen, professor of physics at the University of Iowa, who had described the hazards of microwave ovens as being "about the same as the likelihood of getting a skin tan from moonlight." Osepchuk went on to say that the five-milliwatt emission standard provided a high degree of safety; that in an estimated total of a hundred million hours of microwave-oven use over the past twenty years there had been no validated report of injury to any consumer because of microwave exposure; that there was no scientific basis for believing that cumulative molecular damage could be caused by microwaves; and that the only known possible hazard associated with microwaves resulted from heat.

Osepchuk concluded his testimony by stating that both the scientific and the popular literature contained a great deal of misinformation and nonsense about microwaves, and then he introduced Professor Michaelson, who told the committee not only that there was no substantial evidence of injury to human beings as a result of exposure to microwave radiation within the ten-milliwatt level but also that the scientific and medical communities had not been able to produce any substantial evidence of injury below the level of a hundred milliwatts per square centimeter. To Michaelson, the concept of cumulative effects was based on flimsy evidence; the Soviet data concerning effects of low-level microwaves upon the central nervous system were questionable; and current standards were entirely adequate to protect the public health. "In closing, I would like to make a plea," Michaelson said. "We have reached the point now where we cannot continue to succumb to self-interest groups and individuals who fail to substantiate their claims."

When Michaelson had completed his statement, Senator Tunney quoted a passage from an article entitled "Biologic Effects of Microwave Exposure," which Michaelson and some associates had published in a United States Air Force technical report in 1967 concerning the studies undertaken by the Russians. The passage read:

> The occasional reports of headache, lassitude, stomach-ache pains, sleeplessness, irritability, and other highly subjective symptoms among workers in the vicinity of microwave generating equipment have not been thoroughly investigated. These findings should not be ignored, as similar vague, mild, and undefined symptoms have been experienced in the course of microwave studies in this laboratory. Such symptoms could indicate a basic microwave effect.

When Senator Tunney had finished reading this passage, he observed that after listening to Professor Michaelson's testimony he felt that the professor had changed his mind since writing the article, and asked if this was so.

Michaelson replied that he had indeed changed his mind, and then he explained why. "I have written extensively since then and I have been very fortunate in having had the opportunity to read, study, and survey the literature extensively and intensively in the last several years," said Michaelson, who is a member of the National Academy of Science's Committee on Biosphere Effects of Extremely-Low-Frequency Radiation, which has been set up to determine whether the Navy's proposed Seafarer communications system might prove harmful to human beings, animals, plants, and other organisms. "I have also been very fortunate to be affiliated with many organizations in which these problems are being discussed, and I have been able to critically analyze many, many of the problems, and I feel very secure; in fact, I feel much more confident now than I appear to have been in 1967."

Professor Michaelson was the last witness to testify about the biological effects of microwaves, and when he had finished, Senator Tunney confessed that he was puzzled. "I am somewhat confused by the difference in the testimony that we have had in the past two days, and this is something that I'll have to resolve myself through further study," he said. "I think a person who is not completely familiar with the field would have to agree with me that, in listening to the statements that have been made, there is, in some instances, a one-hundred-and-eighty-degree difference in approach, and I therefore feel that I personally am going to have to do more research and talk to more people who are recognized experts."

If Senator Tunney had attended the four-day International Symposium on the Biologic Effects and Health Hazards of Microwave Radiation, which was co-sponsored by the governments of Poland and the United States and by the World Health Organization, and was held at Jadwisin, near Warsaw, in October 1973, he would have been able to talk with sixty recognized experts from twelve nations, who had met to exchange information and ideas about the microwave problem. He would also have seen some familiar faces. It seems highly unlikely, however, that he would have been able to resolve the confusion he had felt at the hearings. On the one hand, the Senator would have heard John Villforth, director of the Bureau of Radiological Health, state that his organization had "only scratched the surface in developing a biological-effects program with respect to microwaves," and that "even this minimal effort is only being directed at the frequency which is utilized for microwave cooking and for which instrumentation is available." On the other hand, he would have heard Professor Zinaida V. Gordon, the widely respected pioneer in microwave research, say that she and other Soviet investigators had been conducting extensive hygienic, clinical, and experimental studies of the whole range of radio frequencies for more than twenty years, and that there was absolutely no doubt that microwave radiation could have biological effects at intensities far below those necessary for the heating of tissue.

With regard to 180-degree differences of approach, Senator Tunney would have learned that American researchers, in keeping with their long tradition of studying primarily the thermal effects of large microwave exposures, had produced fetal deaths and serious birth defects by irradiating pregnant mice with single two-to-five minute doses of 123 milliwatts per square centimeter, whereas their Soviet counterparts had obtained similar results by irradiating pregnant mice with daily two-hour doses of only 6.5 milliwatts. Concerning the development of cataracts, he could have chosen between a paper submitted by Professor Carpenter, of the Bureau of Radiological Health, who wrote, "As of now, we do not know of a case in which microwave radiation has been the proven cause of a human cataract," and one delivered by Dr. Zaret, who declared that he knew of more than fifty cases with prima-facie evidence of cataracts caused by microwave radiation. And concerning the cumulative effects of microwave radiation in producing cataracts—a concept that was first suggested fifty years ago, by Sir Stewart Duke-Elder, of the Institute of Ophthalmology in London, and later demonstrated in animal experiments by Professor Carpenter—he could have taken his pick of a number of conflicting opinions. Doubts about the validity of the theory were voiced by Michaelson and by Colonel Budd Appleton, of Walter Reed, whereas, it was defended by Dr. Moris L. Shore, director of the Division of Biologic Effects of the Bureau of Radiological Health, and by Dr. H. D. Baillie, a surgeon at the Royal Infirmary of the University of Manchester, who observed that if microwaves produce injury to tissue, one cannot assume that the injury disappears when the power is turned off. And, if he had managed to remain unconfused through all this, Senator Tunney could have picked up some interesting historical tidbits concerning microwaves. He would have learned, for example, that during the Second World War the Japanese Army had investigated the use of microwave radiation as a death ray but that the results of the studies had been destroyed by fire in 1945.

Perhaps the most significant paper at the symposium was delivered by Dr. Maria N. Sadčikova, a senior research worker at the Soviet Union's Institute of Labor Hygiene and Occupational Diseases, who furnished evidence to support the long-held Soviet contention that microwave sickness was a distinct form of occupational disease. Dr. Sadčikova presented detailed clinical observations of the health status of two groups of workers who had been engaged in the regulation, tuning, and testing of microwave-generating equipment of various sorts. The first group consisted of 1,000 workers who had been exposed to power densities of up to a few milliwatts per square centimeter, and the second of 180 workers whose exposure had as a rule not exceeded several hundredths of a milliwatt. Both groups consisted mostly of men under forty who had worked with microwaves for periods ranging from five to fifteen years. When Sadčikova compared the health experience of these two groups with that of a control group of 200 people whose work did not involve exposure to microwaves, she found that among the microwave workers there was a significant increase in neurological complaints, such as heaviness in the head, fatigue, irritability, anxiety, insomnia, and partial loss of memory. In addition, she found that the microwave workers showed a significant increase in cardiovascular symptoms, such as a tendency to have slow heartbeat, reduced blood pressure, and reduced ventricular capacity, and that many of them complained of piercing heart pains that spread to their shoulder blades and their arms. While Dr. Sadčikova did not observe serious cardiovascular malfunction or irreversible neurological changes among the microwave workers, she clearly substantiated the findings of previous Soviet investigations, which had shown that the clinical picture of microwave sickness was characterized by a complex of nervous-system symptoms and of vascular disturbances, including crises of cerebral and coronary insufficiency. She was also able to determine that neurological complaints usually occurred in the initial stages of microwave sickness; that cardiovascular symptoms manifested themselves in the more advanced stages of the disease; and that the symptoms increased in severity and the malady tended to progress in workers whose exposure to microwaves continued, whereas in workers whose exposure ceased altogether the disease was frequently stabilized.

The fact that the workers studied by Sadčikova had been exposed to microwave intensities far below the ten-milliwatt level that had long been considered a safe standard of exposure in the United States for both workers and members of the general population could not have been lost on the American scientists who attended the symposium in Poland. However, except for Zaret, who was considered by many scientists to be a maverick and an alarmist, no American researcher had come right out and said that microwave radiation would prove to be a health hazard for the general population—this despite the fact that investigations conducted both in the United States and in the Soviet Union had clearly shown that intensities of electromagnetic radiation were much higher in the vicinity of television transmitters, television-relay links, and radar stations than elsewhere, and that these intensities might be biologically significant. On the last day of the symposium, however, the possibility that a public-health hazard already existed was raised in bizarre fashion by Zaret, who had also evolved an unusual theory about the effects of non-ionizing radiation upon the heart.

For nearly ten years, Zaret had observed that many of his ophthalmological patients who had worked either with radar or with other microwave-generating equipment were developing cardiovascular disease at an early age. Since studies all over the world indicated that cardiovascular disease is multifactored, and since he was aware of Soviet studies concerning the cardiac effects of microwaves, Zaret wondered if exposure to microwave radiation could be contributing to the occurrence of heart disease in his patients. He attempted to explain how this might happen in an article entitled "Clinical Aspects of Non-Ionizing Radiation," which appeared in the July 1972, issue of the *Transactions on Biomedical Engineering,* a journal published by the Institute of Electrical and Electronics Engineers. Zaret offered a rationale of how low-intensity microwave radiation could cause cataracts to form on the lens capsule of the eye. "As the eye focusses during vision, the elastic lens capsule is constantly under the stress of relative stretch and relaxation," he wrote. "Normally after each stress from stretching there is complete recovery. However, following excessive irradiation, the elastic properties of the capsule may be altered. Eventually this would lead to a mechanical fatigue of the membrane."

After theorizing that structural fatigue of the lens capsule could, in turn, lead to changes in its composition and thus to the development of cataracts, Zaret suggested that elastic-membrane fatigue might also provide a rationale for the biological effects of microwave radiation on other organs. He wrote:

For example, currently there is no acceptable explanation for the delayed cardiac effects occasionally seen following non-ionizing radiation exposure. However, the linings of the heart and its major blood vessels are contained within an internal elastic membrane. The cardiovascular elastic membrane, like the lens capsule elastic membrane, is constantly under the stress of relative stretch and relaxation as it helps to sustain the hydraulic pressure of the circulatory system. Here again, after each stress from stretching there is complete recovery. However, following excessive irradiation, the elasticity of this membrane could also eventually undergo mechanical fatigue and this would ultimately lead to degradation of the elastic membrane's integrity and result in cardiovascular disease. There is much to support this concept because one of the best-known delayed appearing radiation effects is premature aging, which occurs concomitantly with a reduction in tissue elasticity. Certainly all cardiovascular disease cannot be explained in this simplistic fashion, and other predisposing factors must also exist; nevertheless, it is interesting to note that a gross parallel could be drawn between the increased incidence of coronary artery disease and myocardial infarction in urban centers and the increased ambient levels of electronic smog in these environments.

Having drawn this parallel in 1972, Zaret was puzzled when, more than a year later, he read a front-page story in the *New York Times* about the efforts of the Finnish government and the World Health Organization to study and deal with arteriosclerosis in North Karelia and Kuopio, two rural districts in southeastern Finland, whose five hundred thousand inhabitants had been found to experience the highest rate of heart attack in the world. The article, which was written by Lawrence K. Altman, appeared on September 16, 1973—a month before the start of the Warsaw symposium. Part of it read:

> The fact that North Karelia has the highest incidence of heart attacks is a paradox.
>
> Heart attacks have come to be considered a disease of stress in industrialized urban societies. Typically, they are thought of as striking overweight people who seldom exercise, sit behind desks at work, and drive home to watch television.
>
> But North Karelia is a serene lakeland, forested with firs and pines, resembling Maine. Farming and lumbering are the bases of the economy. Hard physical work is the way of life. Yet heart attacks fell robust Finnish lumberjacks like timber.

According to Altman's account, Finnish health officials had decided that increased cholesterol levels, cigarette smoking, and high blood pressure were the most important risk factors involved in the epidemic of heart attacks afflicting the inhabitants of the area. Altman wrote that "the predominant weight of scientific evidence points to the North Karelian diet, which is high in dairy fats and contains few vegetables, as the primary risk factor for the rising number of heart attacks." He then described the efforts of the Finnish government to encourage the inhabitants of North Karelia to cut down on their fat intake, to quit smoking, and to have their blood pressure checked at community screening centers.

After reading Altman's article, Zaret looked at a map that accompanied it, and, struck by the fact that North Karelia was situated along the Soviet border to the northwest of Leningrad, and opposite Lake Ladoga, he found himself wondering if electromagnetic radiation from some large Soviet communications center might be contributing to the incidence of heart attack among the people of the district, who were obviously already at high risk because of their eating and smoking habits. (Six months later, he learned from a former communications-intelligence expert with knowledge of the area that radiation was probably emanating from a powerful over-the-horizon radar complex, whose transmissions were being reflected and enhanced by the surface of Lake Ladoga to achieve long-distance, low-trajectory microwave beams that, bouncing off the layers of the ionosphere, would enable the Russians to detect missiles launched from underground silos in the American Midwest and West.) Since Zaret had been invited to attend the symposium in Warsaw, he decided, on the basis of his hunch, to go by way of Helsinki, where he spent two days conferring with a doctor from the Finnish government's community-health program in North Karelia and with scientists from the electrical-engineering department of the Helsinki University of Technology. While Zaret was in Finland, he learned that Kuopio and North Karelia had not only the highest but also the most rapidly increasing rate of heart attack in the world, and that younger and younger people, including many children, were being afflicted as time went on. He learned in addition that the incidence of heart attack among inhabitants of the two districts rose in direct proportion to how close they lived to the Soviet border. Increasingly certain that his theory had merit, he flew on to Warsaw to attend the symposium, where he took ten of the twenty minutes he had been allotted for the presentation of a paper on microwave cataracts to propose that electromagnetic radiation emanating from the Soviet Union might be a factor in the unusually high rate of heart attack in Kuopio and North Karelia, and to urge that the World Health Organization expand the scope of its existing study of the inhabitants of the two districts in order to investigate this possibility.

Since then, the Finnish government's community-health program of encouraging the inhabitants of North Karelia to quit smoking, to reduce their fat intake, and to undergo treatment for hypertension has succeeded in lowering the heart attack rate for males by forty percent, as well as in stopping the increasing rate of heart attack throughout the district. While these results do not invalidate Zaret's theory they certainly do not serve to strengthen it either. Whether it turns out to be based on fact or fantasy, however, Zaret's theory served as an uncomfortable reminder to the American delegates at the Warsaw symposium and to the scientific community in the United States. After twenty years of knuckling under to the military and after a decade of dismissing and even belittling evidence gathered here and abroad, American scientists were now embarking upon a new era of inquiry, which might well produce some startling results. Preliminary indications that this was so were not long in coming. At a conference on the biologic effects of nonionizing radiation held by the New York Academy of Sciences in February 1974, data confirming the hypothesis that low-level microwave radiation could affect the central nervous system and behavior were presented by Dr. W. Ross Adey and other researchers from the University of California's Brain Research Institute, whose work was supported by the Navy. They demonstrated that exposure to weak electric and electromagnetic fields resulted in a shortening of reaction times and circadian rhythms in human beings, and also in estimates of the passage of time by monkeys, and they were able to correlate these behavioral effects with altered neurophysiological activity and with modified brain chemistry.

Even more striking evidence of possibly adverse effects of low-level microwave radiation on behavior and brain tissue was presented by Allan H. Frey, the biophysicist who had earlier carried out pioneering studies of the ability of human beings and animals to somehow hear or detect microwaves, and whose studies had since been corroborated by other researchers. Frey and his co-workers demonstrated that when rats were given a choice they tended to avoid irradiation by pulsed microwaves having an average power density of only two-tenths of a milliwatt per square centimeter. Frey and his associates also exposed rats to similar levels of pulsed microwave radiation after injecting them with a fluorescent dye that binds itself to proteins in the bloodstream which do not normally pass the blood-brain barrier—a unique capillary system that maintains the brain in a stable environment by preventing certain proteins and other substances from reaching it. When they did, they found that the permeability of the barrier was sufficiently altered by the radiation to allow the dyed proteins to enter the brain.

On the basis of such data, the President's Office of Telecommunications Policy used some circumspect language in its second annual report to Congress on the program for assessing the biological hazards of non-ionizing radiation. The report was sent to Congress in May 1974, and it warned that preliminary indications from scattered experiments suggested that radio-frequency waves might affect the nervous system and behavior, and also normal development and growth processes, "at lower levels than anticipated in the past." After emphasizing that these findings were tentative, the Office of Telecommunications Policy proceeded from the cautious to the obvious, telling Congress that the effects of long-term, low-level exposure to microwaves and other radio-frequency radiation were not adequately known.

If anyone in Congress had cared to find out what was being done to remedy this situation, and by whom, he could have examined the research contracts being let out for the fiscal year 1975 by the dozen or so government agencies whose efforts to study the biological effects of radio-frequency waves were being coordinated by the Office of Telecommunications Policy. He would have learned that, in keeping with the recommendations of the Electromagnetic Radiation Management Advisory Council, and with long-established tradition in this country, a great majority of the projects were being sponsored and supported by the three branches of the armed forces. He would also have got some idea of why the Department of Defense was so eager to study the biological effects of low-intensity microwave radiation even as it continued to claim, as it had been claiming for nearly a generation, that exposure to ten milliwatts was perfectly safe. He would have discovered, for example, that the Air Force was supporting a study of microwave effects on the embryos of zebra fish because it believed that the results might have a major impact on the setting of new standards for exposure to radar. He would have found out that the Army was sponsoring a study of the effects of microwave radiation on the brain tissue of rat embryos because it was "a major developer and user of ground-located devices using microwave beams"; because "the effects on man or animals accidentally irradiated are of considerable concern"; and because "adequate knowledge will allow establishment of improved safety criteria and avoid establishment of excessive restrictions on their use by other governmental agencies." As for the Navy, he would have been informed by the description accompanying the proposal to irradiate human volunteers with microwaves at the Naval Aerospace Medical Research Laboratory, in Pensacola, that "exposure of Naval personnel to microwave radiation is an acute problem," and that "even low doses are likely to reduce the efficiency of personnel in vital duty positions."

While new and much-needed research on the genetic, embryonic, behavioral, and neurological effects of microwave radiation was being undertaken, the old dispute over the role of microwaves in the formation of cataracts erupted again, triggered by Dr. Zaret, who in October 1974 published a case history in the *New York State Journal of Medicine* in which he described the development of typical microwave cataracts in the eyes of the housewife he had mentioned at the Senate hearings and also at the symposium in Poland, whose only known exposure to microwaves came from an oven that was leaking radiation. In an unusual move, the editor of the *Journal* published in the same issue a number of letters commenting on Zaret's presumptive diagnosis that the woman was suffering from microwave cataracts, and on some of his other ophthalmological findings, together with a point-by-point response to these comments by Zaret. Some of the comment was revealing. Confirmation of Zaret's long-held and bitterly disputed contention that microwave cataracts are a clinical entity and that they develop in the posterior capsule of the lens came from Dr. Joseph A. Bouchat, professor of ophthalmology at the Val-de-Grâce Hospital, in Paris, who, together with Dr. Claude Marsol, had made similar observations in the case of a twenty-three-year-old radar technician, and had published his findings, back in 1967, in the *Archives d'Ophtalmologie*. Criticism of Dr. Zaret's article was offered by Michaelson, of the University of Rochester, who had initially written to the editor of the *Journal* urging him not to publish it; by Osepchuk, of Raytheon; by Carpenter, of the Bureau of Radiological Health; by Dr. Donaldson, of the Massachusetts Eye and Ear Infirmary; and by Colonel Appleton, of the Army—all of whom challenged Zaret's contention that there was such a thing as a microwave cataract, and characterized his diagnosis in the case in question as unfounded, and unsupported by medical evidence. Uncertainty about Zaret's diagnosis was expressed by Dr. George R. Merriam, Jr., of the Institute of Ophthalmology of Columbia-Presbyterian Medical Center, in New York, who based part of his doubt on the fact that microwave diathermy had been used at the institute for many years in preoperative and postoperative treatment of the eye. "The usual treatment is about one hundred milliwatts per square centimeter for twenty minutes, and treatments are often given twice a day for up to two weeks," Dr. Merriam wrote. "No adverse effects have been seen."

In his response to Dr. Merriam, Zaret suggested that a follow-up study of patients whose eyes had been treated with microwave diathermy might be valuable. "Although he reports that no adverse effects were noted, perhaps some occurred, but they were not suspected of being related to the radiation therapy," Zaret wrote. "Perhaps also no one has looked into this population grouping for the long-term or delayed effects following an acute exposure regimen of the type described." In light of the fact that for more than twenty years most doctors and scientists, including some military ophthalmologists, had considered 100 milliwatts to be a dangerous, if not damaging, level of exposure to the eyes, Zaret's suggestion appeared reasonable. At any rate, Merriam's disclosure could at the very least be construed as a prime example of the wide discrepancies that apparently existed in the knowledge and the attitudes of various members of the medical and scientific communities toward the biological effects and potential hazards of microwave radiation.

Another example of how, when it came to microwaves, the left hand of the medical profession did not appear to know what the right was doing was provided by Dr. José Daels, of the Department of Obstetrics and Gynecology of the Maria Middelares Clinic, in Ghent, Belgium. Since 1971, Dr. Daels has irradiated 2,000 women with microwaves as they were giving birth, in order to heat the uterine wall and ease the pain of labor. According to Daels, 1,936 of the women described the analgesic effect of the radiation as good. In addition to mitigating the pain of contraction, Daels's patients reported, the radiation produced an agreeable sensation of relaxation. Regarding possible adverse effects, Daels declared in an article published in the July 1973 issue of *Obstetrics and Gynecology* that "no undesirable side effects of microwave heating of the tissues are known," and that "the very rare complications that have been reported have been due to overheating, as a consequence of incorrect dosage." He then proceeded to cite as his authority for these statements an article on the health hazards of microwaves which had been published in the United States in 1959.

During 1974 and 1975, the belated advent in the United States of serious research on the biological effects of low-level microwave radiation was carefully coordinated and watched over by the President's Office of Telecommunications Policy. However, in their third annual report to Congress, issued in April 1975, the OTP people were rather vague about the progress and results of a hundred-odd studies of the problem which were being conducted in various laboratories across the nation. Concerning the warning the OTP had given the previous year that microwave radiation might affect the nervous system and behavior as well as processes of growth and development, it had this to say: "Continuing efforts have developed additional data in those areas. However, at this early stage, the picture is still far from clear. Information is as yet too limited to permit firm conclusions to be drawn." Later on in the report, following a description of experiments showing that low levels of microwave radiation decreased the ability of monkeys to perform tasks, the OTP declared, "There are, nonetheless, substantive indications of effects in the nervous system and behavior at this stage, warranting further investigation." Presumably, they were referring to further investigation that would either substantiate or disprove the firm conclusions that had been drawn fifteen years earlier by the Russians, the Poles, and the Czechoslovaks, whose extensive studies of the effects of long-term, low-level microwave radiation on the nervous system and the behavior of human beings and animals had led them to set standards of exposure to microwaves which were from one thousand to ten thousand times as stringent as our own. However, the authors of the report left considerable doubt about the priority assigned to this kind of investigation, saying that "there is a serious lack of long-term, low-level research due to the time, expense, and commitment required for such work, which is incompatible with the level of resources available for radio-frequency/microwave research in individual agencies at present." Besides blaming limited funds, the report noted that scientists studying the microwave problem were encountering severe problems in determining the doses of radiation necessary to cause biological effects; in understanding the interaction of microwaves with organisms at the macromolecular level; in measuring the amount and distribution of microwave energy absorbed by tissue; and in extrapolating the results of animal exposures to human beings. Whatever the obstacles, though, the 1975 OTP report made one thing clear: after years of claiming that it was extremely difficult, if not impossible, to duplicate Russian experimental studies, American scientists were at last beginning to be able to confirm some of the findings of their Soviet counterparts.

In their fourth annual report, which was issued in June 1976, the OTP people indicated—albeit somewhat reluctantly—that progress had been made in determining the effects of low-intensity microwave radiation on growth and development, and on the blood-forming systems, the immune system, and the endocrine system. After cautioning their readers at considerable length that new data "frequently cause apprehension, can be misinterpreted, and could lead to premature conclusions"; that all newly detected biological effects and changes are not necessarily harmful; and that consideration of new findings "must include the risk/benefits associated with EMR [electromagnetic radiation] itself and in comparison to other factors and known hazards in our lives," the authors of the report got down to specifics. "One important effect that has received increasing attention is the ability of non-ionizing EMR to stimulate division of lymphocyte cells in the intact animal," they wrote, adding that "such effects are of interest because the lymphocytes, which are a type of white blood cells, are an integral part of the body's immune defense mechanism."

In an appendix to their report, the OTP people described a two-day workshop seminar that they and their colleagues on the Electromagnetic Radiation Management Advisory Council had convened in

Washington, D.C., in August 1975, to review the findings of research pertaining to the genetic, hereditary, growth, and developmental effects of microwave and radio-frequency radiation. At the meeting, the results of fifteen research projects were presented by the scientists and investigators who had conducted them. Eight of the fifteen projects showed that low-level radiation produced effects and changes in test animals or genetic material. These changes included birth defects in mouse fetuses; structural defects in darkling beetles that had been irradiated as pupae; the death of zebra-fish embryos at nonthermal radiation levels; delays in the onset of normal cell division in slime mold; and marked chromosomal abnormalities in kangaroo-rat cell cultures. Apparently determined not to alarm Congress, however, the authors of the 1976 OTP report summed up the workshop by stating that the results "were a mixture of positive and negative findings," and that "the largely negative findings with respect to genetic effects thus far are reassuring with regard to the magnitude of risk."

Concerning the genetic effects of microwaves, American scientists who had finally embarked on this aspect of the problem were not playing catch-up with the Soviet scientists as much as with a handful of their compatriots, whose earlier findings had for the most part been ignored. That microwave radiation might have genetic effects had first been discovered back in 1959 by Dr. John H. Heller and some associates at the New England Institute for Medical Research, in Ridgefield, Connecticut, who observed gross chromosomal abnormalities in garlic-root tips that had been irradiated with microwaves at power levels far below those necessary to produce heat. By 1963, Heller and his colleagues had demonstrated that low-power microwave radiation could produce in mammalian cells and in insects mutations similar to those caused by gamma rays, X-rays, and ultraviolet rays. In experiments conducted with male fruit flies they clearly demonstrated that low-level microwave radiation was mutagenic at four different frequencies—in other words, that it could cause genetic damage in the sperm cells of the insects and that these mutations could be transmitted to their offspring. Ironically, when the findings of Heller and his co-workers were published, they received more recognition in the Soviet Union than in the United States, where their data were largely dismissed or disbelieved. In any event, by the late 1960s their research on the genetic effects of microwaves had practically come to a halt for lack of interest and for want of funds.

Similarly ignored were the findings of an epidemiological investigation of radiation exposure in the parents of children afflicted with Down's syndrome, or mongolism, which was conducted between 1962 and 1964 by researchers in the Department of Chronic Diseases at the Johns Hopkins University School of Public Health and in the Department of Pediatrics at the Johns Hopkins School of Medicine, with funds from the Public Health Service. Based on the acknowledged association between Down's syndrome and leukemia, and on the acknowledged association between ionizing radiation and leukemia, the study that the Johns Hopkins scientists undertook assumed that there might be a link between ionizing radiation and Down's syndrome. They proceeded to compare diagnostic, therapeutic, and occupational X-ray exposures incurred by the parents of 216 children afflicted with the syndrome who were born in Greater Baltimore between 1946 and 1962 with X-ray exposures incurred by the parents (including age-matched mothers) of a matched control group of normal children born in Greater Baltimore during the same period. When they completed their study, they found that the mothers of children with Down's syndrome had undergone a significantly greater number of fluoroscopic examinations and more therapeutic radiation than mothers of children in the control group. Therefore, they concluded that ionizing radiation might be a factor responsible for some cases of Down's syndrome. Unexpectedly, they also discovered that although there were no discernible differences in exposures to X-rays or other ionizing radiation on the part of fathers in either group, almost ten percent of the fathers of children with Down's syndrome reported "intimate contact with radar both in and outside of the armed forces," compared to slightly more than three percent of the fathers in the control group. This development surprised and puzzled the investigators, who, although they were not willing to draw any conclusions from it, sensibly recommended in a report published in 1965 in the *Bulletin of the Johns Hopkins Hospital* that "the association between mongolism and radar exposure deserves further investigation."

Incredible as it may seem, neither the Department of Defense nor the Public Health Service saw fit at the time to institute studies to confirm or deny the startling findings of the Johns Hopkins investigators. In fact, four years went by before the military and radiological-health people got around to providing funds for the Johns Hopkins researchers to replicate their original study, to see if they could obtain the same results. And ten years went by before they got around to sponsoring either studies of the mutagenic effects of microwave radiation or epidemiological surveys to determine the incidence of birth defects among the children of men exposed to radar on military bases. By that time, it was 1974, and three years had passed since the Electromagnetic Radiation Management Advisory Council had issued a clear warning to the President that long-term, low-level exposure to microwave radiation could become a critical health problem if genetic effects were involved. No information has yet been made available concerning the surveys of birth defects among the children of military personnel, but the second Johns Hopkins study, which has just been completed, does not show a statistically significant relationship between Down's syndrome and parental exposure to radar. It does, however, suggest that men exposed to the emanations of radar have a significant increase in the number of chromosomal abnormalities in their blood—a finding that, since chromosomal abnormalities can cause birth defects, leaves the whole question of the genetic effects of microwave radiation in human beings open to further investigation.

Whether such investigations will be conducted more vigorously in the future than they have been in the past remains doubtful, in light of the reluctance that people in positions of responsibility for the public welfare obviously feel about pursuing inquiries into the biological effects of non-ionizing radiation which might alarm the public or embarrass the Department of Defense. Beneath this reluctance, of course, lies a deep apprehension on the part of the government and the military-industrial complex about how the citizenry and Congress will react if worst comes to worst and it turns out that exposure to microwave radiation poses a significant hazard to the health of the general population. Not surprisingly, such apprehension at the federal level has, in turn, affected the attitude of many members of the medical and scientific community, who, while trying to come to grips with the microwave problem in the laboratory, are entertaining mixed feelings about revealing the results of their work, either for fear that these will be misunderstood by the public or that money for future research might not be forthcoming. Indeed, among scientists

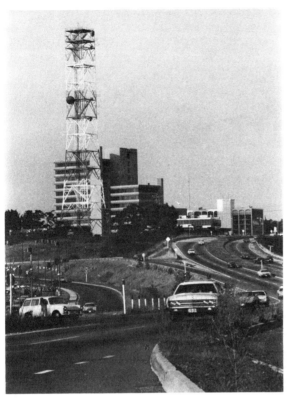

Microwave tower owned by the U.S. Army Communications Command, in McLean, Virginia. PHOTO BY ROBIN TOOKER

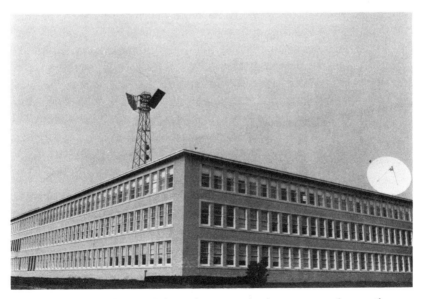

An American Telephone & Telegraph communications tower and a weather antenna that receives telemetry and pictures from satellites, in Suitland, Maryland.
PHOTO BY ROBIN TOOKER

attending the four-day annual meeting of the International Union of Radio Science's United States National Committee, held at the University of Colorado, in Boulder, in October 1975, there appeared to be as much concern about possible press distortion and public misunderstanding of the complex microwave problem as about the potentially adverse health effects of the microwaves themselves. Some of the scientists were concerned that the layman would not readily grasp the difference between biological effects and biological hazards. Others worried that the great potential of microwaves as a tool for studying the electrochemical workings of the brain might go undeveloped if there should be adverse publicity. Still others claimed that misinterpretation of the microwave problem by the press not only was inevitable but had already made the task of the scientific community more difficult. There was also considerable fretting about the damaging effect on public opinion of a number of disability claims that had recently been awarded by the Veterans Administration to former radar technicians who had developed cataracts, and about the outcome of several lawsuits that had been instituted by other ex-servicemen and civilian employees of the armed forces who had been exposed to radar. Yet many of these same scientists also voiced anxiety about the extensive Soviet findings concerning low-level microwave effects, about the lack of adequate funds for microwave research in the United States, and about the absence of any well-integrated program of research within the Department of Health, Education, and Welfare. In fact, several investigators stated that because low levels of microwave radiation were known to affect the nervous system and behavior, the present ten-milliwatt standard was inadequate and would soon have to be lowered. At the same time, a journalist attending the conference was approached on several occasions by scientists and government officials, who suggested that when writing about microwaves he substitute the words "illuminate" and "illumination" for "irradiate" and "irradiation," in order not to alarm his readers unduly.

7

An Unhealthful Post

Within a few months, the worrying about publicity and semantics that went on at the Boulder meeting seemed redundant in view of the news that came out of Moscow. Word in early February 1976 that the Russians were once again beaming microwaves into the American Embassy, on Tchaikovsky Street, not only made headlines blaring the word "radiation" in newspapers all over the world but also touched off a spate of alarming speculation about the health effects of microwaves. Together with a series of contradictory explanations and confusing denials issued by State Department officials, these have combined to keep the story before the public ever since.

According to the first report of the affair, which appeared in the *Los Angeles Times* on February 7, Ambassador Walter J. Stoessel, Jr., had told some of the 125 members of his staff that the Russians were using microwave beams to listen in on conversations inside the embassy, and that such radiation could be hazardous to their health. In the *Los Angeles Times* version, Stoessel informed the staff members that the risk was greatest for pregnant women and that other possible microwave hazards included leukemia, skin cancer, psoriasis, cataracts, and emotional illness. Although Stoessel had assured embassy personnel that the levels of radiation to which they were being exposed were far below the minimum danger levels prescribed by Soviet occupational-health regulations—an irony he appeared not to grasp—he nonetheless offered them an opportunity to transfer to posts outside the Soviet Union. He also urged them in strong terms to keep the matter secret. The *Los Angeles Times* speculated that the attempt to maintain secrecy resulted from fear that public disclosure of the radiation might damage Soviet-American relations during a delicate period when the policy of détente was under strong political attack in the United States. Whatever the reason, there was little doubt that an official lid had been placed on the story. Ambassador Stoessel and State Department officials in Washington refused to comment on any aspect of the *Los Angeles Times* report, and the day after it appeared, when President Ford was asked about it while he was campaigning in New Hampshire, he made his only public statement on the subject. "I do not think it is a matter that should be discussed at this time," declared the President, who did not mention the fact that earlier in the winter he had written a letter protesting the radiation to Chairman Leonid I. Brezhnev. "If it is true, it is a very serious situation."

Rumors circulating among people living and working in the embassy to the effect that they had been exposed to dangerous radiation quickly forced the government to abandon its policy of silence for one of partial explanation and reassurance. While refusing to discuss the situation with reporters, the embassy physician, Major Thomas A. Johnson, of the Air Force, told worried parents that there was little likelihood of any risk to children attending a nursery school in the basement of the ten-story building. A few days later, embassy officials received permission from the State Department to assure all American citizens living in Moscow that no harmful radiation had been detected on the ground floor of the embassy complex, where the snack bar and the medical dispensary are situated, or in the basement commissary. But they refused to comment on the radiation hazard existing on the upper three floors of the building, which contain most of the key offices, including that of the Ambassador. They did admit, however, that medical records of embassy staff members and their families were being reviewed, and that white-blood-cell counts of all

personnel were being taken. Meanwhile, in spite of freezing temperatures, workmen were unsealing rows of double windows throughout
the embassy and installing aluminum screens on the outside, to
deflect the radiation and prevent it from penetrating the building.
The installation of the screens was later said to have been approved
by Secretary of State Kissinger. At the time, the Secretary contented
himself with telling reporters in Washington that the United States
government viewed the radiation as "a matter of great complexity
and sensitivity," and that it had made "unilateral efforts to reduce
the danger."

During the early days of the Moscow microwave crisis, official
sources quoted in newspaper accounts were virtually unanimous in
giving the impression that the Russians were irradiating the embassy
in order to activate eavesdropping devices that had been concealed
in its walls and floors; that the United States government's concern
about possible damage to the health of people working there was
wholly preventive in nature; that the present danger, if any, was
limited to mild irritability and fatigue; and that no adverse health
effects caused by microwave radiation had been observed among
embassy personnel. On February 16, however, the *Boston Globe* reported that Ambassador Stoessel was suffering from a mysterious
blood ailment, resembling leukemia, that was thought to be possibly
caused or aggravated by the radiation. On the same day, an embassy
spokesman made this statement:

> We have seen various stories about the Ambassador's health, all of
> which are inaccurate and misleading. It would not be appropriate to
> comment specifically on the Ambassador's health or on that of any
> other individual. However, the Ambassador feels fine, keeps a busy
> schedule, leads an active life, has not undergone medical treatment,
> and is not at the present time undergoing medical treatment.

Ten days later, it was reported that the Russians had been directing radiation at the embassy not to activate their own listening
devices but to jam American listening devices that had been installed
on the roof of the building. This piece of news appeared in a *New
York Times* story, which also reported, "American officials said they
accepted the Soviet contention that the microwaves were aimed at
the Embassy to disable the sophisticated monitoring equipment and
not to bug the Embassy or to harm American personnel." No expla-

nation was offered as to why it had been deemed necessary to screen the windows of the embassy, but one reason was not hard to infer from a paragraph that appeared in the middle of the *Times* story: "A complicating factor, officials said, was that the current ambassador, Walter J. Stoessel, Jr., had suffered nausea and bleeding in his eyes, although he was reported now feeling better. There is no evidence, officials said, that the illness was directly caused by the microwaves, but there is that possibility."

In addition to amending previous official declarations about the state of the Ambassador's health, the *Times* story of February 26 revealed that during the 1960s and the early 1970s three of Stoessel's predecessors in Moscow (two of whom have died of cancer) had protested to the Russians about radiation hazards at the embassy. That in itself was not really surprising, since earlier Soviet irradiation of the embassy had been reported. However, the fact that the three ambassadors had apparently lodged their protests without informing the embassy staff of the hazards tended to shed light on a story put out by the Associated Press on February 28. According to the AP report, a former administrative officer at the embassy whose wife had died of cancer in 1968 after working there as a secretary had sued the government, claiming that she was a victim of radiation, and had received a settlement of approximately ten thousand dollars, on the ground that she had been given inadequate medical treatment. A further indication that the government considered itself vulnerable to litigation arising from the situation in Moscow came a few days later, when Rowland Evans and Robert Novak reported in their syndicated column that high State Department officials had initially argued against making a public protest to the Russians about the radiation, on the grounds that it would compromise the embassy's electronic-surveillance capability and "might generate damage suits against the government from Embassy employees with claims of illness."

The alerting of the embassy staff early in February to the possible dangers of microwave radiation indicated that the State Department had come to the belated conclusion that the future well-being of its employees in Moscow was more important than its liability for not having informed them about possible microwave health hazards in the past. It is apparent, however, that the State Department seriously underestimated the capacity of its employees in Moscow for being resentful and suspicious of the fact that they had been deceived about such an important matter as their health for so long a time. Indeed, resentment and suspicion fairly jumped out of the pages of a telegram that was sent to Secretary of State Kissinger on February 19 by members of the Moscow chapter of the American Foreign Service Association—a six-thousand-member organization that represents foreign-service officials around the world. The telegram, which was the result of a meeting that had been attended by some forty foreign-service employees and their spouses two days earlier, requested Secretary Kissinger to issue an unclassified written statement providing assurances that there was no evidence of any sort to suggest that any former or present employee at the embassy had encountered health problems linked to microwave radiation. It then requested the Secretary to say whether there had been an unusually high incidence of spontaneous abortion among pregnant women during or after their residence at the embassy; to describe any evidence suggesting that microwave radiation might pose a hazard for pregnant women and their unborn children; and to say whether there had been any legal actions or claims directed against the State Department for health problems resulting from service at the Moscow Embassy. The telegram asked Kissinger to explain why the employees had not been informed of the radiation problem earlier; to disclose when State Department management officials had first become aware of the "potentially harmful effects" of microwave radiation; and to say whether any previous medical tests conducted on embassy employees had played a part in the decision to inform them of the possible hazard. The telegram also asked Kissinger to explain why metal screens had not been put over windows in the embassy much earlier if the effects of microwave radiation could be mitigated by so simple an action.

In view of the obvious legitimacy of these requests, the State Department had little choice other than to make a public announcement in March that it would conduct a full-scale medical investigation of the thousands of embassy personnel and their families who had served in Moscow in the past, as well as those who were serving there now. At the same time, the department sought to allay the anxiety and soothe the anger of its Moscow employees by holding closed briefings that were designed to explain the situation. During the third week of April, Barton Reppert, a reporter for the Washington bureau of the Associated Press, obtained a copy of a confidential State Department paper that had been prepared for these briefings from an official in the department who was concerned about how the situation in Moscow was being handled. The briefing paper said that there was no evidence of a high incidence of spontaneous abortion among women at the embassy, no evidence that the present levels of radiation could produce congenital malformations or have any other effect upon unborn children, and "no known reason to avoid conceiving children under present conditions at the Embassy." It stated that between October 1975 and January 1976 microwave power levels had reached a maximum intensity of eighteen microwatts per square centimeter in certain heavily irradiated areas of the embassy, and that the window screens installed since then "reduce the current microwave signals to a point well below one microwatt per square centimeter but not to a 'zero' level." The screens had not been installed earlier, according to the paper, because before the autumn of 1975 such action had not seemed necessary. As for why embassy employees had not been informed about the radiation sooner, the paper explained that "until last fall, none of the experts who had studied the problem believed that it presented health hazards," and that "under the circumstances it was thought that briefing people on what little we knew of the signal would cause unwarranted apprehension on the part of those assigned to Moscow." The paper also informed embassy employees that "no cause-and-effect relationship has been established between disorders contracted by those in Moscow and their exposure to the electromagnetic field."

There were soon indications that such assurances did not entirely satisfy embassy staff members. Late in April, they were described by one State Department official as being "still very upset about the whole business." Another State Department official in Washington was quoted at the same time as saying that "the way people around here are dealing with this is just hoping that it'll be forgotten." Further suspicion about the State Department's credibility had been voiced earlier in the month by John D. Hemenway, president of the American Foreign Service Association. Hemenway expressed concern that an official cover-up might be in progress and demanded that any group investigating the health situation of embassy personnel exposed to microwave radiation include people without government ties. In a statement of rebuttal issued to the press, Lawrence

S. Eagleburger, Deputy Under-Secretary of State for Management, said that Hemenway's charge of a possible official cover-up was "false and reprehensible," and that "Secretary Kissinger has made clear that our principal concern is for the health and well-being of our employees in Moscow."

By this time, it was clear that whatever the outcome of the controversy between the State Department and its employees in Moscow, a unique population of men, women, and children who had been exposed to low-intensity microwave radiation over long periods of time had been identified. It was also clear that retrospective studies of the health experience of this group of people could yield valuable epidemiological information about the possible hazards of chronic exposure to microwaves. Whether such investigations would be initiated and carried out in good faith by the State Department was, however, another matter, for during the rest of the spring and throughout the summer the information made available to the public concerning the situation in Moscow continued to be clouded by revelations of prior involvement and previous secrecy. For example, it soon came to light that the department's chief medical consultant in the microwave affair was Dr. Herbert Pollack, who had been sent to Moscow to assess the possible microwave health hazard at the embassy even before Ambassador Stoessel told his staff about the situation. Pollack is a member of the Electromagnetic Radiation Management Advisory Council, a professor emeritus of clinical medicine at the George Washington University Medical School, and, it turns out, an old hand at the business of assessing the biological effects of microwaves. Indeed, as a member of the senior technical staff of the Institute for Defense Analyses between 1961 and 1970, Pollack was a leading participant in Project Pandora, the secret study of the effects of low-intensity microwave radiation mounted in 1966, when the government began to be concerned about the health implications of the Soviet irradiation of the embassy in Moscow. The results of Project Pandora, as noted, remained classified for ten years. On May 3, 1976, however, an Associated Press report by Barton Reppert quoted Richard S. Cesaro, who was in charge of Project Pandora, as conceding that some of the scientists connected with the study felt that low-intensity microwave radiation had produced signs of aberrant behavior in monkeys. "My feeling is that we probably should have continued longer with research in that area, and not necessarily concluded it that early," said Cesaro, who is now head of a communications firm in Maryland. "There were a lot of unknowns, and I don't think they were ever really put to bed." Reppert also quoted Dr. Joseph C. Sharp, who had worked on Project Pandora when he was chief of experimental psychology at the Walter Reed Army Institute of Research, as saying that "if certain kinds of restraints could have been lifted, I would have voted to go for more experiments." Sharp, who is now with the National Aeronautics and Space Administration's Ames Research Center, in California, went on to say that "part of the problem with any classified project is that you cannot talk to a wide variety of people and get a bunch of different kinds of ideas. . . . We always felt that we had an arm tied behind our back because we couldn't even talk to our bosses about it."

For his part, Pollack is remembered by several of his colleagues on Project Pandora as being extremely dubious about the possibility that low-level microwave radiation could affect health. In any case, when Reppert reached him at his office in the State Department in May and asked him his present opinion on the subject, Pollack replied, "That's the question they ask me upstairs here, and I can only say one answer. We just don't know." It must be surmised that the State Department has a high regard for Dr. Pollack's experience in studying the biological effects of microwaves and for his assessment of the situation at the Moscow Embassy. It appears, however, that many of the embassy's employees do not. In their telegram to Secretary Kissinger in February 1976, they requested "disinterested expert advice" concerning the potential health problems caused by exposure to microwave radiation "in view of widespread doubt as to Dr. Pollack's impartiality."

Toward the end of May, a new round of revelation and denial got under way when another Associated Press story by Reppert stated that recent tests conducted by electronics specialists from the CIA showed radiation levels in the Moscow Embassy to be considerably higher than those found in earlier tests performed by the State Department, and that an outside telephone line had actually been found to be carrying radiation directly into the office (and, presumably, into the ear) of Ambassador Stoessel. According to the AP report, a State Department source said that Stoessel was "beside himself" with this latest development, and had expressed his concern in classified cables to Deputy Under-Secretary Eagleburger. A State Department spokesman, Robert L. Funseth, responded to the story by saying that Soviet microwave transmissions into the embassy were not higher than those previously measured and by denying that the CIA had conducted any separate tests. However, no one in the State Department denied any part of a Reuters dispatch carried in the *New York Times* on June 26, which revealed that two children of embassy employees had been sent to the United States for further medical study after having been examined by doctors in Moscow. Indeed, a department spokesman named Frederick Z. Brown said that the children had been brought home for treatment of blood disorders. According to the *Times,* Brown went on to say that extensive blood tests of all embassy personnel had failed to establish any connection between blood disorders and the irradiation of the embassy with microwaves.

The news about the children—two three-year-old girls who had been living in the embassy—soon prompted additional disclosures by the State Department. On July 8, the *Times* ran a front-page story beneath the headline "SOVIET DIMS BEAM AT U.S. EMBASSY," which began:

> The United States said today that Soviet authorities in recent months had sharply reduced the level of microwave radiation beamed at the American Embassy in Moscow.
>
> But in its first detailed public account of the situation, the State Department nonetheless rebuked the Russians for continuing the radiation even at the current insignificant level. It said this showed "a lack of concern for living and working conditions of our people in Moscow."

When asked why the Russians were being rebuked if they had cut the radiation levels below those considered by the government to entail a health hazard, Funseth replied that the continued beams caused a psychological problem. According to the *Times* account, Funseth then announced that the State Department had signed a contract with Johns Hopkins University to conduct a survey to determine whether there has ever been any connection between the microwave irradiation of the embassy and the health of past and present embassy employees. Shortly thereafter, it was learned that this study—a three-hundred-thousand-dollar biostatistical and epidemiological survey and evaluation of the medical records and histories of all embassy employees and their dependents over the last ten years—was being directed and coordinated by Dr. Abraham M. Lilienfeld, professor of epidemiology at the Johns Hopkins University School of Hygiene and Public Health, who had also directed the study in the early 1960s which suggested that there might be an association between Down's syndrome and parental exposure to radar, as well as the subsequent study showing a significant increase of chromosomal abnormalities in the blood of former radar workers.

On July 10, in his first news conference in Washington since April 22, Secretary Kissinger defended the government's policy toward the irradiation of the Moscow Embassy, saying that "timidity or concern about our overall relations with the Soviet Union has not been a factor in this." According to an account in the *Washington Post,* Kissinger spoke in guarded fashion, referred without elaboration to "many complicated issues" in the embassy affair, and avoided comment on reports that electronic surveillance conducted by the United States was part of the problem. "We have had to balance various advantages and disadvantages for the United States, and we have had to pay primary attention to the health of our employees," the Secretary declared.

Two weeks later, the Associated Press's indefatigable Reppert wrote a story containing a disclosure so stunning as to make one wonder how readily the men and women working for the State Department in Moscow could be led to believe that the principal concern of the department is for their health and well-being. The story ran in newspapers across the country on July 26, and it revealed that over an eighteen-month period in 1967 and 1968 the State Department had conducted special tests to detect genetic damage in employees returning from Moscow, and that it had not only done so without notifying the employees about the purpose of the testing but had deliberately misled them into thinking that the tests were being made for another reason. According to Reppert's account, analysis of the special tests had been conducted by Dr. Cecil B. Jacobson, of the George Washington University Medical School, who told Reppert that the results had been inconclusive. However, Dr. Thomas H. Gresinger, also a member of the faculty of the medical school, told Reppert that Dr. Jacobson had described the tests to him as showing "funny results—lots of chromosome breaks." Gresinger has since recalled how he first became aware of the nature of the tests that were being conducted on embassy employees returning from Moscow. "I had just finished my residency in gynecology and was starting up a private practice," he said not long ago. "I was teaching at the university medical school, and, to make ends meet, I was also doing consulting work for the medical division of the State Department. One day, while reading Pap smears at the division, I heard some lab technicians joking about some subterfuge that was taking place. According to the technicians, they had been instructed to take buccal smears from the Moscow employees as part of their routine homecoming physical examinations and to tell them that they were being checked for some kind of abnormal bacteria. When I heard the words 'buccal smears,' my ears pricked up. Buccal smears are never used to culture bacteria; they're a scraping taken from inside the mouth and they're designed solely for the purpose of detecting chromosomal abnormalities. Naturally, the next time I went to George Washington I looked up Cecil Jacobson, who was head of the cytogenetics laboratory over there, and asked him what was going on. Jacobson replied that there was a lot of radiation at the Moscow Embassy, that he was looking for chromosome breaks in the returning employees, and that he was finding them in significant numbers."

During the late summer and early autumn of 1976, the furor over the situation in Moscow diminished somewhat, because the attention of the press and the public was focused on the presidential election and its aftermath. In September, however, Ambassador Stoessel left Moscow because of health problems and was reassigned as Ambassador to West Germany, in Bonn, where, according to some medical opinion, his strange blood ailment might prove to be reversible in an environment free of radiation. And on November 12, the State Department issued an administrative notice declaring Moscow to be an "unhealthful post," and announcing that employees stationed there would receive a twenty percent raise in salary as a hardship allowance. According to the notice, the reason for this declaration was "based upon the Department's evaluation of reported environmental conditions regarding sanitation and disease, medical and hospital facilities, and climate." The notice did not make any mention of whether the Moscow climate had changed, nor did it contain any reference to the possibly unhealthful effects of the microwave radiation that was being directed into the embassy. It seemed clear, however, that by this time the department had adopted a policy of commenting on the microwave situation only when necessary, in the apparent hope that the whole affair would eventually blow over and be forgotten.

8

Exaggerated
Reactions

The trouble with the State Department's strategy was that it was bound to keep the department on the defensive. And so it was, for in December 1976 a substantial portion of this book appeared in *The New Yorker,* including the section dealing with the Moscow Embassy up to the time that it was declared to be an unhealthful post. This section appeared in the December 20 issue of the magazine, and it drew an immediate and revealing response from the State Department in the form of a cable signed by Secretary Kissinger and sent to the embassy on the very same day. The cable was described by its authors as "Contingency Press Guidance on *New Yorker* article on Microwaves," and it consisted of nine questions they imagined embassy staff members might ask concerning the article, followed by nine answers that were to be given by department spokesmen in the event these questions were asked. The ground rules for using this conjecture were carefully stated. "There follows contingency press guidance developed for the Department's press spokesman on an 'if asked' basis for questions relating to Paul Brodeur's *New Yorker* article on microwaves (copy pouched)," the cable read. "You may use guidance in briefing Embassy staff but all press questions should be referred to the Department for reply."

The question-and-answer part of the cable read like ventriloquism by satellite control. To the question "Do you have any comment on the December 20th *New Yorker* piece on microwaves?" the spokesman was instructed to reply as follows:

> In terms of the material related to the Department of State and the situation at Embassy Moscow, there is nothing new in this article as far as we can tell. The issues and questions raised are familiar to the expert consultants with whom we have discussed this problem and I think we have covered most of the ground already. As far as the situation in Moscow is concerned, we have stated repeatedly that we have found no evidence that these signals at recorded levels now or any levels in the past have adversely affected the health of our employees. Our own medical studies and the work of Johns Hopkins continues and to date we have no new information that would be cause for alarm. I cannot speak to the article's various allegations concerning other U.S. Government organizations.

The answer to the second question was considerably shorter. The question itself, however, managed to reflect a certain uneasiness on the part of department officials, who, after all, had to imagine that it might be asked to begin with. "Isn't the State Department knuckling under to pressures from military and industrial interests to downplay or even cover up the significance of microwave effects on health?" it read. To this loaded query, the spokesman was to reply "No."

The rest of the cable read:

> QUESTION: What about the former Embassy administrative officer's wife who died of cancer?
> ANSWER: I do not intend to discuss individual cases. I can only reiterate that there is no evidence of any connection with the microwave transmissions in Moscow.
> QUESTION: What about Ambassador Stoessel's health? Has it improved since he left Moscow?
> ANSWER: Ambassador Stoessel is on duty in Bonn and I have nothing to add to my earlier comments.
> QUESTION: What is the latest on the two children who were evacuated for further evaluation in the U.S.?
> ANSWER: As I have said before neither of those cases was con-

nected in any way with the microwave transmissions directed at Embassy Moscow. One of the children returned to Moscow shortly after examination in the States and the other remained in the U.S. to undergo further examinations and treatment. The second case involved a congenital defect of the bone marrow, discovered during the blood test program. Beyond that it is not appropriate to comment on the health histories of specific individuals.

QUESTION: What results are coming from the Johns Hopkins study of Embassy Moscow family medical histories?

ANSWER: The research continues, but it is too early to have any definitive results. We expect to make the findings known when the researchers provide their conclusions to us.

QUESTION: Has there been any recent change in signal strength in microwaves beamed at the Embassy?

ANSWER: The signal activity at Embassy Moscow is monitored continually and the Embassy staff is being kept up to date. The signal strength in all living and working areas of the mission remains a small fraction of a microwatt.

QUESTION: Are we pushing our demands that the signal be turned off?

ANSWER: Our position has been made clear to the Soviets and we continue to insist that the transmissions themselves be terminated altogether.

QUESTION: What about the statement that the strength of the signal at the American Embassy reached 4 milliwatts?

ANSWER: We have never observed levels anything near that high. As we have already stated, the typical maximum levels observed in the period when the signal intensity was at its highest late last year and early this year were in the vicinity of 20 microwatts, one two-hundredth of the figure mentioned in the article. Since then, as you know, the signal strength has been considerably reduced.

Whether the State Department was able to reassure its Moscow employees with this series of evasions and denials of conjectured questions is itself a matter of conjecture. However, the department soon had its hands full with another matter. On January 4, 1977, an administrative notice entitled "Lymphocytosis" was distributed to all embassy personnel and United States citizens living in Moscow. The first three paragraphs read as follows:

> In recent months, the American Embassy Post Medical Officer has observed slightly higher than average numbers of lymphocytes in cell counts in the results of blood tests given at the Embassy. This has

occurred in only about one-third of the individuals tested.

Lymphocytes are one type of white corpuscles found in the blood —a certain level is present at all times in all individuals. Lymphocytosis is the medical term used to indicate only that there are more than average numbers of lymphocytes in a given volume of blood. An increase in lymphocytes is by itself no cause for alarm but actually evidence of resistance. It occurs, for example, during periods of acute viral infection.

The State Department Medical Office, using independent laboratory analysis, has undertaken an additional in-depth review which failed to find any adverse consequences from the lymphocytosis, although the cause remains undetermined. At present it can only be said that there may be a factor in the Moscow environment which produces a benign temporary increase in the circulating blood lymphocytes in some people. There is no connection with microwave radiation directed at the American Embassy.

As might be expected, this latest administrative notice received wide attention in the press, which had previously reported that white-blood-cell counts of all embassy personnel were being taken. However, most of the reports were similar to one that ran in the *New York Times,* under the headline "RADIATION RULED NO PERIL TO AMERICANS IN MOSCOW," and that merely described the contents of the notice. A far more informative article appeared in the *Washington Post,* on January 5, under the headline "BLOOD CHANGES LINKED TO MOSCOW DUTY." It was written by Victor Cohn, who had taken the trouble to contact Dr. Pollack. In spite of the fact that the State Department had assured its Moscow employees that there were only "slightly higher" than average numbers of lymphocytes in their cell counts, Cohn learned from Pollack that in 213 present and past embassy employees and dependents, the average lymphocyte count was *forty* percent higher than the count in other foreign service personnel; that the neutrophil count was fifteen percent higher; and that the counts of eosinophils and monocytes were also increased. Pollack told Cohn, however, that he could be "absolutely sure" there was no connection between the microwave radiation and the abnormal blood counts of embassy personnel because persons heavily exposed to the radiation had blood counts similar to people who were only lightly exposed, as well as to people who had never been exposed. "We're dealing with some unknown factor in the Moscow environment," Dr. Pollack declared. "I don't know what it is, but some kind of viral infection seems most likely." Dr. Pollack went on to say that another possible explanation for the abnormal blood counts was "some parasite like giardia," an organism in drinking water that had been known to cause intestinal sickness in people who had visited Leningrad. For this reason, Pollack told Cohn, the State Department was making further studies to determine whether giardia could be present in the drinking water in Moscow.

Dr. Pollack did not explain to Cohn how he could be sure that some embassy personnel had never been exposed to microwave radiation, and the certainty with which he expressed his conviction that microwaves could have nothing to do with the elevated white-blood-cell counts in embassy employees seems additionally puzzling in view of the fact that Soviet investigators had been observing elevated counts in microwave workers for more than twenty years; that marked changes in white-blood-cell counts, including increases in monocytes and eosinophils, had been reported (albeit later recanted) as far back as 1954 in the group of Lockheed microwave workers in California; and that in June 1976, the President's Office of Telecommunications Policy had issued a report stating that an important biological effect of microwave radiation was its ability "to stimulate division of lymphocytes in the intact animal."

In light of subsequent events, Dr. Pollack's concern about the drinking water in Moscow was rather interesting, for it raised the possibility that the State Department might be casting about for some way to either explain or obscure the reason for the blood abnormalities in its Moscow employees. This possibility became somewhat more apparent on January 15, when a Reuters dispatch appearing in the *New York Times* reported that cyanide and mercury in potentially harmful amounts had been found in the water supply at two Moscow apartment buildings where some Americans were living, and that a memorandum had been circulated among American residents warning them of the possible health hazard. On January 16, a UPI dispatch said that "at one building, the cyanide level was 250 per cent higher than that recommended by the World Health Organization," and that "at another building, the level of mercury was 35 per cent higher than what U.S. Environmental Protection Agency recommends." On the same day, an AP dispatch reported that "seven U.S. families out of about 250 in Moscow live in the two affected compounds," and that the Russians had been requested by the State Department to correct the contaminated water problem. Three days later, buried in the middle of a UPI dispatch that ran in the *International Herald Tribune* under the headline "U.S. EMBASSY TO WIDEN TESTS IN MOSCOW OVER BLOOD COUNT," were the following paragraphs:

> Another recent report, that cyanide and mercury were found in potentially harmful concentrations in the city water supply at two buildings housing seven U.S. Embassy families, was withdrawn yesterday.
>
> State Department officials said in Washington the water samples taken last August apparently had been placed in dirty test tubes.

No explanation for the State Department's precipitous and ill-considered release of the mercury-cyanide story has been given, nor is it known whether the department apologized to the Muscovites for having maligned their drinking water. It seems possible, however, that the department may have jumped the gun on the drinking water story in order to divert attention from the microwave affair. In any case, the department was, as usual, about to be overtaken by events, for on January 21 the following AP dispatch appeared in the *New York Times* and other papers:

> MOSCOW, Jan 21 (AP)—Another child living in the American Embassy building here will be returned to the United States for a medical examination because of a mysterious blood ailment.
>
> The boy, of preschool age, is going home early next week with his parents because of what officials said was a "fluctuating high lymphocyte count." This means more white blood cells than normal.
>
> Last June, two girls living in the embassy were sent to the United States because of unusual blood conditions. As in the case of the girls, the ailment of the boy was said by embassy officials to have nothing to do with microwaves aimed at the embassy for more than a year.
>
> The embassy has not released the names of any of the children involved.

As it turned out, even as the third child afflicted with blood disease was being sent home, the embassy doctor, Lt. Colonel Thomas A. Johnson—a thirty-six-year-old physician with a background in obstetrics—was the subject of a profile written by Peter Osnos of the *Washington Post.* The story appeared in the newspaper on January

22 under the headline "AMERICAN DOCTOR: MOSCOW IMPOSES PSY-
CHIC STRESSES," and began as follows:

> Considering that Americans in Moscow have discovered in the past
> year that they are saturated with Soviet microwaves, drinking water
> contaminated with dangerous parasites, and suffering in large numbers
> from a mysterious blood abnormality, it is understandable that the
> Embassy's doctor should have become a major figure in the commu-
> nity.

According to Osnos, in addition to American officials and their
families, Dr. Johnson had been seeing patients from ninety embassies
in Moscow, including twenty ambassadors who consulted him on a
regular basis. For this reason, Osnos said that Johnson's practice
"resembles that of an old-fashioned country doctor." Osnos then
went on to describe Johnson's general diagnosis concerning the medical complaints of his American patients:

> There is enormous "psychic stress" encountered here, Johnson said
> in an interview the other day: husbands who work much too hard to
> meet the demands of what many regard as "the most challenging
> assignment" of their careers, families who suffer from the ensuing
> "forced separation," a general sense of restrictions and constant sur-
> veillance, a feeling in some cases of "oppression," of being threatened.
> The result, said Johnson, is a high proportion of patients with
> complaints that reflect those stresses: colitis, inflammation of the large
> intestines, ulcer diseases, problems with sleep, tremendous anxieties,
> lack of sexual gratification.

In describing his psychic stress theory, Dr. Johnson appeared to
be unaware of the fact that gastrointestinal problems, insomnia,
anxiety, and decreased libido had long been acknowledged as being
associated with microwave radiation in the medical literature of both
the United States and the Soviet Union. In fact, commenting upon
the disclosure in the early part of 1976 that high levels of radiation
had been detected in the embassy, Dr. Johnson seemed to imply that
the microwaves had induced little more than hypochondria in his
patients. (He was apparently unaware that hypochondria has also
long been known to be an effect of microwaves upon the central
nervous system.) "There was a tremendous surge of complaints,"
Johnson told Osnos. "The microwave crisis was a magnificent place
for people to express all their pent-up frustration and anxiety. From

January to June, I spent a great deal of time counseling, trying to give people a reasonable perspective on the situation, trying to impart a feeling that I was forthright." Indeed, according to Osnos, in order to allay anxiety, Dr. Johnson went so far as to tell his patients that if, as a father of four, he felt that his family were endangered, he would leave Moscow.

Why the medical doctor of a United States Embassy should feel compelled to go to such lengths to try to convince his patients of his honesty is something that Dr. Johnson apparently did not discuss with Osnos, but having already voiced deep suspicion about Dr. Pollack in their telegram to Secretary Kissinger, it seems reasonable to suppose that embassy staff members were reluctant to place their trust in any physician connected with the government. (Indeed, as one embassy wife later put it, "If he [Dr. Johnson] gets his information on microwave radiation from the Department of Defense, it is no wonder that he can't tell us anything significant.")

Wherever he acquired his information about the biological effects of microwaves, Dr. Johnson was apparently in agreement with the State Department's administrative notice of January 4, which declared that the high lymphocyte counts that had been found in fully one-third of his patients were a benign temporary condition and no cause for alarm. However, he was either disinclined or not at liberty to tell Osnos what information he had for considering the blood abnormalities to be benign, or why, for that matter, if there were no cause for alarm, three young children who lived within the embassy building had lymphocyte counts that warranted sending them to the United States for further testing. Dr. Johnson did tell Osnos that he felt his patients had come to terms with the additional hazards of working at the Moscow Embassy. "I haven't seen lately the exaggerated reactions that were commonplace after the initial disclosure," he said.

By "exaggerated reactions," Dr. Johnson was presumably referring to the psychological manifestations of microwave radiation upon his patients, and not to any physiological afflictions (such as blood abnormalities) which the radiation might have induced in them. Indeed, except for a high incidence of colitis and ulcers, which he ascribed to psychic stress, Dr. Johnson gave no indication whatsoever that he felt there had been any unusual physical afflictions among his patients in Moscow. In addition to making no mention of the three cases of young children with blood disorders, he made no mention of the fact that at least one embassy family, who had gone to the United States on leave, had been tested at the Tampa University Medical Center, after their white-blood-cell counts proved to be very high. Nor did he mention the fact that Ambassador Stoessel, whose office faced Tchaikovsky Street (whence the Soviets had been directing radiation into the embassy for years) had suffered bleeding from the eyes, a strange blood ailment, and general poor health which had forced him to leave his post, or the fact that two of Stoessel's predecessors had died of cancer.

As it happened, Dr. Johnson did tell Osnos about two cases of perforated appendixes, which had occurred in high-ranking Americans at the embassy in the winter of 1976 (and which had necessitated emergency flights to Helsinki), as examples of the extreme pressures under which the embassy doctor must operate. What he did not see fit to mention—no doubt because he attached no importance to it— was a rather strange coincidence that was involved in at least four cases of appendicitis, which occurred within a three-month period among people living at the embassy. Three of these cases occurred in the sixth-floor apartment of Brigadier General James W. Wold, the Air Attache to the embassy. The first case was suffered by the Wold family's cook in June 1976; the second case was suffered by the general himself on July 17; and the third was suffered by a daughter of the general in August. As for the fourth case, it was suffered on June 20, 1976, by the wife of the embassy's Political Counselor, who also lived on the sixth floor of the embassy.

It is not known whether Dr. Johnson or any of the medical consultants to the State Department considered this outbreak of appendicitis to be significant, or whether they even wondered if it might possibly be related to the microwave radiation being beamed into the embassy. It is known, however, that high levels of microwave radiation can have serious effects upon the gastrointestinal tract and upon the organs of the hollow viscera, of which the appendix is one. It is also known that General Wold and his family, as well as the Political Counselor and his wife, lived in apartments facing Tchaikovsky Street.

9

Project Pandora
Revisited

How high have levels of microwave radiation been at the American Embassy over the years, and to what extent is the State Department to be believed about the matter? In its classified briefing paper entitled "Moscow Microwave Signal," which was prepared in March 1976, the department employed some carefully qualified, if not deliberately ambiguous, language to describe the intensity of the radiation. Concerning the strength of the microwave beam that had originally been detected in the early 1960s, the department paper said that "at all times it was found to be well below any level associated with known biological hazards." Depending upon one's interpretation of the word "known," that could be taken to mean that the power levels of the Moscow Signal were well below the ten-milliwatt-per-square-centimeter standard that has long been in effect in the United States. Strangely, the briefing paper later declared that "there is general, if not total, unanimity among American experts that exposures below the milliwatt (1000 microwatts)-per-square-centimeter level do not produce hazardous effects," which, of course, could be taken to mean that the power levels of the signal were below one milliwatt.

The briefing paper gave no indication of why the unspecified levels of radiation of the original Moscow Signal were considered serious enough to warrant the time and expense of Project Pandora—the highly classified, three-year research program undertaken by the Department of Defense's Advanced Research Projects Agency (DARPA) to determine whether the signal might have adverse biological effects—or, for that matter, why they were considered serious enough to warrant their being brought up as a matter for discussion at the Glassboro summit meeting in June 1967. The briefing paper went on to claim, however, that from October 1975 through January 1976, "the typical maximum levels measured were up to 13 microwatts per square centimeter," and that "the highest 'maximum point' recorded when both signals were on the air at once was 18 microwatts."

In its contingency press briefing that was sent to Moscow on December 20, 1976, the department instructed its spokesman, in the event he were asked whether radiation levels at the embassy had ever reached four milliwatts per square centimeter, to reply that "we have never observed levels anything near that high." This statement was obviously designed to refute Dr. Zaret's account of how the intensity of the microwave signal was described at a meeting which took place at the Institute of Defense Analysis, in 1965, when Project Pandora was about to get under way. According to Dr. Zaret, the Moscow Signal "was described in detailed technical terms at the meeting," and "was being generated at multiple frequencies and widely fluctuating patterns, and at power densities that never exceeded four milliwatts per square centimeter." Thus the whole matter of radiation levels at the Moscow Embassy boils down to the following: either Dr. Zaret's memory is faulty, or the State Department is lying.

The Department had, of course, already lied to its employees concerning the reason for their being given buccal smear tests. In addition, some rather persuasive circumstantial evidence has recently come to light which indicates that the department may not have been candid when it stated that radiation levels at the embassy had never approached four milliwatts per square centimeter. On March 1, 1977, in response to a Freedom of Information request from Barton Reppert, the Department of Defense downgraded fourteen documents relating to DARPA's Project Pandora from "Secret" to

"Unclassified," and released them to the public. In doing so, the Pentagon obviously decided that after nearly a decade information about Project Pandora was no longer vital to the national security. Whether it was vital to the national security to begin with, or simply part of the Department of Defense's cover-up policy, is open to question. However, an examination of the fourteen documents sheds some interesting new light on the matter, as well as on the question of just how strong the original Moscow Signal may have been.

The earliest of these documents is dated November 1966, and is an evaluation of the microwave-generating equipment and microwave test facility that was being installed at the Walter Reed Army Institute of Research (WRAIR) in order to irradiate monkeys with the Moscow Signal and to determine if it could induce biological and behavioral changes in them. This evaluation was performed by members of the Applied Physics Laboratory at Johns Hopkins University, who found that the microwave generating equipment at the Walter Reed facility was capable of producing a power density of approximately four milliwatts per square centimeter over the S-Band frequency range, with a transmitted power of 250 watts. The reason behind the decision to irradiate the monkeys with four milliwatts was not given in the Johns Hopkins report, or anywhere else in the declassified Project Pandora file, but it is reasonable to suppose that it had to do with replicating the intensity of the Moscow Signal.

The remaining documents in the declassified Pandora file pertain mostly to meetings held in 1968 and 1969, and they go a long way toward confirming this supposition. At a meeting that took place at the Forest Glen Annex of the Walter Reed Army Hospital on December 20, 1968, a special five-member science advisory committee, convened by the Institute of Defense Analysis at the request of DARPA, met to review research techniques and the results of Pandora experiments to date, and to make recommendations for the future of the project. This committee included Dr. Pollack, then a staff member of the Institute of Defense Analysis, and it was unanimous in its opinion that the research techniques employed in the monkey experiments were "sound and acceptable." It was also unanimous in its opinion that "monkeys exposed to the specific 'synthetic Moscow Signal' in field strengths from one milliwatt per square centimeter to four and six-tenths milliwatts per square centimeter showed degradation of work performance after 10-hours-a-day exposure for from 11 days to 21 days." The panel recommended that a program be developed "to determine the immediate or short time effects on humans of the synthetic Moscow Signal," and that the program include chromosomal studies of lymphocyte cells. A few weeks later, the panel learned that chromosomes obtained from the peripheral blood of a monkey irradiated with the Moscow Signal at a field strength of four and six-tenths milliwatts per square centimeter showed marked abberations in forty percent of the cells.

At a meeting that took place at the Institute of Defense Analysis on January 17, 1969, Dr. Pollack reviewed a projected Navy-DARPA study to determine the physiological and psychological effects of radar upon the crew members of the aircraft carrier U.S.S. *Saratoga.* Later, on April 21, the science advisory panel reviewed the results of this study, which was called "Big Boy." The panel learned that the radiation levels on board the *Saratoga* never exceeded one milliwatt per square centimeter even though it had been expected from a naval electronics lab report that there might be levels greater than ten milliwatts per square centimeter on at least eighty percent of the surface of the ship. The committee then discussed blood studies that had been performed on twenty-one crew members from the carrier, and learned that "although two abnormalities were found, they were regarded as in normal range." That the Navy had gone to considerable lengths to keep the crew members of the *Saratoga* in the dark about the purpose of "Big Boy" can be inferred from a terse statement in the minutes of the meeting, which read "Cover story considered appropriate and worked well."

The April 21 meeting ended with the science advisory committee's emphasizing "the need for information on humans in addition to the accelerated animal studies at Walter Reed." The committee urged that "the Walter Reed facility develop a human program," and suggested that "human subjects would be required for six to eight months and that they could be obtained from Ft. Dietrich." The minutes do not record any discussion by the committee of whether or not these human subjects would be fully informed of the possible hazards of their submitting to the proposed radiation.

On May 12, 1969, the committee and researchers from Walter Reed met at the Institute of Defense Analysis to discuss just how to design and conduct the human studies. Among other things, they agreed that the strength of the signal used in the studies should be between four and five milliwatts per square centimeter, which, in spite of the State Department's subsequent denials, obviously provides strong corroboration for Dr. Zaret's claim that the original Moscow Signal was generated at similar intensities. Even stronger corroboration appeared in the minutes of a meeting that took place at the institute on June 18. At that time, the science advisory committee and the Walter Reed people reached the following conclusions about the human studies:

> It was the consensus that the aim should be to duplicate or simulate the Moscow environment as much as appropriate to solve the problem. Since exposure to the Moscow signal tended to be over an eight-to-ten hour period, it is thought that the exposure of subjects to the Special Signal should approximate that time frame.

During this meeting, Richard S. Cesaro, of DARPA, who was the overall director of Project Pandora, reminded the committee that his agency had assigned a high priority to solving the problems posed by the Moscow Signal, and that it was important to do so in fiscal year 1970. Cesaro went on to tell the committee that there was evidence that low-level radiation could penetrate the central nervous system of monkeys, and that it was now necessary to determine how such penetration occurred and what microwave characteristics and biomedical engineering principles were involved. "Such questions relate to whether or not the Moscow Signal is unique and to whether the Soviets have special insight into the effects and use of athermal radiation on man," declared Cesaro, who went on to say that the effects could be physiological, behavioral, and genetic.

As things turned out, the apparently clear direction for future research that was recommended by the science advisory committee and Cesaro in the spring of 1969 soon became clouded with uncertainty. Indeed, during the next few months, a mysterious change of heart and mind seems to have taken place in the people who were carrying out Project Pandora. The first official inkling of this occurred at a two-day meeting that took place at the Institute of Defense Anaysis on August 12 and 13. At that time, Major James T. McIlwain, of WRAIR, suddenly informed the committee that the conclusions drawn from the monkey experiments, which had been conducted at Walter Reed during 1967 and 1968 by Dr. Joseph C. Sharp, may have been erroneous, and that "there is no convincing evidence of an effect of the special signal on the performance of monkeys." Major McIlwain, who had been sitting in on the Pandora meetings as the chief representative of the Walter Reed group for some time, did not tell the committee why it had taken him so long to challenge the validity of Dr. Sharp's work, nor did he provide the committee with a written report of his findings. In view of the new information, however, the committee decided that the Walter Reed researchers "should attempt to resolve the inconsistencies of their conclusions."

Whether the committee really wanted to get to the bottom of the disagreement between Sharp and McIlwain seems somewhat doubtful in the light of subsequent developments. Indeed, it appears far more likely that McIlwain's analysis had been introduced as a convenient way of persuading the committee to withdraw its recommendations for human studies, which, after all, threatened to produce some embarrassing data. In this context, it is interesting to examine some statements made in September 1969 at the Richmond Symposium on the Biological Effects and Health Implications of Microwave Radiation by Dr. Lawrence Sher, of the University of Pennsylvania, who had joined the Project Pandora science advisory panel in the spring. (This was the same Dr. Sher who asked Dr. Marha how he could possibly justify the fact that Czechoslovakian regulations governing exposure to microwave radiation were one thousand times stricter than our own.) At the Richmond symposium, Dr. Sher objected strongly to the use of the term "flaccid paralysis" to describe the limp and unmoving condition of rats that had been exposed to four and six-tenths milliwatts per square centimeter, as well as to the term "clouding of the sensorium" to describe diminished awareness and efficiency in animals irradiated at the same power density.

As it happened, the study whose terminology Dr. Sher was objecting to had been performed by Dr. Don R. Justesen, director of the Neurophysiology Research Laboratories at the U.S. Veterans Administration Hospital, in Kansas City, Missouri, who was conducting experiments under contract to the Surgeon General of the United States Army. It also happened that while he was conducting the study Justesen acknowledged that he had received "continued encouragement and helpful criticism" from Dr. Sharp and Major McIlwain, whom he described as scientific monitors for the Army contract. Therefore, whether he knew it or not, Justesen was obviously performing research for the secret Project Pandora of whose science advisory committee Dr. Sher was a member. Sher, having heard Major McIlwain declare, in August, that there was "no convincing evidence of an effect of the special signal on the performance of monkeys," found himself compelled to object, in September, to the manner in which Dr. Justesen described convincing evidence he had found of an effect of the special signal on rats. Here is how Dr. Sher voiced his objections:

> Lest the terms arouse undue anxiety, flaccid paralysis, which sounds nasty, and clouding of the sensorium happen to me in a private conference room whenever the door is closed and the temperature rises. The clinical significance of microwave effects must be kept in mind. If all or most conventional ovens in the U.S. were today replaced with the available microwave ovens with their attendant possible problems of leakage, I suspect that the clinical effects for the general population would be favorable. My wife burns herself regularly and it is certainly not unusual for ovens, gas operated, to generate very clinically significant problems such as the house catching on fire or other untoward results of cooking.

Few in the audience at the Richmond symposium could have guessed from these facetious remarks that Dr. Sher was sitting on a secret government committee which had been formed to consider the biological effects of low-level microwave radiation upon people living and working in the Moscow Embassy. Like Dr. Sher's wife, however, the embassy people presumably did their cooking with gas ovens. Nor could anyone have guessed that only three months earlier Dr. Sher had heard the director of Project Pandora say that there was definite evidence that low-level microwave radiation could penetrate the central nervous system of monkeys. Certainly Allan Frey had no way of guessing; he responded to the remarks by asking Sher why he didn't go out and buy a microwave oven.

"I would love to have one," Sher replied, "but they are a little expensive." Sher then went on to make a statement about ten-milliwatt exposures that seems puzzling in light of what he had learned as a member of Project Pandora's science advisory committee. "Regarding the figure of ten milliwatts per square centimeter and the papers which we have heard, I have to say that if a person or an animal is exposed to ten milliwatts per square centimeter, a sufficiently sensitive experimental technique must detect some changes," he declared. "Whether this is a change in the partition of biochemical components or a change in galvanic skin response or a change in the quivering of the large toe, a sufficiently sensitive experiment must detect a change. We know that there is energy going into the animal's body and it is reasonable therefore to expect a change."

It may also, of course, be reasonable to expect that Dr. Sher's remarks at Richmond had something to do with his involvement with Project Pandora. In any case, frantic attempts were made in the autumn of 1969 to resolve the differences between Dr. Sharp and Major McIlwain concerning the interpretation of the results of the monkey experiments that had been conducted at Walter Reed. These attempts were unsuccessful, as is evident from a report given to the committee on December 4. The report states that "in Dr. Sharp's view, although most of the experiments produced negative results, certain aspects of the data . . . are suggestive of an exposure effect due to the WRAIR signal." It goes on to say that while "admitting that some changes in the animals' behavior could not be explained by artifacts, Maj. McIlwain believes that there is insufficient consistency in the data to seriously entertain the notion of an exposure effect due to the special WRAIR signal."

Faced with a choice between the two conflicting points of view, the science advisory committee conveniently decided to follow Napoleon's military dictum—when in doubt, do nothing. As a result, Project Pandora came to a rather abrupt end on January 12, 1970, after a final meeting between the committee and representatives of WRAIR and DARPA at the Institute for Defense Analysis. The committee's report of the meeting starts out by saying that "certain events presumed to be threatening to the national interest served as the basis for ARPA's support of Project Pandora," and that funds were given to Walter Reed early in 1965 "to evaluate the threat since it appeared to have strong behavioral and biomedical implications." The report went on to say that preliminary results presented in 1967 "encouraged the belief that the special signal altered primate behavior," and that "cytogenic and histological studies of the brain suggested that comparable energies were damaging to tissue." Influenced by Major McIlwain's subsequent analysis of these results, however, the committee reversed its earlier unanimous opinion that the experiments showed definite behavioral effects in the monkeys.

Indeed, it not only concluded that "no definitive answer to the question of whether the original signal has any effect on the performance of operantly-conditioned monkeys has been provided to date," but also that "the findings thus far can be regarded as negative." And, incredibly enough, the committee reached these conclusions even while admitting in its report that fully five months after hearing his analysis "no written report has been produced by Dr. McIlwain due to the pressure of time."

As for the planned human experiments, the committee decided that "based upon existing information, there is no evidence that any permanent deleterious effects are to be expected." As for the State Department employees and their families at the Moscow Embassy, the committee said that "it may be assumed that continued medical follow-up of personnel exposed to the original signal has been developed, but no details on such a follow-up have been provided."

10

The Cancer
Connection

Clearly, the assumption of the Project Pandora science advisory committee that the State Department's Moscow employees would be followed up medically amounted to nothing more than wishful thinking, unless, in accordance with previous State Department practice, medical follow-ups were performed on these people without their knowledge. In fact, more than six years passed before the department got around to making official blood tests of its Moscow employees, and to contracting with Dr. Lilienfeld and his colleagues at Johns Hopkins for a retrospective epidemiological study of their health experience. Since then, the declassification of the Pandora file has cast doubt upon the State Department's claim that the intensity of the irradiation at the embassy never amounted to more than a few microwatts. It has also, of course, cast doubt upon the department's denial that it ever obliged the military by covering up the significance of microwave effects on health.

During the winter of 1977, sources within the department admitted privately that excessive radiation was emanating from the telephone of former Ambassador Stoessel. It was caused by a high-frequency, one-thousand-watt radio transmitter located on the roof of the embassy above Stoessel's office. When this transmitter was operating, it induced high-frequency signals in the tens of milliwatts in phone lines running to the Ambassador's desk, as well as in phone lines running to other offices in the embassy's political section. Another State Department source has attempted to soften this revelation by claiming that the high-frequency transmitter was never turned on except for a once-a-month test, or in the event that the Russians shut down the embassy's regular communications channel, which runs through the Moscow Post Office. This same source has insisted that there are no other transmitting devices in the embassy, that all other electronic equipment is designed for passive reception, and that no significant radiation could therefore be emanating from within or on top of the building.

If these statements are accurate, they conveniently place all of the blame for the irradiation of the embassy upon the Russians. However, there are a number of reasons for supposing that they may not be true. The passive listening devices on the roof of the embassy are not operated or controlled by the State Department, but by either the National Security Agency or the Central Intelligence Agency. Also, passive listening devices can easily be jammed and rendered ineffective by electronic countermeasures—in other words, by the kind of radiation being beamed at the embassy from the other side of Tchaikovsky Street. In short, it is difficult to understand how passive devices could possibly operate in such a hostile electronic environment unless electronic counter-countermeasures were taken. Otherwise, just how much sense would it make to have placed such listening devices on the roof of the embassy to begin with?

That the State Department is not its own master at the Moscow Embassy should come as no surprise to anyone. It is well known that the official staff of almost any United States embassy contains a large proportion of agents from the Central Intelligence Agency. For its part, the State Department has admitted, at a briefing conducted in August 1976, that all information about the equipment is classified. This does not, of course, let the department off the hook for the biological damage that such equipment may have inflicted upon embassy personnel, or, for that matter, for the damage visited upon them by Russian transmitters on the other side of Tchaikovsky

Street. In fact, the State Department is being sued by a number of its employees, who claim that either they or their offspring have been harmed by the radiation. In part, of course, litigation and the threat of it explain why the department has all along insisted upon the obvious fiction that the radiation levels in the Moscow Embassy never exceeded a few microwatts per square centimeter. By so insisting, the department has simply created another dilemma for itself—in short, how on earth to explain the mysterious blood abnormalities in nearly one-third of its Moscow employees and their families if microwave radiation has nothing to do with it. The solution to this dilemma has not been found, but an interim policy has been formed to deal with it—a policy of diversion and denial.

One facet of this policy has led the State Department to engage in such cat-and-mouse expeditions as the sending of a medical team to Moscow on February 26, 1977, in order to investigate the abnormal white-blood-cell counts. According to a *New York Times* article by Christopher S. Wren, the department had asked the Soviet government back in October 1976 for blood-count statistics on Russian residents of Moscow "to serve as a means of comparison with the situation of the Americans." Wren went on to say that a medical team had been sent to Moscow to obtain this data, and that it was made up of Dr. William M. Watson, head of the State Department's medical division; Dr. Thomas F. Stossel, chief of the oncology division of the Massachusetts General Hospital; and Dr. Pollack. According to the article, Russian health specialists told their American visitors that they could not be of assistance "because no problem existed and because their data had not been analyzed according to American needs." Wren further stated that "the Soviet Union tends to be secretive about statistics that would be freely available in the West," and that "the Russians may also see no advantage in cooperating with a study even indirectly linked to the radiation that has been beamed at the American Embassy, reportedly by electronic devices."

In evolving or passing on these theories, Wren was apparently unaware that white-blood-cell counts are not taken by the American Red Cross or by other blood banks in the United States, and that statistics on lymphocytes do not exist for the residents of, say, Washington, D.C., or for the residents of any other American city. Of course, the Russians just may not have been in the mood to cooperate about anything. President Carter had recently criticized their failure to observe basic human rights, and the State Department had claimed that the Moscow drinking water contained dangerous amounts of cyanide and mercury. According to Wren, the Soviet health officials did see fit to present a basic textbook on hematology to Dr. Stossel—a gesture some diplomats considered condescending. Whether this gesture was an attempt to condescend or to educate is a matter of opinion, especially in light of what two members of the State Department's medical team were quoted as saying during their Moscow visit. Dr. Watson, for example, reported that the lymphocyte counts, which ran forty-four percent above normal in 64 out of 213 American diplomats and their dependents who were tested, constituted a "slight shift." And Dr. Stossel declared that the abnormality, which receded after the Americans left Moscow, "has no known pathological meaning."

The certainty of these two medical doctors about the abnormal lymphocyte counts may well have temporarily reassured the Americans who live and work at the Moscow Embassy. During the early part of May 1977, however, an article written by Keyes Beech, a syndicated *Chicago Daily News* columnist, appeared in newspapers around the country. One version began as follows:

> The State Dept. has given Johns Hopkins University of Baltimore a $250,000 contract to determine whether there is a link between microwave radiation beamed at the U.S. embassy in Moscow and an apparently high rate of cancer among Americans serving there.
>
> Richard Moose, deputy undersecretary of state for management, said the cost of the research project might go as high as $400,000 before it is completed and that it would be a year or more before the results are known.
>
> "But it will be worth it to lower the anxiety level among Moscow Embassy personnel and restore credibility in the State Dept. management by Foreign Service families who felt they have been victimized," said Moose, who visited Moscow six weeks ago.
>
> A separate, nonscientific study is being conducted by an emotionally involved Foreign Service officer whose wife developed breast cancer while they were serving in Moscow, Moose said.
>
> The survey has disclosed that 16 American women who served in Moscow developed breast cancer, Moose said. Two former American ambassadors to Moscow, Charles (Chip) Bohlen and Llewellyn

Thompson, both died of cancer in the past few years.

Zbigniew Brzezinski, Polish-born national security adviser to President Carter, told this reporter in March 1976, in Tokyo, that the cancer rate among Americans in the Moscow embassy was the highest in the world.

He blamed Soviet microwave radiation beamed at the embassy for what appears to be the abnormally high cancer rate.

"But none of this proves anything," Moose said. "We just don't know, but we are determined to find out."

Dr. E. Cuyler Hammond of the American Cancer Society scoffed at the idea that microwaves can cause cancer.

"This is poppycock Buck Rogers stuff," he snorted. "The chances are just about nil, although not impossible. Microwaves are not like gamma rays or X-rays which do penetrate the cells and cause cancer."

Dr. James M. Sontag of the National Cancer Institute at Bethesda, Md., was more cautious. "I wouldn't scoff at the possibility," he said. "It's true that microwaves are non-ionizing and therefore supposedly not carcinogenic.

"But ultra-violet light is also non-ionizing and it can cause cancer," he said. "That's the way people get skin cancer."

Considering all the evidence, Dr. Sontag's remarks about a possible link between microwave irradiation and cancer seem eminently sensible; those voiced by Dr. Hammond do not. Dr. Hammond is Vice-President for Epidemiology and Statistics of the American Cancer Society; he participated in an analysis of the medical effects of the atomic explosions that devastated Hiroshima and Nagasaki in 1945; his large-scale epidemiological studies of more than a million men and women provided a major basis for the conclusions drawn in the 1964 Surgeon General's report on the health effects of cigarette smoking; his statistical analysis of mortality among asbestos workers has provided a major basis for the certainty that asbestos inhalation is cancer-producing; and he, more than most people, should know better than to dismiss out of hand something he has not even bothered to study. One wonders if Dr. Hammond would dismiss as "poppycock Buck Rogers stuff" a suggestion that microwave radiation affects the central nervous system and alters behavior, or that it may cause genetic damage. And what would he say to the fact that when the State Department secretly tested young women from the Moscow Embassy for genetic damage during the late 1960s, it found evidence that such damage had occurred?

In any case, it is a pity that Dr. Hammond did not attend a workshop/seminar convened in Washington on December 15, 1976, by the Electromagnetic Radiation Management Advisory Council. At that meeting, Dr. William M. Leach, chief of the Experimental Studies Branch of the Bureau of Radiological Health's Division of Biological Effects, was invited to discuss research he had conducted at the bureau during the first six months of 1976, together with Professor Przemyslaw Czerski, a visiting scientist on leave from the Department of Genetics at the National Research Institute of Mother and Child, in Warsaw. During 1974 and 1975, Dr. Leach had found that microwave radiation could induce changes in the chromosomes of bone-marrow cells and the lymphocytes of test animals. There was nothing very new in that. Back in 1961, Professor Charles Susskind, of the Electronics Research Laboratory of the University of California at Berkeley, had reported finding cancer of the white blood cells—lymphatic leucosis and lymphatic leukemia—in mice that had been exposed to heavy doses of microwave radiation. As early as 1967, the fact that significant changes could be produced in human lymphocyte cultures by microwave radiation at power densities of only seven milliwatts per square centimeter was reported by Professor Stodolsnik-Barańska, director of the Polish Military Institute of Aviation Medicine, who described these findings at the Warsaw symposium in 1973. For his part, Professor Czerski—a renowned hematologist and geneticist—had told the Warsaw symposium that there were "easily demonstrable and easily quantified microwave effects" on the lymphocytes and lymphocytic systems of mice, rabbits, and guinea pigs which had been exposed to low doses of radiation.

In the work they performed together at the Bureau of Radiological Health, Professor Czerski and Dr. Leach found that within six to eight days after single, five-minute exposures to continuous-wave microwave radiation having a power density of from fifteen to twenty milliwatts per square centimeter, lymphocyte counts in groups of irradiated animals rose one and a half times as much as those in control groups of animals that had not been exposed to the radiation. (The fact that all of the animals were cooled so that their body temperatures either rose only slightly, or did not rise at all, or in some cases even dropped, strongly indicated that the effect of microwaves on their white blood cells was not caused by heating.) Even more alarming, up to twenty percent of the normal lymphocyte cells in the irradiated animals underwent blastic transformation, which means that the cells grew in size and divided in two. In lymphoblastoid transformations something has gone biologically wrong, and at the December 15 meeting in the Office of Telecommunications Policy, Dr. Leach took note of this. Leach told his audience that he believed the cell changes observed in the irradiated animals could either be associated with an immune response in reaction to a foreign antigen, or the result of the loss of a cell's ability to control its own division.

Leach then said something that caused several people in the audience to put their hands over their ears. "We have a word for that," he told his listeners, who included Dr. Stossel and Dr. Pollack. "The word is cancer."

11

The Genetic
Time Bomb

Behind the State Department's worried denials that microwave radiation could have anything to do with the blood disorders afflicting its Moscow employees lies the deeper anxiety in high government circles that the radiation to which tens of thousands of civilian and military personnel have been subjected has inflicted genetic damage upon them. Anxiety about the genetic effects of microwaves first came out into the open in December 1971, when the Electromagnetic Radiation Management Advisory Council—a nine-member group that includes Dr. Pollack—warned that "the consequences of undervaluing or misjudging the biological effects of long-term, low-level exposure could become a critical problem for the public health, especially if genetic effects are involved."

The council did not, of course, sound this warning on the spur of the moment. It knew very well that a decade earlier Dr. Heller had found that microwave radiation generated at levels far below those necessary to produce heat could cause gross chromosomal abnormalities in garlic-root tips, and that low-level radiation could cause genetic mutations in mammalian cells and in insects. It knew of the 1964 findings of Dr. Lilienfeld and his colleagues at Johns Hopkins concerning the apparent association between radar exposure and Down's syndrome. It knew from data presented at the Richmond symposium of 1969 that microwave radiation had induced chromosomal abnormalities in kangaroo-rat cell cultures, and that the researchers who conducted these studies had found that "the types of chromosome aberrations observed in this study are the same as those induced by ionizing radiation in other organisms including humans." And at least one of its members knew about the secret tests for genetic damage that the State Department had been running on its Moscow employees. As for the genetic problem, the official minutes of the Project Pandora meeting of April 21, 1969, are revealing. For one thing, they clearly show that although DARPA was aware of the implications of the five-year-old findings of Dr. Lilienfeld—that "eighteen out of twenty-five mongoloid children had fathers who had been exposed to radar"—the agency was only just then getting around to giving consideration to financing a study to further investigate them. But it is the following paragraph, from the minutes of the April 1969 meeting, which constitutes the "smoking gun" of the State Department's genetic cover-up:

> Dr. Pollack reported the studies of Dr. Jacobson at George Washington University who has studied young women returning from embassy in Moscow (State Dept. contract). One hundred and forty blood samples were examined over a four-year period of time. Four of them reportedly showed serious chromosomal abnormalities.

Following its 1971 warning about the possible genetic consequences of microwave radiation, the Electromagnetic Radiation Management Advisory Council, together with the OTP, the Department of Defense, and other governmental agencies continued to learn about genetic changes induced by microwaves. In 1973, at the Warsaw symposium, Professor Stodolsnik-Barańska described chromosomal abnormalities in irradiated test animals, and suggested that microwaves might well have mutagenic effects. In 1974, Professor Czerski reported similar findings at the New York Academy of Science's meeting. And in August 1975, when members of the council and the OTP met to review the findings of research pertaining to the genetic, hereditary, growth, and developmental effects of microwave and radio-frequency radiation, they learned that in eight out of fifteen projects, low-level radiation had produced effects and changes in test animals or genetic material.*

In light of all this, it is small wonder that the classified briefing paper issued by the State Department in March 1976 was cautiously worded on the question of genetic damage caused by microwave radiation. Indeed, the briefing paper showed the department tip-toeing into the delicate subject of genetic damage like some kindly obstetrician into a maternity room. "Pregnant women and their unborn children are, of course, always considered as a vulnerable category of persons in terms of preventive health in general, and it is advisable to minimize exposure to any deviation from a normal environment," the paper declared. Having covered itself in this coy fashion, the department proceeded to assure its Moscow employees that there was "no known reason to avoid conceiving children under present conditions at the Embassy." Gathering the courage of its convictions, the department then stated categorically that "there is no evidence in the medical and scientific literature that these levels of radiation would have any effect upon unborn children."

The validity of these assertions, as well as the veracity of the State Department, will now be tested in the courts. A number of former Moscow employees whose wives have given birth to malformed babies are either suing, or are about to sue, the department for damages. (One cannot help but wonder how the department will attempt to explain in court the sub rosa tests for genetic damage it administered to young women returning from Moscow in the sixties.) Whatever the legal resolutions, however, since the Pandora meetings, the government and the military have systematically suppressed information about the genetic effects of microwaves in human beings and covered up a number of potentially embarrassing situations in which such effects have been observed. Perhaps the quintessential example of this policy has been the Army's handling of the genetic problem at its huge helicopter-pilot training center at Fort Rucker, Alabama.

---

*On February 10, 1977, the council heard Dr. Ezra Berman, a veterinarian at the EPA Health Effects Research Laboratories, describe the results of some animal experiments he had recently conducted. Berman found that when pregnant mice were subjected to microwave radiation having a frequency of 2.45 gigahertz and power densities ranging from 3.4 to 28 milliwatts per square centimeters, they delivered litters in which there was a significant increase of a birth defect known as exencephaly, which is hernia of the brain.

The Fort Rucker affair began in the winter of 1971, when Dr. Peter B. Peacock, professor and chairman of the Department of Public Health and Epidemiology at the University of Alabama, together with some colleagues, undertook to study the incidence of congenital malformations in Alabama. These statistics are recorded on a county-by-county basis at the Birth Defects Center maintained by the University's School of Medicine. Upon examining these records, Peacock and his co-workers discovered that between July 1969 and November 1970, there was a significant increase in certain birth defects in seven out of the state's sixty-seven counties. This increase was particularly noticeable in the counties of Dale and Coffee—adjacent counties located in the southeastern corner of Alabama. Indeed, Peacock and his colleagues found that during the seventeen-month period, seventeen white children suffering from congenital clubfoot had been delivered in these two counties. The expected number of children with this affliction had been less than four. They also learned that the rate of children born with congenital anomalies of the heart was significantly higher in Dale County than in other parts of Alabama. In July 1971, they published their findings in the *Journal of the American Medical Association of the State of Alabama.*

During 1972, a follow-up investigation undertaken by Dr. Peacock and an assistant yielded the astonishing fact that all seventeen of the children with congenital clubfoot had been delivered in the Lyster Army Hospital at Fort Rucker. As might be expected, Peacock concluded that something might be wrong in the environment at Fort Rucker. He also suspected that the causal factor could be microwave radiation since the base was known to have a heavy concentration of radar.

To investigate the matter more thoroughly, Peacock enlisted the support of the Southern Research Institute—a private, nonprofit organization located in Birmingham. In November 1973 the institute completed a detailed report for the Environmental Protection Agency. The first paragraph of this document, entitled "Congenital Anomalies and the Use of Radar in Military Bases," read as follows:

> This report summarizes the findings of the first phase of a three-phase study designed to investigate possible relationships between incidence of congenital anomalies and exposure of parents to mi-

crowave radiation of X- and S-Band radar at military bases. The findings of the first phase of the study leave little doubt that a serious health problem is manifesting itself in the offspring of military personnel of Fort Rucker, Alabama, and that additional investigation, such as proposed for Phase II, which seeks to identify the causal factors, is justified. Congenital anomalies occur at a significantly higher level at the Lyster Hospital, Fort Rucker, than at other hospitals, including other military hospitals, in the state.

As for the possibility of human exposure to microwave radiation at Fort Rucker: "There are 46 radar installations located within 30 miles of the base, which comprise one of its particularly unique characteristics."

After making some statistical adjustments, the researchers declared that "clearly, during the period 1968–1972, an abnormally high rate of anomalies occurred in births at the Lyster Army Hospital." They also said that, in addition to clubfoot, these excess defects included cleft palate, as well as anomalies of the heart, genital organs, and circulatory and respiratory systems.

While investigating the incidence of birth defects, the institute's investigators undertook to compare the fetal death rate at Lyster Hospital at Fort Rucker with the fetal death rate at the regional hospital at nearby Eglin Air Force Base, in Florida—an installation also known to have massive concentrations of radar—and to compare these rates, in turn, with fetal death rates at three hospitals located on military bases with far less radar equipment. When they did so, they found strong evidence of an abnormally high fetal death rate at Lyster and a nearly identical fetal death rate at the regional hospital at Eglin. These rates were far higher than those at the other military hospitals. Not surprisingly, they considered this "additional evidence that a health problem may be associated with radar."

However, while the institute's statisticians were corroborating the fact that an unusually high level of birth defects had occurred in the military population at Fort Rucker, they also turned up evidence suggesting that the apparently high rate of clubfoot that had been found by Peacock might come from reporting differences between staff doctors at Lyster Hospital and those at civilian hospitals elsewhere in Alabama. "This finding appears to corroborate earlier comments of several physicians in the Birmingham area who claim to record only the more serious incidences of clubfoot because of the

social stigma attached to that anomaly," they wrote. "Such an influence is not likely to be so pronounced in military hospitals."

On January 28, 1974, the Southern Research Institute sent the final
report on the first phase of its proposed study of birth defects at Fort
Rucker to Mrs. Edie Tompkins, then assistant director of the Environmental Protection Agency's Division of Health Effects Research.
The institute informed Mrs. Tompkins that the second phase of the
study "is now being proposed for activation," and that it "is designed
on the premise that incidence rates of congenital anomalies in the
Lyster Army Hospital are abnormally high." The second phase of
the study would include an examination of birth certificates, medical
records, military 201 files, and radar inspection reports "in an effort
to identify the pertinent factors leading to the high rates." A third
phase, if it proved necessary, would endeavor to obtain additional
information through personal interviews with patients and physicians.

A funny thing happened to the institute's proposal to activate the
second phase of the study of birth defects at Fort Rucker—it never
got off the ground. The chief reason for this was simple enough: the
United States Army Medical Research and Development Command
refused to accept the premise that the rate of birth defects at the
Lyster Hospital was abnormally high. In fact, the Army claimed that
the Southern Research Institute had not demonstrated that a problem existed to begin with. As a result, the second phase of the
institute's proposed study turned into a two-year reexamination of
its 1973 report on the first phase, which, of course, had been a detailed
reexamination of the initial findings made by Dr. Peacock in 1971 and
1972. To compound the Catch-22 aspect of all this, the Army refused
to provide the institute with the medical records, 201 files, and radar
inspection reports that might have enabled the institute to prove its
case for the second phase. During 1974 and 1975, staff members of
the institute engaged in a series of negotiations with the Army,
including a session with a team of officials from the Medical Research and Development Command. These negotiations proved
fruitless, however, and in the end the institute was forced to try to
justify the need for a study of radar and congenital anomalies by
returning to square one—a reexamination of the birth certificate data
that had led to Dr. Peacock's original conclusions.

This reexamination was directed by John A. Burdeshaw, a statistician who replaced the statisticians who had conducted the institute's first assessment of the situation at Fort Rucker. After nearly two more years of studying the problem, Burdeshaw's conclusions were the subject of a report that was given the somewhat watered-down title "Factors Associated with the Incidence of Congenital Anomalies: A Localized Investigation." The report was dated March 31, 1976, and was sent to Mrs. Tompkins at the EPA in April.

In his reexamination, Burdeshaw extended the time period of Peacock's earlier study by investigating the incidence of birth defects in Alabama over the period extending from July 1968 to December 1972. Since the Lyster Army Hospital was suspected of having a significant increase in birth defects, its rates were compared with those of forty-six other hospitals in Alabama, including the twenty-two largest hospitals in the state. When Burdeshaw finished analyzing the data, he found that he had compiled evidence both for and against the conclusion that there was an unusually high incidence of birth defects at Fort Rucker. Among the evidence mitigating against such a conclusion was the fact that between July 1968 and December 1972, Coffee and Dale counties ranked sixth and eighth, respectively, among the sixty-seven counties in Alabama in terms of overall anomaly rates. Also, while the Lyster Army Hospital and the Air Force regional hospital at Maxwell Air Force Base, in Montgomery County, had the highest birth defects rates out of the forty-seven hospitals surveyed, five other hospitals had rates that were not much lower. A third finding was that other birth defects studies—particularly one conducted at the Mayo Clinic—showed anomaly rates that seemed to be consistent with those at Lyster Hospital. And, finally, there was evidence that the high incidence of birth defects at Lyster might have been due partly to overreporting on the part of certain physicians on the staff.

Two contrary observations, however, stood out. First, it was highly significant that the hospital at Fort Rucker and the hospital at Maxwell Air Force Base showed the highest birth defects rates out of forty-seven hospitals sampled throughout all of Alabama. Not only were both of these installations military aviation centers, but their rates could not easily be explained by alert reporting alone, because birth defects rates at two nonaviation military bases in Alabama were far lower. Second, Burdeshaw found an odd geographical pattern. Thirteen out of the seventeen counties with birth defects rates in the upper twenty-five percent range lay within a contiguous band that ran from the southeastern-most corner of the state in a west-northwesterly direction and ten out of the twenty counties in the southeast quadrant of the state had birth defects rates in the upper twenty-five percent range. Not surprisingly, Burdeshaw concluded that although this phenomenon "may involve more than a 'military base' explanation," it was also "more than can be explained by chance."

Toward the end of the institute's report to the EPA, there were two paragraphs that clearly showed how uninterested the Army really was in looking into the cause of birth defects at Fort Rucker. The first read:

> In the early phases of this study, it appeared that the rates in the Fort Rucker area were considerably higher than elsewhere in the state, and plans were formulated to obtain data that might aid in explaining the high rates. These data were mainly medical and occupational items measured on military personnel and their spouses, who were stationed at Fort Rucker during the time interval being studied. However, when permission to obtain certain items of information was requested of the Office of the Surgeon General (OSG), Department of the Army, it was denied, although never formally.

The second paragraph carried another indictment:

> Late in the study, a map was furnished to the Institute of a nine-county area of southeast Alabama and neighboring parts of Georgia and Florida on which navigational radar sites were indicated. Also included with the map was a classification of types of installations according to certain operational characteristics, such as power, frequency, and beam direction. Approximately 15 or 20 installations were active during the four and one-half year period under study. Had this information been received earlier, it may have been possible to determine the approximate areas that are subjected to hazardous amounts of non-ionizing radiation from these radar sites, and to determine thereby whether these areas have higher than normal incidence of congenital anomalies.

In spite of the conclusions of the institute's report, the EPA seized upon it as justification for not looking any further into the birth defect situation at Fort Rucker. Indeed, Mrs. Tompkins has stated flatly that Dr. Peacock's assessment of the incidence of birth defects at Lyster Hospital "did not hold up," and that the situation was a "clear case of over-reporting." Mrs. Tompkins also said that once Burdeshaw found the incidence of birth defects to be high in a belt of counties in southeastern Alabama, the clubfoot and other defects reported at Fort Rucker "completely disappeared as a factor." Both Dr. Peacock and the investigators at the Southern Research Institute disagree strongly with this conclusion.

During the two years that the Southern Research Institute was conducting a hamstrung reexamination of its own previous findings for the EPA, another development further complicated the cloudy Fort Rucker affair. This development began back in the autumn of 1973, when Dr. Peacock left the University of Alabama and came to New York City as medical director of the American Health Foundation—a private nonprofit organization—and professor of public health at Cornell University. Radiation was still of concern to Dr. Peacock, and in the spring of 1974 he and the American Health Foundation submitted a technical proposal to the FDA's Bureau of Radiological Health to study the problem from a new angle. The proposal was entitled "Radar and Congenital Malformations" and it contained an interesting interpretation of the situation at Fort Rucker. After referring to the fact that seventeen cases of clubfoot had been reported in Dale and Coffee counties during 1968 and 1969, Peacock described his subsequent study as follows:

> A follow-up investigation undertaken by W. Satterwhite under the direction of Dr. Peacock yielded the interesting finding that these children had all been delivered in the military hospital at Fort Rucker, Alabama, and their fathers were helicopter pilots. A review of the local situation at Fort Rucker revealed that these pilots had been heavily exposed to radar. Unlike fixed-wing pilots flying in from a reasonable altitude these helicopter pilots were exposed for most of their working days while flying at relatively low altitudes.

In his proposal to the Bureau of Radiological Health, Dr. Peacock tried to remove the new study of radar and birth defects from the tangle of controversy that had enmeshed the Southern Research Institute's attempts to investigate the situation at Fort Rucker. He suggested that it be based upon the records of helicopter pilots and fixed-wing pilots, who had been stationed at Fort Dix, New Jersey, between 1968 and 1970. Peacock went on to suggest that such records include the age and race of these men; an occupational history that would indicate the number of months each had spent as a pilot and the amount of exposure to radar he had incurred; data on whether any of the children fathered by these men since 1968 showed congenital malformations and, if so, what type; data on environmental levels of radar exposure in the neighborhood of the base; and medical histories and information concerning the mothers of children fathered by the two pilot groups since 1968. He then wrote the following analysis and discussion of his proposal:

> If exposure of men to radar does increase the likelihood of congenital malformations among their children we have no idea how such malformations are produced. It is known that certain congenital malformations do show a seasonal distribution and this suggests that heat may be a possible mechanism with a short-term effect operating at the time of conception but possibly having no residual chromosomal effect. If radar does operate this way then one should find that children conceived while their fathers were exposed to radar would show an increased incidence of congenital malformations while children conceived after their fathers returned to civilian life should show no continued excess. On the other hand, if radar acts like ionizing radiation by producing chromosomal breaks, there may be some continued effect over the rest of the presumptive father's life which would show in children conceived after the father had returned to a life where he did not have an excess of radar exposure. It is also possible that the mother might be exposed in some as yet unidentified manner, either from her husband (as has been reported with asbestos) or from the environment of the base. Hopefully, the helicopter and fixed-wing pilots will be sufficiently alike in most regards, including the residences of their wives, to eliminate most of these alternative variables as possible causes of any differences that may be found.

Dr. Peacock's study proposal and his assessment of the problem must have struck the FDA's Bureau of Radiological Health as both scientific and sensible. After reviewing it, they provided funds to carry the program out. At that point, however, the bureau and the American Health Foundation found themselves in the same position as the EPA and the Southern Research Institute. They faced, in short, unyielding opposition from officials of the Army Medical

Research and Development Command (AMRDC), who claimed that there was no evidence of a genetic problem to begin with. By the late summer of 1975, Dr. Peacock must have felt that he had walked into a minefield. On August 19, he sent Brigadier-General Kenneth R. Dirks, commander of the AMRDC, a map showing the county-by-county distribution of the cases of clubfoot recorded in Alabama between November 1968 and October 1970, as well as a detailed listing from the birth defects registry showing that seventeen out of the twenty-one cases of clubfoot that were recorded for Dale and Coffee counties during this period had occurred in the Lyster Hospital at Fort Rucker.

General Dirks was apparently unimpressed with this documentation, or, for that matter, with the American Health Foundation's study proposal. In a letter written on September 3, 1975, he turned down the foundation's request for access to the medical records of Army pilots on the basis that its proposed methodology was inadequate. On September 24, Dr. Peacock wrote to General Dirks. "It seems, I hope unintentionally, that you have missed the point of our proposed investigation into a possible relationship between congenital malformations and being a helicopter pilot," Dr. Peacock said. "We have never claimed that a relationship between congenital malformations and radar is 'proven,' otherwise this would have been published, but we do feel strongly that sufficient suspicion has been raised to require—nay, demand—an adequate and detailed investigation."

As for the charge that his proposed methodology was inadequate, Dr. Peacock had this to say to General Dirks:

> We accept that the details of the methodology may not have been filled out—this could very well have been your contribution—but the overall design was developed, reviewed, and approved by the best civilian epidemiologists in this country with a significant record of productive work. I am in no position to estimate the qualifications of those who were your reviewers on this occasion.
>
> May I urgently suggest that you re-open this issue. It appears that it is not really your right to decide whether or not this study needs to be carried further—unless you wish to lay yourself open to the (hopefully unjustifiable) charge that you are placing the possible interests of the Armed Services ahead of the interest of those Americans who

might be exposed to an excess risk. One would hate to make a political issue of this.

Dr. Peacock's reluctance notwithstanding, the way the Army had handled the genetic hazard posed by exposure to radar obviously did constitute a political issue. Indeed, microwaves had been a political issue ever since the military and the government had decided to cover up the problem more than fifteen years before. Within a few weeks, however, Dr. Peacock appeared to have come to this conclusion himself, for on October 16 he wrote a letter to Senator Abraham Ribicoff, of Connecticut, which read in part as follows:

> I have always admired the way you were prepared to take on powerful and entrenched interests when it seemed this was for the benefit of the citizens of our country. It would be deeply appreciated and, I think, of service to our country, if you could take a look at some material I have prepared and take appropriate action. As you will see, the FDA has funded a research program to investigate possible risks to which helicopter pilots are exposed, but the Army is protecting itself by playing coy.
>
> I am attaching a series of documents which are, I think, self-explanatory. In summary, we found a remarkable excess of congenital clubfeet among children born in the U.S. Lyster Army Hospital at Fort Rucker, Alabama. The 12 cases delivered in that hospital in 1969 were one-quarter of the total cases for the state of Nebraska and one-eighth of the total number reported from the city of Atlanta (I have named these two areas because the Federal Government uses these registries to estimate the national statistics). While this excess could have been due to chance, this was sufficiently unlikely that further investigations seemed warranted. In looking at what characterized helicopter pilots the item that stood out was their exposure to radar during the training program. Both the EPA and FDA were interested in these findings and after going through their review panels, FDA funded an investigation to check this out in another area to see whether these findings stood up when rigorously tested under other conditions. After initially indicated interest and possible support, the Army suddenly closed the door, suggesting that they might be concerned about the outcome of the investigation.
>
> I have no personal financial interest in this study. The contract shows me as receiving 5% of my salary from this investigation—this was at the urgent request of the FDA which asks its Principal Investigators to have some financial commitment—but even this is no

longer the situation since I have resigned from the Foundation (I am still very happy with the ideals and leadership of the Foundation) to go back into private practice. I do not care who undertakes this investigation, or even who receives the credits—if any—should my suspicions be justified, but I am most concerned that the investigation should be carried out to protect the unborn children of our young men in the helicopter service. No reply to my last letter has been received from the Army.

At the same time that he wrote to Senator Ribicoff, Dr. Peacock made efforts to get some of the material supporting his position into the hands of Ralph Nader's group. It is not known what, if anything, Senator Ribicoff or the Nader people did, but it seems likely that the Army got wind of Peacock's action, for it suddenly pulled a dramatic switch in tactics concerning the American Health Foundation's study proposal. At a meeting on November 10 at the AMRDC headquarters in the Forrestal Building, in Washington, D.C., Army officials made no further mention of deficiencies in methodology; they did, however, inform representatives from the Bureau of Radiological Health and the American Health Foundation that the Privacy Act, which had been passed by Congress on December 31, 1974, would prevent them from furnishing the foundation with information about birth defects in the children of Army aviators. According to the minutes of this meeting, the Army reminded the bureau people that "under New York State law a contracting government agency is also negligent if their contractor is in noncompliance with Federal Law (i.e. Privacy Law)."

Frustrated by this latest tactic, the foundation and the bureau attempted to enlist the support of the Navy and the Air Force in carrying out a study that would be based upon voluntary participation on the part of military aviators, who would be asked to answer a questionnaire on the incidence of birth defects among their children. Just why the foundation and the bureau assumed that either the Navy or the Air Force might be more interested in finding out about the problem than the Army is not clear. It is clear, however, that both the Navy and the Air Force turned the proposal down. The Navy's rejection was made by Captain Paul E. Tyler, director of the Electromagnetic Radiation Project Office of the Naval Medical Research and Development Command, who, in 1971, had been instrumental in cancelling the Navy's contract with Dr. Zaret. "The questionnaire as presently constructed will give no indication of radar exposure since the identification of either a helicopter or fixed-wing pilot per se and their total flight hours has no correlation with radar exposure," Tyler wrote in a letter to the American Health Foundation on December 30, 1975. "How will radar exposure levels be estimated?"

This objection was also vintage Catch-22, of course, since the Navy, as well as the Army and the Air Force, had for years refused to release the only inspection reports that could possibly have revealed the radar exposure levels to which military aviators and other personnel had been subjected. Later in his letter, Captain Tyler said that "the questionnaire, except for a question concerning X-rays, does not include any other unique aspects of military aviation versus other occupations which, if there is really an increase in birth defects in this group, could also be causal factors." The captain, who is a medical doctor, did not say what these other possible causal factors might be, and he certainly was not about to list radar among them. Indeed, Captain Tyler apparently was eager to extend the presumption of innocence to radar. In the last sentence of his letter he made the somewhat redundant point that Dr. Peacock's study "certainly does not indicate that radars per se were the cause of his findings," which—Catch-22 again—was the very point that Peacock had made all along in his futile attempts to initiate a thorough investigation of the cause of the abnormally high rate of birth defects at Fort Rucker.

During the winter of 1976, the FDA's Bureau of Radiological Health made a few half-hearted attempts to keep the study of radar exposure and birth defects alive, but a stop-work order was issued in February, and by June the American Health Foundation's proposal was considered dead by everyone involved. Since then, efforts have been made by the foundation to identify certain occupational groups whose members have been exposed to microwave radiation, in order to investigate the incidence of birth defects among their offspring, and at present it appears likely that a study of birth defects in the children of microwave diathermy machine operators may be undertaken.

As for the credibility of the Department of the Army in the Fort Rucker matter, it is interesting to note that during the two-year period in which they engaged in negotiations with the Southern Research Institute and the EPA, on the one hand, and with the American Health Foundation and the FDA, on the other, officials of the Medical Research and Development Command never let on to either group that they were dealing with the other, or that they were considering two separate study proposals, until they had effectively neutralized each of the proposals separately. Thus, through a combination of cat-and-mouse, sheer stonewalling, suppression of data, and sly manipulation did the Army manage to thwart scientific research on the genetic effects of microwaves proposed by the two regulatory agencies of the federal government charged by Congress to protect the public health from the threat of microwave radiation.

These days, the Army medical people in Washington, D.C., appear hopeful that the Fort Rucker affair will remain a closed book. They either avoid the subject or discuss it in only the most guarded terms. One colonel, who was a medical officer at the base during the late 1960s, flatly denied knowing anything about the incidence of birth defects there. Another colonel, who had also been a medical officer at Fort Rucker, brought up the high incidence of birth defects Burdeshaw had found in the belt of counties in the southeastern part of Alabama, in order to advance the notion that the whole business might be chalked up to consanguinity.

Still other people interested in covering up the Fort Rucker affair have claimed that if there was any excess of birth defects among the children of helicopter pilots it was probably due to the effects of vibration, although there are virtually no medical studies of any reliability to show that this might be the case. The fact that some of these stories have originated with the Army's Aeromedical Research Laboratory and its Aviation Medicine Research Division—both of which, amazingly enough, are located at Fort Rucker—raises serious doubt about the military's capacity to be objectively involved in scientific research, and whether it should even be allowed to act as a direct funding agency for such research.

Such a smokescreen as that laid down by the Department of the Army invariably tries to conceal one artful dodge too many. In the case of the Fort Rucker cover-up, the needless artifice consists of a report whose omissions are so glaring that it can only be construed as a deliberate effort by the Army to mislead the Bureau of Radiological Health. On November 10, 1975, the Army Medical Research and Development people informed the bureau that the Privacy Act would prevent them from making the medical records of military aviators available to the American Health Foundation. At that point, an official of the bureau requested that the Army furnish information on microwave radiation levels at Fort Rucker so that the bureau might at least have some way of determining whether helicopter pilots had actually received greater exposures than pilots who flew in fixed-wing aircraft. Colonel Charles Dettor, Deputy Chief of Staff for Research at AMRDC, agreed that such information would be useful, and promised that an environmental survey of Fort Rucker would be made.

As things turned out, the Army did not get around to making the survey until the spring of 1976, and did not furnish the Bureau of Radiological Health with a copy of the results until September of that year. By then, of course, the proposals to study birth defects at Fort Rucker had been withdrawn. The survey was carried out between April 19 and April 23 by the Laser Division of the Army Environmental Hygiene Agency, which is located at the Aberdeen Proving Ground, in Maryland; it was coordinated with the commander of the Aeromedical Research Laboratory at Fort Rucker; and the report of it was approved and signed by four agency officials. The report began by saying that radiation field intensities encountered at the Cairns Army Airfield at Fort Rucker "in general, were many orders of magnitude less than the established permissable exposure levels." It went on to say that the primary site for testing was a grassy knoll known as "Chinook Hill," located at the northwest end of the airfield, and that it was selected because it was two or three feet higher than the surrounding terrain, and thus "provided the least obstructed path to most of the radiating sources at Cairns Army Airfield." The report then listed the radiating sources as an AN/FPN-40 Ground Controlled Approach Radar; an ASR-5 Surveillance Radar; and an AN/FPS-77 Weather Radar. A map of the airfield accompanied the report and showed the exact location of the three radars.

According to the report, the purpose of the survey was to measure the intensity of microwave radiation that might be encountered at ground level by personnel in the vicinity of the airfield. "In case of a pilot overflying the area of the airfield, the levels would not be expected to be greater except for emanations from the AN/FPS-77 radar," the report declared. "Tests at ground level were not made directly in the main beam of this system, whereas an aircraft could fly through the main beam encountering greater field strengths, possibly approaching that received from the ASR-5 radar."

Having raised this possibility, the authors of the Army report did not indicate what levels of radiation might be encountered by an aircraft flying through the main beam of the ASR-5, or, for that matter, through the main beam of the AN/FPN-40 Ground Controlled Approach Radar. According to their report, these measurements would have to await the completion of subsequent tests that "will be performed on airborne platforms such as helicopters while flying typical airfield departures and approach patterns." The report went on to state that "areas to be monitored would include the aircraft cockpit between pilots, with equipment being set up aft of the cockpit and the surveillance antenna aimed at the space between the pilots," and that "antennas could be aimed out through open doors to monitor the fields the aircraft was intercepting."

As might be expected, the radiation measurements provided by the Army, as well as its plans for future tests at Fort Rucker, were accepted in good faith by the people at the Bureau of Radiological Health. They had no way of knowing that the 1976 survey of microwave radiation levels at Cairns Army Airfield bore little relationship to the radiation levels encountered by helicopter pilots at Fort Rucker between 1967 and 1972. It was rather like equating a census report made on Eniwetok after the inhabitants had been evacuated with a population count made in the years before the atoll was designated as a nuclear testing site. If the bureau had been less trusting, it might have asked for the microwave radiation survey of Fort Rucker that had been conducted by the Army Environmental Hygiene Agency in May 1971. The bureau could then have performed an interesting study in comparative literature, starting with the opening paragraph of the 1971 survey, which read as follows:

> On May 18–19, 1971, a survey was made of the microwave facilities located at Fort Rucker, Alabama. The microwave-generating sources available for survey were one ASR-5 surveillance radar, ten AN/FPN-40 radar sets, and eleven microwave cooking ovens. Measurements were made only on radars at airfields within the immediate vicinity of

Fort Rucker. Upon arrival at Fort Rucker it was learned that nine auxiliary airfields located in the upper part of the state had AN/TPN-18 radar sets for surveillance and final approach opertions.

Unlike the 1976 survey, the 1971 survey described the radiation levels generated by the AN/FPN-40 Ground Controlled Approach Radar in considerable detail. According to the report, this radar set generates beams of pulsed high-frequency energy from two separate antennas—an azimuth antenna, which sweeps from side to side, and an elevation antenna, which moves up and down. The report went on to say that the azimuth antenna radiates a maximum power density of nearly thirteen milliwatts per square centimeter, which decreases to less than ten milliwatts at distances beyond 170 feet, and that the elevation antenna radiates a maximum power density of nearly fourteen milliwatts per square centimeter, which decreases to less than ten milliwatts at distances greater than 230 feet. As for the nine AN/TPN-18 radar sets located at auxiliary airfields, the report said that they performed the same function as the AN/FPN-40; that their azimuth antennas radiated power density levels greater than ten milliwatts out to a distance of 80 feet; and that their elevation antennas radiated power levels greater than ten milliwatts out to a distance of 35 feet. The report described the hazards for personnel who operate the AN/TPN-18 as follows:

> The feed horn radiates toward the reflector a power density of approximately 2000 milliwatts per square centimeter at a distance of three inches from the feed horn. The elevation antenna normally drifts down to its lowest elevation, and the power is automatically switched to the azimuth antenna when operating in the track mode and the antenna drive is disabled. However, if due to a malfunction, or if manually held, the elevation antenna is not allowed to drift down, power is still fed to it. Under these conditions, it is quite easy for personnel to inadvertently stand in this hazardous area and the radiation is at eye level. The power density is so high that even while the antenna is scanning, the area is hazardous.

Thus, in the autumn of 1976, did the Army lead the Bureau of Radiological Health down the garden path, indicating that helicopter pilots at Fort Rucker had only been exposed to radiation emanating from one Ground Controlled Approach Radar, when, in fact, they had been exposed to the radiation of at least nineteen such devices. But to more fully comprehend what the exposure of these men really entailed, and to further understand the extent to which the Army pulled the wool over the bureau's eyes, it is helpful to know something about the helicopter-pilot training program during the Vietnam war.

To begin with, some 16,000 helicopter pilots were trained by the Army between 1967 and 1972. Most of these men received their preliminary training at Fort Wolters, in Mineral Springs, Texas. They were then sent for advanced training either to Fort Rucker or to Fort Stewart, near Savannah, Georgia. At the peak of the program in 1969, some 200 helicopter pilots were graduated every other week from Rucker, and another 100 or so from Fort Stewart. According to men who were stationed at these bases, about half of the pilots were second lieutenants; half were warrant officers; and more than fifty percent of them were married.

There were two phases of training for student pilots at Fort Rucker. First, there was a two-month period during which they learned to hover and to fly by instrument in TH-13 Bell helicopters, similar in appearance to the traffic helicopters one sees during rush hour in large cities. Then there was a four-month period during which they spent a great deal of time making radar approach landings in tiny, two-seater TH-55 helicopters, which are manufactured by Hughes Aircraft, and which resemble mosquitos. In both of these training phases, student pilots and their instructors flew at relatively low altitudes—usually between 500 and 1500 feet—in helicopters whose cockpits consisted of clear plastic bubbles extending down to the floor pedals, which enabled the occupants to see straight ahead, out to either side, the sky above their heads, and the ground beneath their feet.

As for their exposure to radar, what better way to ascertain this than to talk with some of the pilots who trained at Fort Rucker between 1967 and 1972. *"Radar!"* said one of them recently. "Hell, there was radar all over the place. Why, there was a radar set in practically every cow pasture in Alabama, Georgia, and northern Florida, in those days, and we must have set down in most of them. We used to spend hour after hour landing and taking off from those places. Usually, there'd be some tech sergeant down there, teaching a bunch of recruits how to operate the set. Some days, we practiced radar approach landings a dozen times or more. Then, when we graduated to the big Huey's, we started the whole process all over again."

As for the field strengths of the radar beams through which they flew, another former pilot had this to say: "I don't know much about field strengths, but I can tell you we didn't fly *through* those beams, we flew straight *down* them."

There was apparently no mention of the hazards of microwave radiation. "Everybody was sure we were on our way to get killed in Vietnam," one pilot declared. "It wouldn't have been nice to worry us about radar."

If one thing seems evident from all of this, it is that Dr. Peacock was eminently correct when he wrote in his 1974 study proposal that the helicopter pilots at Fort Rucker had been heavily exposed to radar "while flying at relatively low altitudes." Indeed, it seems evident that by flying straight down powerful microwave beams while sitting in wrap-around plastic canopies that were transparent to microwaves, these 16,000-odd men must have been thoroughly irradiated day in and day out, week after week, during their training period at Fort Rucker. It also seems evident that student radar operators and technicians must have worked in an environment saturated with microwave radiation. In fact, practically everybody living or working in the vicinity of Fort Rucker must have encountered an extraordinary amount of microwave radiation. Yet during all the years it spent thinking up excuses for not making the medical records of Fort Rucker personnel and their offspring available to independent scientific researchers, the Army not only hid the fact that these exposure levels existed, but also attempted to underreport them. Concurrently, it encouraged the notion that the abnormally high incidence of birth defects at the Lyster Hospital was a question of overreporting.

The clearest fact to emerge from the whole sorry Fort Rucker affair is, of course, that the Army set about to cover up the microwave exposure experienced by thousands upon thousands of pilots, instructors, ground personnel, and dependents who were stationed there. The Fort Rucker cover-up does, however, provide an interesting object lesson. It shows the lengths to which the military establishment will go to ignore the genetic effects of exposure to microwave radiation. Above all, it provides a warning in bold relief to the Congress and to the American people. A national policy which gives the Department of Defense the power to control or thwart scientific research on the biological effects of microwaves is a policy that allows the fox to guard the chicken coop and makes test animals of us all.

12

Irretrievably
Messed Up

As might be expected, the policy of the government toward the possible health hazards posed by low-level microwave radiation—a policy that, by and large, has ranged from evasion and obfuscation of the problem to outright suppression of medical data relating to it —has had many complicated ramifications. The fact that this cover-up has been invoked in the name of national security has made it a relatively easy one to justify and to carry out. It has also provided a convenient umbrella for the vast electronics and defense industries, since the government felt obliged to set the same standard for both civilian and military personnel.

As a result, there have been disastrous consequences for some of the employees of the military-industrial complex. One example is provided by the health experience of a number of workers who were involved in the Air Force's electromagnetic-pulse, or EMP, project. EMP is a multimillion-dollar testing system that was devised in the sixties by the Air Force Weapons Laboratory and operated under contract with the Air Force Space and Missile Systems Organization primarily by the Boeing Company, of Seattle. Its purpose was to simulate the pulses of radiant energy accompanying nuclear explosions and to determine the effects of the electric fields of those pulses on the warheads and guidance-and-control systems of the nation's thousand-odd Minuteman intercontinental ballistic missiles in underground silos. In spite of the fact that little was known about the biological effects of chronic exposure to pulsed electric fields, Boeing and the Air Force conducted extensive EMP tests on missile sites between the autumn of 1968 and June 1972, using ground-based pulse generators as well as huge airborne pulsers (called big zappers by the men who worked with them), which were carried aloft by Army H-47 Chinook helicopters. As early as 1971, Boeing was aware of two cases of leukemia and one case of skin cancer—all three occurring in men in their thirties or forties—among a group of seventeen technicians who had been conducting EMP tests at missile sites near the towns of Brady and Cascade, in Montana.

In April 1972, however, Boeing filed a petition with the Department of Labor's Occupational Safety and Health Administration (OSHA) requesting promulgation of a standard for exposure to EMPs which would be identical to one the Air Force had proposed several months earlier. The standard allowed an exposure level fifty to a hundred times as high as the level employed by the company. The petition informed the administration that "such action, if approved, will permit Boeing and other private employers to continue to support programs vital to the national security without having to individually establish the propriety of their activities with regard to fulfillment of their duty under Section 5 (a) (1) of Public Law 91–596." Public Law 91–596 is the Occupational Safety and Health Act of 1970, and Section 5 (a) (1) requires each employer to furnish his employees with "employment and a place of employment which are free from recognized hazards that are causing or are likely to cause death or serious physical harm to his employees." After more than three years had passed, the Occupational Safety and Health Administration turned down the petition. In this decision OSHA was advised in the matter by representatives of the Department of Health, Education, and Welfare's National Institute for Occupational Safety and Health (NIOSH) and by the members of the American National Standards Institute (ANSI) subcommittee that had been set up to determine safe levels of human exposure to electromagnetic radiation. The grounds were that "the need for a standard regulating employee exposure to EMPs has not been shown" and that "the scientific information necessary for the development of a standard currently does not exist."

Some of the advice that enabled OSHA to come to this conclusion was ambivalent to say the least. For example, after meeting with representatives of Boeing in September 1972, Gerald J. Karches and Dr. Wordie H. Parr, of NIOSH, wrote a report saying that "there is no basis for linking the cancer cases to EMP nor is there any justification for assuming EMP was not a factor." The two NIOSH officials went on to tell the Boeing people that there was not enough information available to set a meaningful standard, and that "since there were very few individuals involved in this work and no evidence was apparent that EMP produces harmful effects, that developing criteria for standards would have a low priority." At the same time, they recommended that Boeing "limit exposures to the lowest practicable levels, either by distances or engineering controls."

As for the three armed services, all assured the ANSI subcommittee verbally and in writing that there was not enough data on the biological effects of EMP to justify the setting of a standard. Perhaps the most revealing attitude was expressed by Captain Tyler, director of the Navy's Electromagnetic Radiation Projects Office, in a memorandum to the committee on August 4, 1972. "Recommend that attempts be made to delay setting of standards until more experimental data is available," the captain wrote. "If standards must be set now, then try for as high a level as possible. If adverse effects are determined in the future, it is far easier to further lower the standards than to relax them."

Incredibly, only one scientist out of the dozen or so who were queried expressed concern about the lack of preventive medicine implicit in such advice, and, unlike Captain Tyler, he was not a medical doctor. He was Leo Birenbaum, secretary of the ANSI subcommittee, and a member of the Department of Electrical Engineering and Electrophysics of the Polytechnic Institute of New York. "We are all speculating," Birenbaum wrote to Sava I. Sherr, chief of the Standards Office of the Institute of Electrical and Electronics Engineers, Inc., on July 20, 1972. "I feel it is very important to realize that these are all intelligent speculations. There is inadequate biological data on experimental animals from which to draw well-based conclusions. Research is needed here. Let us hope that as we exchange clever letters, as we are now, that not too many people's lives are being irretrievably messed up by using too high an EMP tolerance limit."

Meanwhile, two more cases of cancer had occurred among people who had been exposed to EMPs at missile sites in Montana. An Air Force safety officer in the EMP program, who had been stationed at Malmstrom Air Force Base, in Great Falls, had developed leukemia and died of it, and a twenty-nine-year-old guard employed by Boeing at one of the sites had developed bladder cancer. Moreover, a family of four who lived on a ranch close to a missile site where EMP tests were conducted had developed a variety of complaints that provide an eerie echo of the symptoms first reported by the Russians in their early examinations of workers exposed to the emanations of radar and other electromagnetic devices. The family's complaints include loss of hearing, loss of memory, loss of hair, loss of appetite and weight, premature aging, low blood pressure, blood disorders, blurred vision, thyroid problems, dizziness, fatigue, and headaches. These people have made claims against the Air Force for damages. In addition, two of the cancer cases are scheduled for hearings in Workmen's Compensation Court.

As it happens, a call for research on electromagnetic pulse had been sounded as far back as July 1970 at the Technical Coordination Conference on EMP Biological Effects, which was sponsored by the Lovelace Foundation for Medical Education and Research, in Albuquerque, New Mexico. In addition to a number of officials from the Air Force, this meeting was attended by representatives of Boeing, including its director of occupational medicine, Dr. Franz Bartl. Also attending were people from the Bell Telephone Laboratories, in Whippany, New Jersey, where a great deal of EMP research was being performed for the government; the Stanford Research Institute of Menlo Park, California, makers of EMP test equipment; and the EG & G Company (which stands for Edgerton, Germischausen, and Greer) of Albuquerque, manufacturers of electromagnetic pulse generators.

The Lovelace Foundation conference was chaired by Dr. Frederic G. Hirsch—the same Dr. Hirsch whose diagnosis of cataracts in the eyes of a microwave technician working for the Sandia Corporation had caused such a furor back in the early 1950s—and it was Hirsch who summarized the conclusions reached at the conference concerning the need for EMP studies. "In order for such studies to be done, support in the way of funding will be required and cooperation established between investigators and agencies operating pulsers," he wrote. "Research into the chronic effects need not be elaborate or expensive in order to be meaningful and useful; until this is done, nothing more than conjecture will be available for those who must answer questions, establish guidelines, and make decisions which may have far reaching legal and physiological ramifications."

In the seven years that have passed since Dr. Hirsch's remarkably prophetic summary, very little has been learned about the biological effects of electromagnetic pulse. This is because very few studies of EMP have been undertaken, and also because those studies that have been undertaken have been financed and controlled by the Department of Defense, which—Catch-22 again—has been only too glad to let the whole matter remain conjectural. During this period, the DOD has been working frantically on some highly classified programs designed to perfect the use of EMP as a weapon against nuclear ballistic missiles. The ramifications of this super-secret project will be discussed later in this book. For the time being, however, in order to understand the intellectual climate which enabled the military to thwart research on the biological effects of weapons systems, we will take a closer look at the Lovelace Foundation's meeting on EMP back in the summer of 1970.

Surprisingly, the published proceedings of the Lovelace meeting do not contain a single word about the use of EMP to simulate the intense pulses of radiant energy that accompany nuclear explosions. Instead, Dr. Hirsch opened the meeting by describing "the apparent similarity between an electromagnetic pulse and the electrical field charges that accompany a lightning stroke." Dr. Hirsch told his audience that "when a thunderstorm is building up, field strengths of perhaps twenty thousand volts per meter exist under the storm cloud," and that "when a lightning stroke occurs, a pulse of as much as three million volts per meter is generated." He went on to say that lightning strokes can generate substantial electric field strengths for distances up to several kilometers. "Since we have all, at one time or another, been proximate to lightning strokes, we have been in fields whose intensities were several hundred thousand volts per meter without being aware of it," he declared. Reminding his listeners that "there are several reports in the literature which document the psychological disturbances experienced by people who were quite close to a lightning bolt but not actually hit by it," Dr. Hirsch proceeded to tell them that, after being exposed to EMP, albino rats that had been trained to run through a maze exhibited a temporary "disruption of the maze-running ability characterized by a prolongation of running time, a hesitancy of decision making points, and an ultimate refusal to run after several pulses."

After reporting that EMP apparently had no behavioral effects upon a pair of monkeys, Dr. Hirsch called upon a colleague, Dr. Alfred Bruner, to describe the results of a third test. "In another experiment, we simultaneously exposed four Dalmatian dogs to several EMPs on a single day," Dr. Bruner said. He then made a statement that sounded eerily similar to the one made fifteen years before by Dr. Barron, of Lockheed, who, before recanting them, had called "paradoxical and difficult to interpret" some significant changes observed in the white-blood-cell counts of workers exposed to microwave radiation. "We had a biostatistical expert take a look at the blood data and he thought there were a couple of them that showed a significant difference from pre-to-post exposure," Dr. Bruner declared. "However, since there was no consistency in these, we were inclined to regard all the data as showing no significant change."

As for the attitude of the Air Force toward the possible health hazard of electromagnetic pulses, Dr. Bruner described this as one of tolerant amusement. Then a Lieutenant Colonel Portasik, who was chief of electromagnetics at Kirtland Air Force Base, in Albuquerque, expressed his own tolerant amusement when asked about exposures at the EMP test facility. "A lot of us walk in that region all the time," said Portasik. "It's funny how we will have visitors come out and the facility will be pulsing away. The people don't really know what's going on and they're nice and calm. But when we start talking about the field levels to which they are being subjected and say 'Well, here we are in about one thousand volts per meter,' then all of a sudden the 'tingling' starts."

Shortly after the colonel delivered his lighthearted theory about the role played by imagination in EMP effects, a Captain Evans, listed in the conference program as director of occupational medicine at Kirtland Air Force Base, described a study he had made of fifteen men who had worked at the EMP facility for periods ranging up to two years. According to Captain Evans, physiological tests of these people showed nothing out of the ordinary. "The only changes we found were in talking to these individuals subjectively," Evans continued. "About four of them reported easy fatiguability since they had been at the facility." Evans then described some other changes that had occurred among two men who had worked close to the electromagnetic pulser for approximately eight hours. "These two individuals reported on the same day extreme fatiguability, extreme irritability, real arthralgia, aching of the joints when they moved, and mild frontal headaches," Evans said. "They snapped at everyone and were extremely tired that evening. They both went home, got eight hours of sleep, and felt perfectly well the next day as far as we know."

The genetic effects of EMP were first raised during a discussion period, and were dealt with as follows:

> QUESTION: I have heard a rumor that people working in an EMP environment have been having babies all of the same sex. Is there anything to this?
>
> LT. COL. PORTASIK: I think that this phenomenon has just about had it, because after twelve in a row where the people had all girls, the thirteenth one was a boy.
>
> DR. HIRSCH: Well, at the same time, over at one of our local elementary schools, every teacher that had a baby had a child of the same sex. They finally broke that string at seventeen. I can't quite equate dipoles and third grade teachers very well.

Later in the conference a Dr. Williams, who was listed as being affiliated with EG & G Company, and with the University of New Mexico, discussed the genetic problem in more scientific fashion. "I would ask if there have been any chromosomal changes in animals before and after exposure," said Dr. Williams, who subsequently made some suggestions for future research. "I still think that things that occur over a long period of time don't accumulate in a vacuum," he declared. "They reside someplace, occurring in some cell structure. This is my suggestion: measure the electric field intensity inside the nerve tissue, look for small changes to provide answers for guys who work for EG & G who will have all girl babies, and look for intracellular changes. Electrical energy appears to break down building blocks and if there are no changes there, I don't think changes will occur."

At this point, Dr. Bruner admitted that the animal experiments conducted by him and Dr. Hirsch were not "the best kind of experiments" and were poorly funded. He went on to say that he would like to test some animals living a long time under the pulser. "We would include several different species so we could look for changes in offspring and perform chromosomal and biochemical studies on them," Dr. Bruner declared. "We could have some monkeys and also we could do some more behavioral work. We do think that the thing that has to be done next is chronic, long-term exposure."

As things turned out, only one or two of the kind of studies suggested by Dr. Williams and Dr. Bruner ever got done. The reason was simple. As with the proposed studies of birth defects and radar, the military did not want to know if there was anything biologically harmful about EMP. Indeed, for reasons it presumed to be of national security, the military felt it could not afford to learn that EMP might be hazardous to human beings. As a result, just as Leo Birenbaum had feared might happen, people's lives got irretrievably messed up. The reason for that was also simple. Human beings, not rats and monkeys, were in effect used as test animals in inadvertent experiments involving chronic, long-term exposure to electromagnetic pulses.

Another example of how the military-industrial complex has used national security to thwart inquiry into the biological effects of electromagnetic radiation occurred at a Philco-Ford Corporation plant in Philadelphia, where during the late 1960s two men in their thirties, who had been among a group of twenty-three technicians testing microwave-generating equipment for a highly classified Army operation called Project Tempest, developed brain tumors. In December 1970, officials of the Pennsylvania Department of Environmental Resources, who had learned of the brain tumors by chance, visited the plant and tried to investigate the situation, but were told by a Philco-Ford supervisor that no information about Project Tempest could be given out unless security clearances were obtained through proper channels.

Describing this encounter in a report a few days later, Dr. Shiro

Tanaka, the chief of the department's Plant Health Services Section, quoted the supervisor as saying that Tempest testing was a special type of project measuring "something coming out of existing equipment at the energy intensity of microvolt range." Dr. Tanaka then wrote, "I felt something like touching an unidentified object through ten layers of thick blanket." In a subsequent report, he pointed out that the male death rate from brain tumors in Pennsylvania was three and a half for every hundred thousand men in the population, and that two cases in a group of twenty-three men was "almost twenty-five hundred times as many as expected."

In March 1971, a story in *Medical World News* said that the equipment the twenty-three technicians had been working with "appears to be an electronic detection system ordered by the National Security Agency, which monitors worldwide communications." The article quoted Edward J. Baier, who was then director of the department's Division of Occupational Health, as saying that the entire matter had been placed under heavy security. It also quoted officials of Philco-Ford as insisting that radiation was no problem in the plant; that the two cases of brain tumor were no more than a "statistical curiosity"; and that fears among electronics workers were caused by rumors.

Any chance for an inquiry into the biological effects of Project Tempest was taken care of at a meeting held in Baier's office in Harrisburg on July 31, 1971. In addition to Baier and Dr. Tanaka, the meeting was attended by three officials from the National Institute for Occupational Safety and Health, including Herbert Jones, chief of NIOSH's Physical Agents Branch, and Vernon E. Rose, Assistant Director for Health and Surveillance. Also present were three officials from the FDA's Bureau of Radiological Health, including Henry J. L. Rechen, of the Division of Electronic Products, and Dr. Andrew C. Wheeler, a special assistant to John Villforth, the director of the bureau, who had sent Baier a telegram requesting a statement about the alleged brain tumors in the Philco-Ford workers. The most influential attendee, however, was undoubtedly Lieutenant Colonel Herbert E. Bell, of the United States Air Force, who was a staff assistant to the Assistant Secretary of Defense for Health Environment.

In his report of the meeting, Baier said that "the National Institute for Occupational Safety and Health (NIOSH) was very much interested in cases such as these since they are charged with this type of investigation under the federal Occupational Safety and Health Act." As for what NIOSH would actually undertake to do, Baier, who later would become deputy director of the institute, had this to say:

> In essence NIOSH will aid us in a review of all personnel who were employed at the plant—a cursory evaluation of the health status of present and former employees. They will also aid us in any environmental measurements which will need to be made although at the present time there is no instrument sensitive enough to detect some of the radiations present. NIOSH will also conduct further investigations in plants in other states where similar projects are carried out.

The statement requested by Villforth about the brain tumors, was described by Baier as "a format for answering questions posed by the press," and read as follows:

> 1. To date no cause and effect relationship between the work environment and the cases of brain tumor has been demonstrated.
>
> 2. Pennsylvania's occupation health program in conjunction with the National Institute for Occupational Safety and Health will continue programs into the potential occupational hazards of the work environment.
>
> 3. Representatives of the Department of Defense and the Federal Bureau of Radiological Health concur and will continue to assist with their expertise to contribute to the pursuit of these studies.

Since then, no information has been made public by NIOSH, by the Bureau of Radiological Health, by the Commonwealth of Pennsylvania, or by anybody else concerning the health experience of the men who worked for Philco-Ford on Project Tempest. Indeed, the whole matter has simply and conveniently been swept under the rug. It is known, however, that during the sixties and early seventies Philco-Ford manufactured components of the Integrated Wide-Band Communications System (IWCS), which consisted of immensely powerful, 250,000-watt microwave transmitters, powerful amplifier tubes, thirty-yard-wide receiver antennas, and a variety of multiplexing gear for sorting out signals on various channels. It is also known that the National Security Agency has deployed this system in many countries around the world—Ethiopia, Iran, Turkey, Cyprus, and Thailand are just a few—in order to detect, record, and send back to the United States telecommunications and radar signals transmitted by Communist nations. In addition, it is known that Tempest testing is simply an unclassified term referring to routine and periodic tests that are conducted both in the factory and in the field on such communications systems, in order to determine whether the equipment may itself be radiating signals containing compromising information of value to an enemy. Indeed, such organizations as the National Security Agency, the Defense Communications Agency, the Central Intelligence Agency, the Army, the Air Force, and the Naval Electronics Systems Command undertake Tempest testing on a large scale.

Why, then, did Lieutenant Colonel Bell not inform the Harrisburg meeting that if NIOSH did not possess instruments sensitive enough to detect the radiation emanating from such communications systems, the Department of Defense surely did? Was it because the colonel was there to keep everyone else in the dark? And did these people, in turn, not want to be kept in the dark? Definitive answers to these questions are not known. Nor is it known whether Tempest testing can be conducted without irradiating the brains of the unsuspecting people who perform it; or how many men and women have been involved in Tempest testing over the years; or, for that matter, how many other people have been exposed to radiation from IWCS and similar systems while installing or operating them, and what their health experience has been. (Such information will undoubtedly be considered highly classified by the various organizations that use this equipment.) It is known, however, that during an eleven-month period in 1967 and 1968 three men in their forties and fifties who were members of a Philco-Ford group of about twenty technicians engaged in setting up IWCS microwave-generating equipment on the border between Thailand and Laos and Cambodia dropped dead of coronary attacks.

13

An Aggressive
Study

Still another example of how the military-industrial complex has managed to ignore the hazards of electromagnetic radiation occurred at the Naval Air Station at Quonset Point, Rhode Island, where three civilian employees among a group of eight technicians who were engaged in the overhaul and repair of Tactical Airborne Navigation equipment (known as TACAN), which is similar to radar in operation, either have developed cancer or have died of it since 1970. One of these men died of lung cancer in 1970; another died of cancer of the pancreas, lungs, and liver in 1973; and the third man, who left the Naval Air Station in 1973 to work on TACAN for the Federal Aviation Administration, has been found to have cancer of the pancreas, lungs, and liver.

The fact that the man who died of cancer of the pancreas was only thirty-one years old, and that the man who is ill with the disease is only thirty-five, is highly unusual. Ninety-nine percent of all reported cases of pancreatic cancer occur in people over forty, and most of them occur in people in their fifties and sixties. But the fact is that these two men worked side by side at a test bench at the Quonset Naval Air Station for several years. It is believed that no two cases of pancreatic cancer occurring among men working in such close proximity have ever been reported before. Equally disturbing is the way this situation is being handled by the Navy and by NIOSH. After learning of the two cases of pancreatic cancer, in the autumn of 1975, the NIOSH people in New England made a survey of the problem in their area and recommended in a report dated January 13, 1976 that an "aggressive study" be undertaken of the hazards of occupational exposure to microwave energy, and that future microwave surveys at military installations be coordinated with officials of the Department of Defense. On July 13, 1976, Dr. John F. Finklea, the director of NIOSH, finally got around to writing a letter to George Marienthal, Deputy Assistant Secretary of Defense for Environment and Safety. The letter expressed concern over the TACAN situation, and informed the Secretary that "we would be pleased to meet with appropriate personnel to review the information currently available to us and to explore the possible courses of action to follow up in this matter."

Just what such coordination and review might entail became clear at a two-hour meeting on August 12 at the headquarters of the Navy's Bureau of Medicine and Surgery, in Washington. According to a bureau report dated August 17, this meeting was held to discuss "alleged carcinogenesis resulting from exposure to microwave radiation." It was attended by six officers from the Bureau of Medicine and Surgery, three of whom were physicians; by Captain Tyler, of the Naval Medical Research and Development Command; by three officials from NIOSH, including Dr. Parr, who by this time had become chief of the institute's Physical Hazards Effects Branch; by a statistician from the National Academy of Science's National Research Council; and by Lieutenant Commander Peter S. Labyak, of the President's Office of Telecommunications Policy. Labyak seemed to be representing both the President and the Naval Electronics Systems Command. The report went on to say that searches of the medical literature undertaken by Captain Tyler and Dr. Parr revealed "no prior evidence that microwave exposure is related to development of cancer." The next paragraph of the report read as follows:

> At the heart of the TACAN instrument is a klystron tube which not only produces microwave radiation but also ionizing radiation in the form of X-rays. Considerable shielding and other safety devices make X-irradiation of users negligible and microwave radiation is below maximum permissible levels. Should the shields be removed and the instrument energized during a repair procedure, exposure to X-rays would be possible. The F.A.A. prohibits such practice. The work procedures at [the Naval Air Station at] Quonset Point are not known at this point.

The possibility that X-rays might be involved in the cancers that had developed in the TACAN workers shed an ominous new light upon the situation. A number of studies have suggested that the adverse biological effects of either microwaves or X-rays can be enhanced in combination with the other. However, the Navy's real worry became abundantly clear in the very next paragraph of the report, which described some comments made by Captain Tyler, who has proved to be nothing if not consistent in his efforts to downgrade the biological hazards posed by microwave radiation. "Captain Tyler emphasized the problem of compensation awards in the area of radiation exposure, particularly microwave exposure, on the basis of poor scientific evidence or no scientific evidence whatsoever in support of the claimant," the report continued. "The conferees took due note of this."

According to the report, the conferees ended the meeting by agreeing that "NIOSH would alert the Navy of any F.A.A. decision" in the case of the former civilian employee of the Navy who is suffering from pancreatic cancer; that NIOSH would obtain a detailed description from this man of his work practices while he was employed by the Navy and by the FAA; that the Navy would "endeavor to identify TACAN repairmen at all Navy Air Rework Facilities," and to obtain information on deaths among civilian workers at all Navy Air Rework Facilities; that representatives of the Navy's Environmental Health Center and NIOSH would tour all such facilities "to measure microwave/X-ray levels and observe work practices of those exposed to microwave/X-ray, including TACAN repairmen"; and that this would be done in a way "to avoid alarming TACAN workers unduly."

Whether it was ethical for the National Institute for Occupational Safety and Health—an organization charged by Congress with the responsibility of conducting research to protect the safety and health of American workers—to agree to alert the Navy about a case that was obviously heading for litigation, and that involved a terminally ill man with a wife and child, is something that needs looking into by Congress. But there are other aspects of the TACAN situation that require clarification. It is not clear, for example, why the work practices at the Quonset Naval Air Station were unknown to the Navy, let alone why NIOSH should be called on to obtain a detailed description of them. It is known, however, that the patient in question gave an account of these work practices to representatives of NIOSH back in November 1975. This account included the following facts: he and his fellow-employees at the Naval Air Station often worked on unshielded TACAN power tubes; the Navy shipped these tubes in packages containing no warning that they could emit X-rays; but TACAN power tubes packaged and shipped by the FAA did contain such warnings. It is also known that as early as August 1960, at the fourth and final Tri-Service conference on the biological effects of microwave radiation, Colonel George M. Knauf, the conference chairman, had told an audience that included high-ranking officials from the Army, the Navy, and the Air Force and representatives from some of the largest electronics companies in the nation that there was a "vitally important problem of X-ray exposure" in the operation of high-power tubes used in radar, and that "a recent unfortunate accident has again emphasized the need to keep this area of personnel risk in the foreground in our programs of personnel instruction." This accident involved several technicians at a General Electric Company test facility near Lockport, New York, who were irradiated with X-rays generated by the klystron tube of a radar that GE was developing under contract to the Air Force.

Starting in the 1960s, manuals issued to Navy personnel contained warnings that high-voltage tubes used in radar could also produce X-rays. Indeed, NAVMAT P-5100—a manual issued by the Naval Materiel Command in June 1967—listed a number of precautions that should be taken in order to protect radar repairmen from this hazard. One of them reads as follows: "When bench testing X-ray–producing electronic devices be sure that adequate X-ray shielding is provided to protect all personnel in the testing area." As if this were not a sufficient call for caution, NAVELEX 0101,106—a manual issued by the Naval Electronics Systems Command in August 1971

—said that "the high voltage tubes used in the generation, amplification, and shaping processes associated with microwave and radar transmissions are inadvertent producers of X-radiation," and that when radio-frequency power is applied in these tubes the X-ray emissions "can reach 800 milliroentgens per hour, an extremely dangerous level."

However, whether the Navy has any real intention of protecting its personnel and its civilian employees from the hazards of microwaves, X-rays, and other electromagnetic radiation seems somewhat doubtful. Consider a Bureau of Medicine and Surgery instruction sent on March 28, 1974, to all Navy ships and stations having medical personnel. The instruction announced that henceforth the bureau's Radiation Effects Advisory Board would act as a consultant to the Surgeon General in the evaluation of "alleged or true radiation exposure to personnel injury involving claims against the government." It further ordered that "no local authority shall make any statement or release any information regarding the evaluation of radiation or radioactive contamination-related injuries, actual or alleged, without consulting the Radiation Effects Advisory Board." The reason given for the order provides a classic example of the motives of the military-industrial complex in suppressing information about the health hazards of electromagnetic radiation:

> In the past, responsible medical department personnel have made statements or signed certificates which indicated a causal relationship between radiation exposures and physical defects that could not be substantiated by existing facts or documents. This has led to unwarranted public and employee concern and apprehension. Merely including radiation exposure information in association with personnel injury or illness may be misconstrued by a patient or the public as indicating causal relationship. The resulting public apprehension could seriously jeopardize the military and civilian nuclear power programs. Therefore, in all illnesses or injuries allegedly associated with radiation, the significance of any radiation exposure shall be carefully evaluated and documented.

As for the combined Navy-NIOSH study of the radiation exposures and health experience of TACAN repairmen at the Navy Air Rework Facilities, it was allowed to drag on interminably after first being proposed in August 1976. During September and October of that year, the Navy collected information on the number of deaths and disability retirements that had occurred since 1972 among the twenty-seven thousand or so civilian workers employed at Air Rework Facilities at Alameda and San Diego, in California; at Jacksonville and Pensacola, in Florida; and at Norfolk, Virginia; Quonset Point, Rhode Island; and Cherry Point, North Carolina.*

The Navy also collected information on the number of deaths and disabilities that had occurred among TACAN repairmen at all these Air Rework Facilities. However, at a meeting that took place at the Bureau of Medicine and Surgery on November 17, 1976, the Navy informed NIOSH that it did not have information on the causes of death and disability among the men. Moreover—shades of the Army's cover-up of the Fort Rucker affair—the Navy informed NIOSH that since the death-and-disability listing contained the names, social security numbers, and occupational and demographic backgrounds of individuals, it could not be released under the Privacy Act. For their part, the NIOSH people tried to claim that they had not been able to acquire specific details on TACAN work practices at the Quonset Naval Air Station from Robert W. Engell, of Ellington, Connecticut—the former TACAN repairman suffering from pancreatic cancer—even though their own reports clearly indicated that Engell had already given this information a year earlier.

As for the Federal Aviation Administration, it was not only Engell's last employer, but a major user of TACAN equipment, and was naturally very interested in the outcome of any study of the health experience of TACAN workers. Indeed, the FAA was represented at the November 17 meeting by Dr. O. C. Hood, chief of its Aeromedical Division, who, according to the minutes of the meeting, declared that the radiation emanating from TACAN is so "soft" that repairmen would have to be leaning directly against the energy source in order to receive enough ionizing radiation to stimulate carcinogenesis in the pancreas. Unfortunately, the minutes do not

---

*In this regard, it is interesting to note that in August 1976 the Comptroller General of the United States issued a report to Congress on hazardous working conditions in federal agencies, which revealed that when officials of the Occupational Safety and Health Administration inspected the Naval Air Rework Facility at Alameda, they found 198 violations of mechanical hazards standards; 245 violations of fire and electrical standards; 33 violations of housekeeping standards; and 12 violations of health standards.

record what reaction those in attendance gave to this remark by Dr. Hood. One cannot help but wonder if it was not intended more as some kind of legal statement to put the Navy on the spot than as a medical opinion. After all, Dr. Hood must surely have read (or at least been told about) a long article on microwaves by Jonathan Winer, which appeared in the *Boston Globe,* less than four months before, on June 25, 1976. In that article, Engell described the radiation exposures to which he and his friend, who died of pancreatic cancer at the age of thirty-one, were subjected while repairing radars at the Quonset Naval Air Station. "The radiation-emitting equipment was eight inches away from our bellies for eight years," Engell told Winer. "I have no idea how much radiation I was exposed to. But I was never warned beforehand. When I asked about it, health officials assured me everything was okay."

During the winter of 1977, there was further indication that a cover-up of the TACAN situation was in progress. On February 27, the *Hartford Courant* carried a story by Nancy Pappas, who charged that the Navy and NIOSH had failed to carry out their agreement to study the radiation exposure and health experience of the TACAN repairmen. Pappas's story ran beneath the headline "NAVY WON'T INVESTIGATE X-RAY LINK TO CANCER," and part of it read as follows:

> Last week a NIOSH spokesman said no measurements had been made yet because of delays in arranging with the Navy for visits to air stations.
> The spokesman also said the health research is being handled by the Navy's Environmental Health Center in Cincinnati.
> But the center's commander, Capt. Thomas Markham, said last week he had no plans to do health research on TACAN repairmen. He said the center only planned, as does NIOSH, to measure the tubes' radiation levels.
> Further, he said, the Navy still has "only hearsay evidence" that the Connecticut man has cancer. He charged that the man refused, on his lawyer's advice, to provide his Navy medical records.
> The cancer victim's lawyer said last week the Navy never sought his client's records. "If they want them, they're welcome to them," he said.

No one knows what possessed Captain Markham to suggest that Engell might not be suffering from cancer. However, on September 22, 1976, Dr. Henry M. Williams, of the Herblein Radiation and

Oncology Center, in Hartford, Connecticut, had informed William A. Felsing, Jr., acting director of NIOSH's Office of Extramural Coordination and Special Projects, that an operation showed Engell "was found to have a primary pancreatic carcinoma with liver metastases." Also, on January 18, 1977, Felsing had sent the pathology report on Engell to Captain D. F. Hoeffler, director of the Navy's Occupational and Preventive Medicine Division, claiming that the letter from Dr. Williams "was not received in my office until sometime around the first of December."

On March 17, 1977, Engell's lawyers filed a $4,500,000-suit for personal injuries and damages in federal district court in Hartford against six electronics equipment suppliers, claiming that "as a result of his exposure to defendant's electronic tubes, equipment, and products, plaintiff Robert Engell was diagnosed as having cancer." Named as defendants in the suit were the International Telephone & Telegraph Corporation, the Raytheon Corporation, Varian Associates, Teledyne Ryan Aeronautical and Teledyne Inc., Rockwell International Corporation, and the General Dynamics Corporation. Since it would be difficult to imagine six firms any closer to the heart of the military-industrial complex than these, it is not surprising that the Department of Defense viewed the situation with alarm. Indeed, the department felt the need to take cover. On March 23, Deputy Assistant Secretary Marienthal fired off a memorandum to the Assistant Secretary of the Navy for Installations and Logistics, requesting that the Navy take the lead in looking into the alleged increased risk of occupational cancer among TACAN repairmen, and declaring with consummate understatement that "the results of the first two meetings indicate that there is a need for further investigation."

Meanwhile, on March 22, a third meeting between the Navy and NIOSH took place at the Bureau of Medicine and Surgery, in Washington. It was also attended by representatives of the Army, the Air Force, the Federal Aviation Administration, and the President's Office of Telecommunications Policy. At the outset of this meeting, Felsing noted that his organization had been "unable thus far to proceed with an epidemiologic investigation of the TACAN repairmen," but that an "aggressive approach" was being planned in order to give a NIOSH epidemiologic study team access to the required personnel and medical records. (Felsing might have used different language had he remembered that more than fourteen months had passed since the NIOSH people in New England had urged their superiors to undertake an "aggressive study" of the TACAN workers and the hazards of occupational exposure to microwaves.) At the March 22 meeting, Felsing went on to say that "it is not known at this time whether the available records on NARF employees and TACAN repairmen will be of sufficient scientific quality to guarantee success in a prospective or retrospective evaluation," and that "conditions of the Privacy Act will have to be met."

The report of the meeting noted for the record that there were approximately fifteen to twenty TACAN repairmen at each of the six Naval Air Rework Facilities, and went on to make the reassuring observation that "this is an extremely small number when compared to the approximately 6,300 other electronics repairmen and the 27,-500 total civilian NARF employees." What the report conveniently omitted, however, was the troubling fact that while there may be only fifteen or twenty TACAN repairmen at each of these facilities at any one time, hundreds upon hundreds of the Navy's apprentice-electronic mechanics (not to mention how many Army and Air Force personnel) have been exposed to TACAN through their being required to take six hundred or so hours of service and training on TACAN operations.

The rest of the meeting appears to have been the usual mixture of ignorance, self-interest, and incompetence. Two officials from the Naval Air Command noted that NAVAIR publications on work-safety practices dealt primarily with microwave radiation, and, apparently unaware of NAVMAT P-5100 or NAVELEX 0101,106, claimed not to know whether other Navy publications dealt with the risks of X-radiation emanating from unshielded power tubes. Two officials from the President's Office of Telecommunications Policy—Janet Healer and Lieutenant Commander Labyak—stressed their office's concern with the adverse publicity being given to the TACAN issue, and called for prompt and aggressive measures to resolve the issue as soon as practicable.

As for the FAA, Dr. Hood expressed the opinion that the proposed epidemiological studies of TACAN workers would probably not produce any useful correlation between microwave exposure and cancer on the grounds that "such an association should have become apparent long ago in view of the fact that radar/TACAN-like navigational instruments have been in use since the 1940's." Since Dr. Hood had already dismissed the possibility that TACAN workers

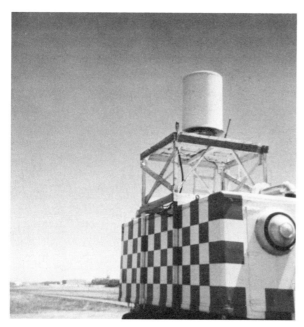

Mobile TACAN trailer by side of Runway 6 at Bradley Field.

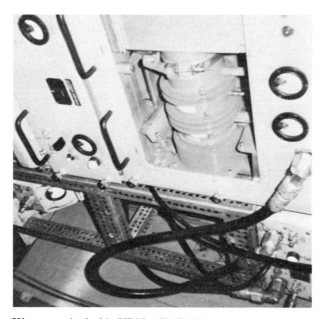

Klystron tube inside URN-3 TACAN transmitter.

might be endangered by X-radiation, he evidently felt they had nothing to worry about. While it is difficult to believe that the chief of the Aeromedical Division of the FAA could be so ill informed, Dr. Hood apparently did not know that the difference in power output between the radars of the 1940s and those of recent years is tantamount to the difference, say, between the beams of a flashlight and a lighthouse.

The FAA is the employer of several thousand air traffic controllers and eight thousand electronics technicians, all of whom are occupationally exposed to microwave radiation. It was therefore only natural for the FAA to claim that microwave and X-ray emissions from its equipment were negligible, and to hope that the belated medical investigations now being undertaken will not show any correlation between microwaves and cancer, or, for that matter, between microwaves and any other diseases.

Hope is one thing, however, and knowledge is another. The question is what the FAA people knew about microwave exposure and microwave disease, and when they knew it. As it happens, there can be little doubt that high officials of the administration have known for years that microwave radiation posed a serious health hazard to their employees and to other people working in the aviation environment. For example, during the early 1970s, the FAA allowed a retrospective study of cataracts in airline pilots to be conducted for Project Pandora—a study that showed a significant increase in the development of cataracts in these men. It also sent representatives to a meeting of the Armed Forces Epidemiology Board that was expressly convened to discuss the biological hazards of microwave radiation. Indeed, at this meeting, held on April 1, 1971, in Room 341 of the Walter Reed Army Institute of Research, a ten-minute presentation of the study of cataracts in airline pilots had been given by none other than Dr. Pollack.

FAA technicians were being heavily exposed to microwave radiation and the FAA could scarcely have failed to deduce this from even the most rudimentary examination of the 1971 report by the Electromagnetic Radiation Management Advisory Council. In addition, they had been informed of it in detail during the winter of 1976 by Robert Engell. When the Quonset Naval Air Station was closed down in 1973, Engell had gone to work for the FAA as an electronics

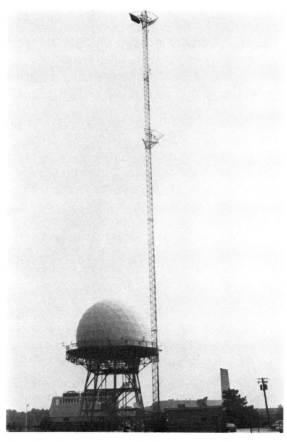

A radome housing an FAA air route surveillance radar at the Airway Facility Sector, in Suitland, Maryland. Tower on right controls and directs aircraft in flight.
PHOTO BY ROBIN TOOKER

technician. From June 1973 to July 1974, he had worked for the Airway Facility Sector (AFS) at the regional airport in Rapid City, South Dakota—there are hundreds of such sectors all across the United States—and from then until the spring of 1976, he had worked at the AFS at Bradley International Airport, in Windsor Locks, Connecticut. When Engell learned in October 1975 that he had developed cancer of the pancreas at the incredibly early age of thirty-three, he strongly suspected that radiation was the cause, since Donald Cadieux, a close personal friend with whom he had worked side by side for eight years at the Quonset Naval Air Station, had died of the same cancer in 1973, at the age of thirty-one. However, when Engell undertook to warn his FAA supervisors at Bradley about the danger of radiation emanating from TACAN and other microwave equipment, he was ignored. Then, on February 18, 1976, he wrote a letter to the Hartford office of the Department of Labor's Occupational Safety and Health Administration, which began as follows:

> I am presently employed by the Federal Aviation Administration (Department of Transportation) at Bradley International Airport in Windsor Locks as an Electronics Technician. Due to the seriousness of my condition and the likelihood of others also being affected at the numerous Airway Facility Sectors (AFS) throughout the country, I believe your office should be made aware of the strong possibility that there are unsafe levels of microwave radiation at various facilities and that immediate measures be taken.
>
> Below, I will attempt to outline what I believe to be a serious threat to my life and others employed by the F.A.A., also exposed to microwave radiation.

Engell then went on to describe his work at Bradley on remote transmitters (RTR). These are line-of-sight, 300-megahertz radiating antennas, and they are located at all major airports in order to provide communication between airport control towers and airplanes. "It is necessary to maintain microwave radiation antennas at this facility on four towers, approximate heights of which are 75 feet," Engell wrote. "These towers must be climbed and [at the top] there are four to five radiating antennas. It is necessary to spend a large part of one working day in checking these out for operations during which time there are 60 watts to 80 watts of power being transmitted at the person working on same. This is an extremely high level of power which can cause serious biological and somatic effects on the human body."

After noting that a fellow employee who had worked with him on remote transmitter towers at Bradley during 1975 had been given medical retirement for stomach cancer, Engell turned to the subject of Tactical Airborne Navigation Equipment (TACAN), writing as follows:

> This piece of Electronics Navigational equipment, of which there are two facilities in this sector at Windsor Locks and in Glastonbury, is used to guide every properly equipped plane to the airport to which they are going. It radiates a signal from the ground to the aircraft in

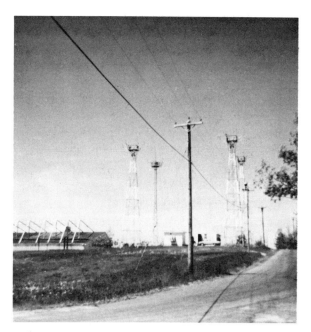

RTR towers at Bradley Field, Windsor Locks, Connecticut.

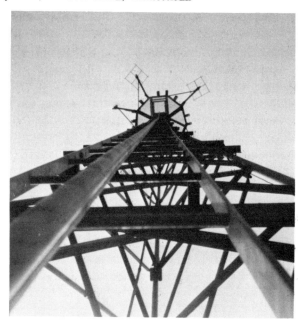

RTR tower from ground level showing two VHF transmitting antennas.

the air. This equipment is located at the airport in a USAF trailer at Windsor Locks and is on a scheduled periodic check for proper operation, or if it had become inoperable. It is not possible to determine what has gone wrong when it is not turned on, so it is necessary for the person trouble-shooting to be exposed to microwave emissions. It contains radioactive high-power klystron tubes that are replaced by the technician and transmits in the frequency range of 1000 megahertz, which is at a wave length of 30 centimeters. This energy will penetrate the human body at extremely deep levels according to the latest government manual on the subject.

Later in his letter, Engell referred to the lack of response he had received when he tried to warn his FAA employers that the microwave-generating equipment they were using might be dangerous. "In the past I have questioned the safety of this equipment and have effectively been ignored," he wrote. "There is a total lack of interest, insofar as I can conclude, in the individual health of the technicians. The medical office at F.A.A. Regional Headquarters has informed me that no medical records are maintained on technicians, but are on controllers."

Engell then recommended that some simple protective measures be taken. Indeed, these measures were not only simple but so obviously sound in terms of basic preventive medicine that one can scarcely imagine why the FAA and its Aeromedical Division had not implemented them long ago. "When there are potential radiation hazards, should not employees be equipped with shielding which would not allow these rays to penetrate their bodies?" Engell wrote. "There should also be signs posted for minimum approachable distance. (10 feet in the USSR.) It is interesting to note that there are no Danger or Warning signs at any of the F.A.A. facilities, warning the technicians of radiation danger which seems to be quite a simple procedure. These precautions would seem to me to be quite simple when compared to the life of ONE person."

14

Well Aware
of the Hazards

In keeping with established governmental tradition, the Federal Aviation Administration tried to counter the charges Engell had made in his letter to OSHA with a memorandum of denial. Among other things, the memo stated that "although we have a military TACAN at the Windsor Locks location, it is not one of Mr. Engell's responsibilities. We do, however, understand that one of his major responsibilities while working for the U.S. Navy at Quonset Point was the servicing of TACAN equipment." In addition to trying to shift blame to the Navy, this statement contained a semantical dodge so transparently specious as to border upon mendacity. Whether Engell was technically "responsible" for the TACAN at Bradley International Airport is, of course, neither here nor there. What is pertinent is something that the FAA knows full well—that Engell's name appears on FAA work sheets as having logged hundreds of man-hours of time repairing and servicing TACAN equipment at Bradley. Having neglected to mention this, the FAA memo went on to say that none of its employees could be harmed by radiation from either TACAN or RTR equipment if they adhered to FAA regulations, and to claim that the administration "is well aware of the hazards of both X-ray and microwave radiation and takes immediate and effective means to protect its employees." The memo concluded by claiming that "in view of the facts contained above, we find that the allegations in the referenced complaint are without merit, and that no corrective actions are required."

Incredible as it may seem, there is every indication that the FAA has taken itself seriously and not instituted any corrective actions to reduce the radiation hazards described by Engell. Possibly this is because the administration fears that such action would be an admission of prior negligence. Whatever the reason, there is plenty of indication that many FAA employees do not share the administration's complacency about the situation. In October 1976, the president of the Federal Aviation Science and Technological Association (FASTA) wrote a letter to William T. Coleman, Jr., the Secretary of Transportation, referring to Engell's complaint and asking for an immediate investigation of the health hazards posed by microwave-radiating equipment "even if it requires a complete shutdown of the system." In November, Secretary Coleman wrote a reply in which he claimed that Engell's complaint "was carefully evaluated by the F.A.A.," and that "based on that evaluation and a study which had been recently completed for the F.A.A. by the National Bureau of Standards, it was concluded that an F.A.A. employee would be exposed to harmful job-related radiations only if he violated safety regulations or bypassed safety interlocks."

Coleman's attempt to place the blame and liability for radiation exposure and injury upon FAA employees may well have been motivated by legal considerations. The fact that he did so as a member of the cabinet of the President of the United States, however, goes to show how high the cover-up of microwave hazards has reached. In order to understand just how utterly inaccurate Coleman's reply was, it might be helpful to quote from a letter that was written to the president of FASTA by one of Engell's fellow technicians at Bradley International Airport, after the FASTA newsletter had published Coleman's reply. It read in part as follows:

> I am writing in regards to an article appearing in the FASTA Newsletter, Volume 2, Number 10, dated December 1976. The article

in question is concerning "Radiation Exposure."

I can assure you that this subject is very disturbing to all of us technicians here at AFS-817, Windsor Locks, Connecticut, since it has a direct effect on us. We find the response you received from Mr. Coleman lacking in investigative areas and in contradiction to established F.A.A. Procedures for maintaining Air Navigational Aids/Radar.

To begin with, I refer you to para. 2 of the response and I quote "it was concluded that an F.A.A. employee would be exposed to harmful job-related radiations only if he violated safety regulations or bypassed safety interlocks." One of the mandatory maintenance checks of a TACAN, specifically a model RTN-2, is to check the Average and Peak Power monitors. To do so, as directed in F.A.A. Orders and Manufacture Instruction Book, a technician must reduce the 24,000 volt power supply to a value which will cause a monitor alarm. To reduce this high voltage a technician must bypass a cabinet interlock, open a cabinet door, reach in among RF wave guides and above a Klystron Power Tube and physically rotate a High Voltage control. Also, on this same TACAN equipment, many of the tuning procedures require access to this same cabinet area. It is impossible for a technician to adjust or tune this equipment any other way.

Another example is related to a Radar beacon, type ASR-3D, manufactured by the Bendix Corporation. This type of equipment employs a radioactive tube, type 5749. This tube is a thyatron and is used to trigger a magnetron. Adjustment of this tube's circuit requires an interlock to be bypassed and a technician to be brought in very close proximity to the tube while adjustments are made by the technician.

So much for what William T. Coleman, Secretary of Transportation of the United States, knew about the radiation hazards of FAA employees for whom he was responsible. Further indication that FAA employees were worried about the situation appeared in an article that ran in the Oberlin, Ohio, *News-Tribune* on December 30, 1976, under the headline "MICROWAVES? NO HAZARD FOUND HERE." According to the article, the FAA's control center on East Lorain Street was not polluting Oberlin with microwaves because "The towers at the F.A.A. are not radar but communications relay towers, which are to radiation what spigots are to waterfalls." The article went on to say that "the towers are 75 feet high and are rated at 100 milliwatts," and that "Paul Ciprian, F.A.A. airways facilities sector chief here, said radiation on the ground around the towers is just about zero." Although the spigots-to-waterfalls analogy was no doubt reassuring to the citizens of Oberlin, it does not seem likely that it would provide much comfort to FAA technicians such as Robert Engell. While maintaining the radiating antennas on these towers, these men have obviously been subjected to microwave radiation far in excess of the government standard. Indeed, the article in the *News-Tribune* made oblique reference to this possibility:

> Inside the F.A.A. organization, the grapevine is ahead of both the government and the *New Yorker* magazine piece. "I'm afraid to look at it," an F.A.A. man said of the article. "I've already told my wife to sue the government when I die, no matter what—a broad band lawsuit."

As for radiation hazards in FAA operations elsewhere in Ohio, the article read as follows:

> Brecksville, for instance, has a long-distance F.A.A. radar scanner. While the Oberlin relay towers radiate 1 watt, the Brecksville radar radiates four and a half million watts of microwave energy.
> It is so strong that even the F.A.A. was concerned about people driving past it on Rt. 82; if a heart-attack patient wearing a pacemaker were "zapped" by the Brecksville radar, the device might be stopped or desynchronized on the spot. An F.A.A. official said that concern was determined to be unfounded. Ground-level radiation tests have been done near the radar, he added, but he did not know the results.
> Frank Trebets, sector field office chief at the Brecksville F.A.A. radar, said that he and his staff wear dosimeter devices to measure X-ray and gamma radiation produced in generating the radar signal but that the strength of the microwave signal itself had not been measured at ground level.

Since the article did not say how far the FAA's powerful Brecksville radar is from Route 82, there is little way of knowing whether the concern that radiation emanating from it could interfere with cardiac pacemakers is well founded. However, Air Force Regulation 161-42, which was issued on November 7, 1975, does list half a dozen radars whose cardiac pacemaker risk-distance ranges from 1000 to 1700 feet. According to the regulation, risk-distance is defined as the distance in feet from the radar "beyond which none of the cardiac pacemakers tested are likely to miss more than ten beats per minute."

As for the ophthalmological hazard posed by microwave radiation, the FAA never saw fit to publish or release the results of the retrospective study showing an increase in the incidence of cataracts in airline pilots, which was conducted for Project Pandora. However, other evidence has emerged to show that people working in an aviation environment run a significantly increased risk of developing cataracts. Dr. Zaret believes that many of these cataracts may be caused by microwave radiation, and he has written as follows about one such case for the *British Journal of Ophthalmology:*

> Case 9 was a commercial airman having been certified in 1965 at age 30, and flying since then as a flight engineer, copilot and pilot. In 1971, at age 37, the patient first noticed that his vision became fuzzy due to glare when light was shining directly into his eyes. However, it was not until late in 1972 that he was found to have an early stage of cataracts but, as he was still able to see 20/20 with each eye under the contrived dark room conditions of the visual acuity test, he was approved for flying. He was not disqualified from flying until September 1973 when he failed the examination because vision then was reduced to 20/40 in his right eye; nevertheless, his left eye was still capable of 20/20 despite the stage of cataractous change clearly evident in Fig. 1.

In addition to suppressing and ignoring information on the incidence of microwave-induced cataracts in the eyes of airline pilots, the FAA has been keeping very quiet about their occurrence in the eyes of air traffic controllers, even though this situation obviously poses an incredible danger to human life. The Department of Labor has awarded compensation to two former air traffic controllers for work-related cataracts. However, Dr. Zaret has diagnosed six cases of microwave cataracts in air traffic controllers. In a letter entitled "Cataracts in Aviation Environments," which appeared in *The Lancet*—a leading English medical journal—on February 26, 1977, Zaret described one such case as follows:

> The earliest symptom of radiant-energy cataracts is often transient visual problems, such as looking through a misty fog or wet glass, symptoms which can antedate objective signs by years. For example, one of the air-traffic controllers, during a five-year period between 1967

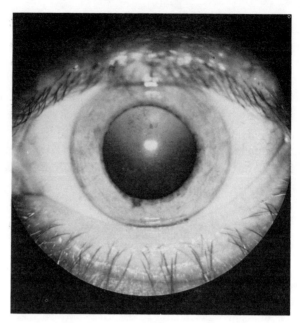

The eye of an airline pilot with 20/20 visual acuity whose posterior capsule has become studded with small opacities. PHOTO BY MILTON ZARET

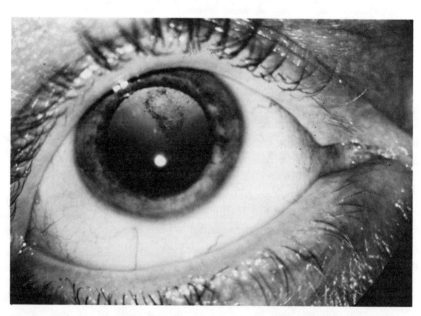

The eye of a microwave technician with 20/20 visual acuity, whose posterior capsule shows a later stage than in the photograph above of cataractous change. At this stage, there is a collection of fluid bubbles on the posterior capsule. PHOTO BY MILTON ZARET

and 1972, experienced many episodes of wrongly identifying aircraft or losing others on his radar plot. Several times mid-air collisions were prevented only by the intervention of colleagues. Throughout this period numerous ophthalmological examinations and an extensive physical and neurological evaluation failed to reveal the diagnosis. The earliest sign of lens opacification appeared in his left eye in 1970; but it was not until 1972, when visual acuity was still correctable to 20/20 in the right eye and reduced only to 20/30 in the left, that he was diagnosed as having an incipient cataract and finally disqualified as an air-traffic controller.

Ophthalmological tests for certifying the visual status of operational aviation personnel are inadequate. Careful slit-lamp inspection of the lens capsule and evaluation of entopic glare function should be added. In addition to improving air safety, this will permit early diagnosis and removal from further exposure.

Dr. Zaret has described this same case in even more detail in the article for the *British Journal of Ophthalmology:*

> While actively controlling 12 to 15 aircraft in 1971, without realizing he could not see them on the radar scope, the patient lost the position and flight pattern of two military jet aircraft in his sector. Fortunately an associate controller noticed that the patient was having difficulty, recognized the danger, and intervened immediately. Still other examples occurred in 1972 when on each of two successive shifts the patient wrongly identified two aircraft on the radar scope and in each instance unwittingly directed them into potential mid-air crash patterns.

Not surprisingly, the FAA and its medical experts have been as silent about Down's syndrome among the offspring of airline pilots as they have about cancer and cataracts among people working in an aviation environment. The fact is, however, that mongolism among the children of airline pilots may be unusually high, and—as with Fort Rucker—a study to determine the exact extent of these birth defects was proposed, opposed, and then dropped in the early 1970s.

Here is the way it happened. Back in 1970, Dr. Irvin Emanuel, of Seattle, then assistant professor of preventive medicine at the University of Washington, had as a patient an airline pilot who had fathered a child afflicted with Down's syndrome. Since this pilot knew several other airline pilots with children suffering from Down's syndrome, he checked around and discovered what appeared to be an extraordinary number of airline pilots in the area who had fathered children with this devastating birth defect. Based on this admittedly informal and limited investigation, Dr. Emanuel undertook to make a crude estimate of the incidence of cases of Down's syndrome among the children of the fifteen hundred or so airline pilots who lived in the Seattle area—a terminal point for flights to the Far East as well as for over-the-Pole flights to Europe. He came up with an estimate that the number of cases might be twice the expected number.

With approval and some financial support from the local chapter of the Airline Pilots Association, Emanuel and two colleagues then designed a study and put together a questionnaire to determine more precisely the extent of the problem. Their plan was to send three copies of the questionnaire to all married air crew members living in the Seattle area, asking them to fill out one copy and to distribute the other two copies to a pair of married couples living in their neighborhoods, who were not air crew members but who would be willing to answer the questionnaire. (In order to make sure that these couples would be selected at random, the questionnaire was to be distributed to them solely on the basis of the location of their houses or apartments with respect to those of the air crew members.) The first paragraph of a letter drawn up to accompany the questionnaire read as follows:

> Through an informal and limited investigation, we have recently become aware that a number of local air line pilots have had children with Down's syndrome (Mongolism). Other birth defects have also been identified among pilots' children. We feel that there may be an abnormally high number of birth defects among children of air line pilots. In order to accurately determine whether this is true, the Department of Preventive Medicine, University of Washington, is doing a study with the cooperation of the various local councils of the Air Line Pilots Association.

Since the subject of the proposed study was so sensitive, the last part of the letter assured the recipients that all information would be treated "with the same confidentiality as a physician's record or a hospital record." Before the questionnaire went out, however, the local councils of the Air Line Pilots Association withdrew their support; and the study was never conducted. "Something went wrong," Dr. Emanuel said not long ago. (He is now Director of the University of Washington's Child Development and Mental Retardation Center.) "We never did find out exactly what happened, or why. We asked but we never got a good answer. I was later given to understand that officials of the national Air Lines Pilots Association were against the study, and that they told the local councils not to go ahead with it. I also heard that the medical consultant for the national association was very much opposed to the study."

15

The Tip of
the Iceberg

The pattern of the microwave cover-up is unmistakable. And so is the reason that the federal government, the military, the vast electronics industry, and all of the academic and research institutions financed by the military–electronics industry complex have been standing on their collective head to avoid conducting meaningful epidemiological studies of the health hazards posed by microwave radiation. People in the military–electronics industry complex don't want to know the extent of the problem. If they knew about it they might have to admit they knew about it, and then might even have to do something about it, which would cost a lot of money both in terms of litigation and preventive measures. This is not to say, of course, that people in the government and in the military–electronics industry complex don't know a lot already about the microwave hazard. For twenty years, in order to enlarge their arsenals and enhance their profits, they have engaged in a massive cover-up of a whole spectrum of microwave biological effects, hoodwinking the Congress and the American people. Here is the top of the tip of the iceberg—some important things they knew and when they knew them.

In 1954, Dr. John T. McLaughlin, a surgeon in Glendale, California, treated a Hughes Aircraft Company radar repairman who had unwittingly exposed himself to the beam of a radar transmitter. An article by Dr. McLaughlin, "Tissue Destruction and Death from Microwave Radiation (Radar)," appeared in *California Medicine* in May 1957, in spite of Howard Hughes's efforts to obtain a court injunction against its publication.

Dr. McLaughlin began by pointing out that microwave penetration in tissue "is to some extent a function of frequency, and one of the advantages of microwave diathermy is that deeper tissues can be heated more efficiently." He went on to say that cellular injury or death occurred when tissue temperature was maintained at 5°C above the normal blood temperature. "Tissue temperature even a few degrees above body temperature is dangerous," he wrote. "Irreversibility depends upon the duration of the hyperthermic episode. The higher the temperature, the shorter the time necessary to cause cell death. Tissues respond to heat denaturation with an aseptic inflammatory reaction and subsequently are prone to infection. Local temperatures of 64°C will cause tissue necrosis and gangrene at the site."

Dr. McLaughlin observed that "not all areas of the body are equally well equipped with mechanisms for regulating their temperature by means of a change in flow of blood," and that "the chambers of the eye and the contents of the hollow viscera, such as the gallbladder, urinary bladder and lumen of the gastrointestinal tract are relatively avascular and largely devoid of effective mechanisms for regulation of temperature." He then cited an experiment which showed that when rabbits were irradiated with electromagnetic waves, visceral temperatures were elevated even when oral and rectal temperatures remained normal. "The elevation was particularly pronounced in the relatively avascular hollow viscera," McLaughlin wrote. "In these experiments, when only the abdomen was irradiated, it appeared that death was preceded by a syndrome resembling that noted in burns and traumatic shock."

Having outlined the scientific background, Dr. McLaughlin then got down to the case at hand, describing it as "a report of a case in which the patient died from tissue destruction caused by absorption of microwave energy." The first part of the case report read as follows:

> A 42-year-old white man, while working, stood directly in the beam of a radar transmitter, within ten feet of the antenna. In a few seconds he had a sensation of heat in the abdomen. The heat became intolerable in less than a minute and he moved away from the antenna. Within 30 minutes he had acute abdominal pain and vomited. When medically examined, an hour after the exposure, he was in a state of mild shock. The blood pressure was 90/30 mm. of mercury and the radial pulse rate 72 with auricular fibrillation.
>
> Upon abdominal examination generalized acute tenderness was noted, with decided muscle spasm and rebound tenderness. There were no peristaltic sounds. Leukocytes numbered 10,300 per cu. mm. —82 percent neutrophils, 5 percent eosinophils, 10 percent lymphocytes and 3 percent monocytes.
>
> In an x-ray film of the abdomen, there was no evidence of free air under the diaphragm. A specimen of urine was unobtainable.
>
> The patient denied any history of symptoms suggestive of gastric disease. He had had rheumatic endocarditis in childhood and had had a mitral commissurotomy one year previously. Since the cardiac operation the patient had been taking digitalis. Whether he had been fibrillating before the present episode was not known.
>
> The patient was immediately admitted to hospital. Additional x-ray films did not show free air in the peritoneal cavity. The stomach was greatly distended and there was a small amount of gas in the colon, pooled in the cecum and ascending colon. The general appearance of the abdomen was considered consistent with acute peritonitis. X-ray films of the chest showed considerable cardiac enlargement with elevation of the left diaphragm.

After describing the analysis of the patient's blood, Dr. McLaughlin said that the diagnostic possibilities considered were abdominal blood clot or a perforated peptic ulcer, and that the decision was made to operate. During surgery, it was discovered that the entire abdominal wall and the lining of the abdominal cavity were dusky red and that "the portion of the small bowel that could be seen was beefy in color." According to Dr. McLaughlin, all visible surfaces were covered with petechiae—small crimson, purple, or livid spots that can accompany severe fever. "The appendix appeared gangrenous," he wrote. "It was removed."

Following the operation, the patient did reasonably well for a time. On the fifth day, however, diarrhea and abdominal distension occurred, suggesting bowel obstruction, and on the tenth day evisceration of the abdominal wound took place and the patient went into profound shock. Emergency surgery was performed immediately but it proved unsuccessful. "The portion of the bowel at the point of penetration lay in the left side of the abdomen at the level of the umbilicus," Dr. McLaughlin wrote. "A six inch segment of bowel was resected and the abdomen was closed. The patient continued in shock and died in 24 hours."

According to Dr. McLaughlin's article, the pathologist's report on surgical specimens taken from the patient indicated peritonitis in the small intestine, and the autopsy report revealed the spleen to be twice its normal size and to have undergone recent obstruction and hemorrhaging. Swelling was noted throughout the small bowel, and red lesions were found in every square centimeter of the intestinal lining. In addition, the adrenal glands were found to be remarkably small.

In the final section of his article, Dr. McLaughlin said that the diagnosis was intestinal inflammation of undetermined type, adrenal gland atrophy, and rheumatic heart disease:

> In this very perplexing case multiple sections were made of the small intestine particularly, in order to evaluate the sequence of events and the direction of spread of the inflammatory process. The most critical problem was whether or not the enteritis [intestinal inflammation] which involved the entire wall of the intestine, was simply a neighborhood reaction from the peritonitis. If that were the case, the perforation of the small intestine was unexplained. However, the very definite and diffuse mucosal inflammation of a small round cell type and the lack of dense continuity with the plastic peritoneal exudate strongly suggested that peritonitis was secondary to enteritis.

Because of these findings, Dr. McLaughlin was able to declare that his patient had died from tissue destruction caused by absorption of microwave energy:

> In the case here reported, the sudden onset, with sensation of unbearable heat, the cooked, hemorrhagic appearance of the small bowel and the pathological reports all point to the local absorption of heat in the umbilical and hypogastric regions with some generalized whole body radiation effect appearing in the myocardium, liver, and spleen. The

hemorrhagic infarcts of the spleen were similar to those seen by the author in two other patients who were exposed to sufficient microwave radiation to cause pathological changes in the tissues.

Dr. McLaughlin's observations should have been sufficient reason to launch an investigation of the extent to which people working with radar in both the armed services and the electronics industry might be suffering from the effects of heavy exposure to microwave radiation. But no—Catch-22 again—this could not be done. In his article Dr. McLaughlin gave the reason. "The frequency and power factors of the microwave radiation to which the patient was exposed were unavailable because of security regulations," he wrote. "It was enough to cause a painful sensation of heat in the abdomen, however, and when heat can be felt, the tolerable level has been exceeded."

Security regulations? Outright suppression is what it amounted to. In fact, these so-called security regulations were nothing less than a hoax pulled by a military-industrial complex that had developed acute myopia because of the Cold War.

The military knew perfectly well, for example, that during World War II seamen on the brutally cold Murmansk run used to warm themselves in the radar beams. And people in the electronics industry knew that during the 1950s the sensation of heat from microwave-generating equipment was commonly felt by workers in radar manufacturing plants from one end of the country to the other. For example, in the old RCA factory known as Building Number 3, in Camden, New Jersey, where some 1200 workers were engaged in the manufacture of E-4 and E-6 fire-control radars for aircraft, people walking in the aisle between the test section and the assembly section of the plant could often feel heat generated by radiation emanating from the sets that were being tested.

Further, an article entitled "Health Hazards from Microwave Radiation," which Dr. McLaughlin published in *Western Medicine* in April 1962, contains these clinical observations:

> In observing a large number of persons engaged in the manufacturing of microwave equipment who were exposed intermittently for various periods to microwave radiation, 115 were noted to exhibit various degrees of abnormal capillary fragility as manifested by the Rumpel-Leede test. The only cases examined were those who sought medical advice for the reasons outlined below. These represent only

a small percentage of the total number exposed, and no effort could be made to determine what percentage of the exposed population might have been affected.

Field strength, frequency, and power factors are unavailable for security reasons. Exposure ranged from 1 to 3 hours daily at distances from 1 ft. to 50 ft. from the antennae. Each of the examined persons had experienced the sense of warmth that is a result of microwave exposure. Headache and a warm feeling when exposed are such common findings that they are accepted as a normal occupational hazard in this type of work. Unfortunately, many, in ignorance, allowed considerable heat to be generated in their bodies in order to achieve a therapeutic diathermy effect.

The Rumpel-Leede test was accomplished by maintaining the blood pressure cuff on the arm at a point midway between systole and diastole for 3 minutes and then counting the petechiae in a 4 cm. circle in the anticubital fossa [forearm].

Dr. McLaughlin went on to say that the number of cases of abnormal capillary fragility defied the statistical occurrence of the primary causes of purpura—a disease caused by blood leaking out of its normal channels, and marked by livid spots on the skin or mucuous membranes. "There was no common exposure to the known causes of purpura such as organic arsenicals, gold salts, benzol, or sedormid," he wrote. "Thiurea and sulfonamids were eliminated. None of the patients were exposed to ionizing radiation; such a group constituted a different clinical picture. The only possible etiological factor common to all the cases was the exposure to microwaves." According to McLaughlin, three hundred controls were established in persons undergoing routine physical examination. One case of purpura was found in this group, and he had been exposed to microwave radiation in his previous employment. In addition to observing purpura in people who were occupationally exposed to microwaves, Dr. McLaughlin found three cases among one family who lived adjacent to an area where radar sets were tested. "None had any other microwave exposure, and they were completely unaware of the cause of the purpura," he wrote. "Examination of the test area showed them to be in the test pattern at a distance of at least 100 yards."

After describing four cases of microwave-induced capillary fragility, failure of adequate blood clot retraction, and abnormal bleeding,

Dr. McLaughlin ended his report on a note of sober reflection and recommendation:

> Microwaves are a potential health hazard and will continue as such until adequate studies point to the amount of such energy the human may safely absorb. In addition to amounts of energy, this safety standard must consider frequency which, in this range of the spectrum, is an important factor. Penetration and absorption of microwaves are both functions of frequency, hence power is not the only element of danger to be considered. The amount of energy to which one is exposed is important, but we must speak in terms of the amount of energy being absorbed and at what depth in the body absorption occurs. The answers to these and other important questions can only be arrived at by giving due consideration to frequency. A standard of how much energy one may safely absorb per square centimeter will be inadequate unless we can state the total amount of energy he may absorb and in what period of time.

Dr. McLaughlin went on to point out that "since some of the undesirable effects of microwave exposure are from the heat created, there will be different safety levels for different organs, since the capacity for cooling varies in different parts of the body; muscle and bone can obviously be heated with a greater margin of safety than the brain or the lens of the eye." He then made the following assessment of the public health problems posed by electromagnetic radiation:

> Today the average human is exposed to a multiplicity of frequencies of the electromagnetic spectrum which were undreamed of 2 decades ago. Infrared and ultraviolet modalities are common accessories in the average home, school and place of business. Ionizing radiation has emerged from its protective shell and Geiger counters are now toys for children. There is a proved synergism and antagonism between various forms of radiation; therefore, any safety program must consider the interaction of the various forms of energy and prepare to cope with this extraneous factor.
>
> Microwaves are part of our way of life, and exposure is not limited to military personnel, nor persons engaged in the fabrication of this equipment. It would behoove us to establish a definite clinical and pathological pattern of exposure and make this information and knowledge available to every physician, since they are the ones who

will examine and treat the majority of the affected patients. Simultaneously, a satisfactory method of treatment would be a valuable addition to the physician's armamentarium.

Dr. McLaughlin ended his article by observing that as of 1962 experimental work had merely demonstrated the danger of exposure to microwave radiation in the radar-frequency range, and that "until further information is available, this form of energy should be afforded the same respect as other energetic radiations such as x-rays, gamma rays, and neutrons."

In light of what is now known about the biological effects of microwave radiation, Dr. McLaughlin's observations in the so-called California case of 1954, together with the eminently sensible recommendations he made in 1962, fairly take one's breath away. What happened, then, as a result of these observations and recommendations? Nothing. Why? Because Dr. McLaughlin's fellow physicians and scientists—both military and civilian—decided at the time of the first Tri-Service Program that the California case could be dismissed either as unproved or as involving gross heating of the hollow viscera, and that Professor Schwan's whole-body heat dissipation theory and the ten-milliwatt standard would take care of everything.

In arriving at this decision, the medical and scientific community was encouraged mightily by the military and the electronics industry, who were only too glad to be rid of McLaughlin's troublesome conclusions. They hastened to get on with the four-year Tri-Service Program that would validate the ten-milliwatt standard, which, in turn, would allow the proliferation of microwave devices to proceed unimpeded. Nonetheless, McLaughlin's work had to be discounted. And so, at meeting after meeting, it was discounted as being scientifically invalid, irrelevant, and poorly rationalized. Indeed, such criticism was repeated so often and at so many meetings that by the middle of the 1960s, a whole new generation of microwave scientists —totally financed by the military–electronics industry complex and marching in intellectual lock step—simply passed on the belief that McLaughlin's work was invalid, like acolytes who automatically chant the litany of orthodoxy.

What happened to Dr. McLaughlin also happened, of course, to

Dr. Zaret. And in this manner were two early prophets of the biological hazards of microwaves neutralized by the military–electronics industry complex. They had dared to suggest that microwaves—the radiation that the military conceived of as indispensable to the national security, and that the electronics industry conceived of as travelling at the speed of light in a straight line to immense corporate profits—might be hazardous to human health.

It is important to examine the long-range consequences of such a policy of suppression. For example, what has been its effect upon the health of tens of thousands of the nation's workers? To be sure, McLaughlin's California case concerned a patient whose hollow viscera were massively exposed to a high level of microwave radiation. But even so, the often repeated claim of the military–electronics industry complex that the biological consequences of such exposure have no bearing upon possible health hazards for the general public is totally without foundation.

The consequences of heavy exposure to any agent that poses a health hazard should be taken by an enlightened society as a warning that there may well be a need for preventive measures at much lower levels. The annals of occupational and environmental medicine are filled with examples of the necessity for this approach. Asbestos, vinyl chloride, and saccharine come to mind immediately. All of these substances are known to produce cancer in test animals at high doses. Asbestos and vinyl chloride produce cancer in test animals at low doses as well, and tests are under way to determine whether this will prove to be true of saccharine. Unfortunately, in the case of asbestos, the test animals have literally been hundreds of thousands of asbestos workers around the world. Indeed, the National Institute for Occupational Safety and Health has estimated that of the one million current and former asbestos workers alive today in the United States, some three hundred and fifty thousand can be expected to die of asbestos-induced cancer. In the case of vinyl chloride, warnings about its being a powerful liver-cancer-producing agent in rats were ignored in the United States until the same cancers developed in the human beings who were engaged in its manufacture. As for saccharine, in spite of a recent Canadian study indicating that men who use artificial sweeteners have up to sixty percent greater chance of developing bladder cancer than men who do not use them, the Congress has voted to delay the FDA's proposed ban of this compound.

In all of these examples, of course, Santayana's dictum—those who cannot remember the past are condemned to repeat it—can obviously be applied, just as it can be applied to the microwave situation. For instance, if instead of dismissing the California case out of hand, the medical and scientific community had undertaken to thoroughly investigate it and similar incidents involving heavy exposure to microwave radiation, at the very least preventive measures and protective work practices might have been instituted, and young men like Robert Engell, who is only thirty-five years old, might have much longer lives ahead of them than they do now. And does it not seem possible that Dr. McLaughlin's observations in the California case might have some bearing on the curious incidence of appendicitis attacks—the appendix being part of the hollow viscera —which, in three months, afflicted four people living in the Moscow Embassy in sixth-floor apartments facing Tchaikovsky Street?

16

Some Intense Exposures

A fine example of what can happen when doctors fail to appreciate medical history was published in the *Journal of the American Medical Association* on July 22, 1968—eleven years after McLaughlin published his findings in the California case—by two medical doctors in the Air Force's Aerospace Medical Division, who examined a thirty-one-year-old man referred to them for evaluation of infertility. Part of their report read as follows:

> The patient was a repairman at a weather radar installation where he had been employed for four years. He frequently performed maintenance on the radar antenna while the equipment was in operation. He did not wear protective clothing. On occasion, while working near the microwave beam, the patient noted a sensation of warmth, although he received no visible burns. Two years before the present studies, in 1963, the patient was seen medically for the first time during a fertility investigation. At that time, the physical examination was normal, but the sperm count was 9,500,000. In 1964, testicular biopsy showed a marked decrease in spermatogenesis with atrophic tubules, appearing

open and empty, populated only by Sertoli's cells. Some tubular lumens showed necrotic debris. . . . In July 1965, the patient was referred to Wilford Hall USAF Hospital. He complained of irritability and mild insomnia occurring during the preceding year, but specifically denied any history of decreased libido, previous testicular inflammation, or familial history of gonadal dysfunction.

In further describing this case, the two Air Force physicians said that it was "the first case in which microwaves appear to have been a factor in the induction of male infertility, without demonstrable improvement eleven months after the last exposure." (One wonders if they knew that during World War II—fully twenty-five years before they published this statement—rumors that microwave radiation could cause infertility were so widespread in the Navy that radar operators were often called upon to dispense "treatments" to shipmates who felt obliged to make themselves sterile before going ashore on liberty.) The two Air Force doctors also wrote that "the ordinary precautions currently in use near microwave transmitters appear adequate to preclude excessive exposure such as this patient experienced." They had no way of knowing, of course, that whatever these "ordinary precautions" may have been, they were certainly not adequate, say, to protect Robert Engell and his fellow workers at the Quonset Naval Air Station, or the dozens of Air Force radar technicians who developed cataracts after serving on radar surveillance planes, or the unborn children of the helicopter pilots who trained at Fort Rucker. But the Air Force physicians reached almost dizzying heights of optimism in the final paragraph of their report. "Our patient was exposed repeatedly to microwave power densities more than 3,000 times the currently accepted safe level established by the U.S. Air Force . . . and, furthermore, wore no protective garments," they wrote. "Such exposure raises the question of biologic damage." Raises the question of biologic damage? In fact, if their patient had really been exposed to a microwave beam with a power of 30,000 milliwatts per square centimeter, his testicles would literally have been cooked. These two doctors apparently were unaware that radar men had been known to pop popcorn and fry eggs at such power levels.

Still another case involving occupational exposure to microwave radiation in the 1960s sheds some interesting light on the question of just how much power is needed to produce damage to sperm cells and genitalia. It was published in the March–April 1969 issue of the *American Industrial Hygiene Association Journal* by Vernon E. Rose and two colleagues from the Bureau of Occupational Safety and Health, who, together with a member of the Ohio Department of Health, made a clinical study of microwave-oven repairmen. In an introductory section to their report, Rose and his co-workers wrote as follows about their subject:

> A review of the literature indicates some concern with consumer exposure to energies from microwave ovens, mainly because of faulty door seals, but only one case involving an oven repairman has been recorded. That case involved an oven repairman who turned on the unit with the door open. He subsequently filed a claim for injury specifying burns in the region of the lower abdomen and possible sterility. The latter claim was denied. The exposure of this occupational group as compared to the consumer must be assumed to be greater, and consequently, a greater likelihood of overexposure is possible.

After noting that the development of microwave ovens "has increased to the point that models are being developed for use in the home," Rose and his colleagues got down to a case-history discussion. The first part of it read as follows:

> A 40-year old white man was first seen in November, 1967, with complaints referable to the skin, eyes, and genitalia. He has been the supervisor and chief repairman of automated vending machines and microwave ovens for over 5 years in a firm specializing in such devices. Periods of exposure to microwave ovens during repair work were frequent, varying from few or no hours per day to most of a working day.
>
> Skin problems began in August, 1965, with an acute, transient scrotal and groin dermatitis that lasted a few weeks. Since the summer of 1966, he has had about twelve episodes of a rash on his lower abdomen and right thigh. The affected area would itch and burn, and it appeared to be blotchy and red, with "bumps" and "cords" under the skin. Lesions faded without scarring after 4 to 6 weeks. The areas involved were the closest portions of his body to the working level of the microwave ovens. He claimed that sometimes he sensed heat on the skin involved when he repaired these ranges.
>
> For the past 1 to 2 years he has noted failing vision, and has had

to wear glasses for the first time. Although he does not recall eye irritation directly related to the repair of microwave ovens, he has experienced "burning" of the eyes in the past 2 years.

Since March, 1966, he has noted the development of indurated nodules in his penis, leading to deviated and painful erections, and finally, to impotence.

Other than an allergy to penicillin and a peptic ulcer of the stomach, under medical treatment with antacids since 1965, his health has been good. He abstains from alcoholic beverages and smokes a pipe only.

In the medical evaluation section of their report, Rose and his co-workers said that an eye examination revealed "no evidence of cataracts, retinal abnormalities, or increased intraocular pressure," in the oven repairman. "Biopsy of the active lesions on the right thigh on November 9, 1967, revealed an inflammatory reaction, related primarily to the blood vessels, at all levels of the skin down to subcutaneous fat," they continued. "The blood vessels were encroached upon and distorted due to edema and the mixed infiltrate of lymphocytes, eosinophiles, and polymorpho-nuclear leukocytes." In addition to this, a sperm count and bilateral testicular biopsy revealed that the man was sterile, and that a number of his Sertoli cells were abnormal.

After describing the patient's work practices, which included repairing microwave ovens with the safety interlock system disengaged, Rose and his colleagues said that "in following this procedure, the repairman's face and body are approximately 24 inches from the magnetron," and that "the repairman works this close to the oven so that he can observe its operation and note the occurrence and location of any malfunction or short circuiting." The investigators then measured the intensity of the microwave radiation to which the repairman was exposed under these conditions, and found that at a distance of twenty-four inches from the magnetron the power density was twenty milliwatts per square centimeter at face level, and eighteen milliwatts per square centimeter at the level of the abdomen.

To their credit, Rose and his colleagues recommended that microwave-oven repairmen be protected from such exposures by copper mesh screening that would "intercept and absorb the microwave energy," and reduce the power levels to less than five milliwatts per square centimeter. They did not, unfortunately, appear to be particularly alarmed that the oven repairman exhibited these abnormalities after exposures to a microwave radiation power density only twice as high as the power level then considered safe for consumers. Indeed, Rose and his co-workers did not appear convinced that the medical problems exhibited by their patient could even be caused by microwave radiation. "This man has Peyronie's disease, or plastic induration of the penis," they wrote. "This condition has been reported frequently since its description by Peyronie in 1743, and has not heretofore been ascribed to microwave energy exposure. Therefore, its relationship to such energy might be only fortuitous. The impotence associated with reduced spermatogenesis and altered Sertoli cells might also be coincidental. However, we cannot discount a true causal realtionship to microwaves."

As for the patient's skin problems, Rose and his colleagues noted that they "suggest a relationship with incident microwave energy," and that "similar experimentally-induced microwave damage has been seen in animals and in the viscera (intestinal organs) in the fatal human case reported by McLaughlin." But it is in the final paragraph of the section of the report entitled "Conclusions" that Rose and his colleagues managed to achieve a dizzying obtuseness:

> Seven co-workers of the subject were examined on November 13, 1967. Their exposure to microwave energy ranged from the insignificant (since they worked 10 to 20 feet from these ovens) to several hours a day of direct exposure while they repaired the radar ranges for varying periods up to 5 years. Four had visual complaints ranging from tiredness, watering, and burning to decreased acuity, but these were not always related to the work environment. No gross ocular abnormalities were seen, but slit-lamp examinations for cataracts were not available. There were no skin or genital complaints, nor were abnormalities of these areas seen.

It can only be inferred from this that Rose and his co-workers either did not know about (or had little regard for) the Russian studies concerning the ophthalmological hazard of microwaves, and Dr. Zaret's contention that only slit-lamp examination could reveal early evidence of microwave damage to the eyes. Just what possessed Rose and his colleagues to be so sanguine about the results of their investigation is not known. In the summer of 1971, however, Rose represented NIOSH at the meeting called by Edward J. Baier, of the Pennsylvania Division of Occupational Health, to look into the question of the brain tumors that had developed in men engaged in

Tempest testing at the Philco-Ford plant in Philadelphia, and concurred with the sanguine statement put out by the division about the matter. Also, in the winter of 1977, Rose, who is now director of NIOSH's Division of Criteria Development and Standards, and Dr. Finklea, director of NIOSH, spent several hours discussing the microwave problem with a high official in the Defense Intelligence Agency. The level of concern existing at the top echelons of NIOSH over the hazards posed to workers by microwave radiation had been summed up admirably in the following memorandum from Baier (now deputy director of NIOSH) to Finklea and Rose on October 26, 1976:

> Frank Worden, Western Electric, called today concerning problems in electronics plants. Apparently the experiences in Ohio, Pennsylvania etc. which we've been looking into are being tagged "Electronics Disease."
>
> I discussed this with Elliott Harris and asked him to send his bibliography on microwave exposures to Frank.
>
> Apparently Western Electric is looking at all forms of radio-frequency, microwaves, vibration etc. to see if there are human effects. I bring this to your attention in case you are asked about the "new" disease.

Clearly, it is important not only to determine who knew what and when about the biological effects of microwaves but *how* he went about interpreting it. An interesting case in this regard involves a fifty-six-year-old radar repairman who has been blind and deaf since 1970, and a number of people who were called upon to determine how his condition came about. Here is a substantial part of the report of the Department of Labor's examiner, who rejected the repairman's claim that his injuries were caused by radiation:

> Claimant Thomas E. Montgomery was born on June 19, 1921. In 1942, at age 21, he was hired by the U.S. Army Signal Corps at Barksdale, Louisiana to serve as a learner radio mechanic. From 1948 to 1955, he was employed by the Baltimore Signal Depot. He served as a radar repairman. While at that location, he was promoted to radar repair lead foreman and on August 15, 1954, he transferred to the Tobyhanna Signal Depot. He continued to be lead foreman of radar repairers at Tobyhanna Signal Depot.
>
> Claimant alleges that he suffered loss of hearing and blindness as a

result of exposure to radiation while employed at Baltimore Signal Depot and Tobyhanna Army Depot. The claimant said, in an undated letter received at this office on May 28, 1971, that the beginning of his present disabilities occurred in 1949 at which time he was accidentally exposed to intense microwave energy. As a result of his exposure, claimant became dizzy and noticed a loss of hearing in his right ear. He was examined at the Army dispensary but examination failed to account for dizziness and some loss of hearing. Claimant was advised to consult his private physician.

Claimant has been examined by a number of specialists in ophthalmology and otolaryngology. None of these examiners express rationalized medical opinion to connect claimant's blindness and loss of hearing to his employment. The most recent medical opinion report submitted by claimant is from Dr. Naomi Gerber. It does not add any significant medical information to indicate that claimant's disabilities are attributable to his condition of employment. Dr. Horner, Deputy Medical Director, states in his memorandum dated May 15, 1974 that "the conclusions presented by Dr. Gerber are essentially speculative and do not constitute rationalized medical opinion."

Dr. Gerber, it turns out, is a physician who is chief of the Department of Rehabilitation at the National Institutes of Health, in Bethesda, Maryland. In the autumn of 1973, she examined all of Montgomery's medical records, as well as a detailed personal account of his occupational exposure to microwave radiation. After reviewing the retrievable medical literature on the biological effects of microwaves, Dr. Gerber made a fundamental assumption: Montgomery's blindess and deafness could not be attributed to any existing disease process such as diabetes, renal disease, vasculitis, or serious atherosclerosis. She then suggested that it was entirely probable that the patient's blindness and deafness were related, and were the result of thermal injury caused by his exposure to microwave radiation.

Dr. Charles E. Horner, also a physician, was the Deputy Medical Director of the Department of Labor's Employment Standards Administration. Here are the last two paragraphs of Dr. Horner's memorandum of May 15, 1974:

I do not believe that the conclusions reached by Dr. Gerber, after review of pertinent medical literature, constitute rationalized medical opinion to connect claimant's blindness and loss of hearing to his employment. The conditions with which he is afflicted, although of unknown etiology, were well known clinically long prior to the use of microwave radiation and are described in standard textbooks. I do not find evidence in the file to connect these conditions with his employment.

As might be expected, Dr. Horner expressed his opinion of the Montgomery case at far greater length than this. Here is his review of the case file, dated April 25, 1972. Among other things, it contains an interesting interpretation of the phenomenon of coincidence.

It is apparent that claimant has been exposed to varying amounts of microwave radiation over a period of many years. In common with most of the cases of exposure to microwave radiation in the early days of radar, there is no documentation of the amount or intensity of exposure. His claim is related to loss of vision and of hearing.

Loss of hearing in the right ear occurred in 1949 following an exposure to presumably intense microwave energy. The loss of hearing took place several hours later and was accompanied by nausea and vertigo. There is no record of the amount, intensity, or duration of the exposure. This is not surprising since at that period little or no attention was paid to these factors due to ignorance of the effect on human beings. In 1970, a similar episode took place and he lost the hearing in his left ear. The impression at that time was thrombosis of the auditory artery. No specific causative factor has been found for the deafness in either ear. Apparently the episodes of sudden hearing loss about twenty years apart are similar and considered to be on a vascular basis. In the case of the first episode concerning the right ear there is no evidence to connect this with his accidental exposure on the same day except the time sequence. There is certainly nothing to connect a similar episode on the left side with microwave exposure some twenty years before. It would seem that exposure to energy sufficient to bring about coagulation of the blood and thrombosis in the branches of the auditory artery would produce some local heat effect on the ear itself or side of the face in the case of the original right ear episode. No mention is made in the file as to the presence or absence of heat sensation or as to the position of claimant's head in relation to the energy source. If he was working generally facing the energy source it would be reasonable to suppose that the effects would be apparent in both ears. These comments are not made in an effort to quibble over minutiae but simply to present factors considered in evaluating the claim. In general, as far as I can determine, hearing loss of this nature occurring a few hours after intense exposure has not been noted. This is certainly true for a similar hearing loss in the opposite ear some twenty years later.

Visual loss due to cataract formation secondary to microwave exposure has been extensively documented and although still slightly controversial, has been generally accepted by workmen's compensation bodies. The visual loss in this case has been felt to be due to repeated retinal hemorrhages with vitreous degeneration secondary to retinal hemorrhages and retinitis proliferans and chronic glaucoma. This is felt to represent a case of Eale's disease which is a syndrome of recurrent hemorrhage into the retina and vitreous affecting mainly males who usually show no evidence of systemic disease. No mention is made of cataract formation in the extensive ophthalmological information in the file. It would be expected that an individual exposed to excessive amounts of microwave energy as claimed in this case would show cataract formation. This cannot be absolutely established as there are apparently individuals with considerable exposure to this type of radiation who do not form cataracts. In general, however, absence of cataracts in this case would be a factor tending to question the extreme amount of radiation exposure claimed.

In summary, the file does not contain sufficient medical evidence to support claim of loss of vision and hearing due to conditions of employment.

As things turned out, Montgomery was eventually awarded compensation for job-related injuries in spite of Dr. Horner's reluctance to connect them with microwave radiation. To its credit, the Department of Labor referred the case to Dr. Zaret, who described Montgomery's exposure to radar in an article entitled "Blindness, Deafness and Vestibular Dysfunction in a Microwave Worker," which appeared in *The Eye, Ear, Nose and Throat Monthly,* in July of 1975:

> The patient's state of good health continued until sometime in 1949 when he was involved in a known accidental exposure, typical of the type associated with microwave trouble-shooting and believed to be the most severe of his career. The incident involved the patient and a co-worker who were testing a mobile-van-mounted target tracking radar. While the co-worker was absent from the test area, the patient noticed a malfunction in the automatic tracking system. He switched off the radar, climbed to the roof of the motor van, inspected the antenna dipole, and found it faulty. The co-worker returned and,

unaware that the patient was on the roof of the van, turned on the radar transmitter preparatory to making more tests. The patient, unaware that power had been restored, was exposed to intense microwave energy at a distance of less than two feet. A few hours later, he became dizzy and noticed a hearing loss in his right ear. Several days passed before the patient recovered from the sensation of dizziness. However, within a two-week period, the hearing loss progressed to a complete irreversible deafness in his right ear. He also developed a severe persistent equilibrium disturbance, exhibited by difficulty in walking a straight line because of veering to the left, due to dysfunction of the vestibular apparatus of his right ear.

In the concluding section of his article, Dr. Zaret pointed out that repeated diagnostic examinations of Montgomery by many physicians had excluded all possible known causes for his blindness, deafness, and dizziness except microwave radiation. Zaret ended with an assessment of the case that seemed all the more eminently sensible and understated coming from a physician who, for nearly ten years, had been under savage personal and professional attack from military physicians, from scientists whose work has been financed by the military, and from various representatives of the microwave-oven industry. "Some readers may never accept a microwave relationship as having been established for this case," Zaret wrote; "others may accept it with zealotry. Nevertheless, it behooves all of us in the health maintenance professions to become better informed about the biological effects of hertzian radiation and to remain alert to its potential especially when dealing with what appear otherwise to be idiopathic disease processes."

The patient in this case could in fact speak very well for himself. He had this to say to Jonathan Winer, of the *Boston Globe,* about the condition that has left him deaf, blind, and virtually unable to walk because of damage to his inner ears: "The term microwave and the term radiation have never been mentioned in my civil service compensation, although the award says 'job-related injury.' What else caused it then?" As it happens, Montgomery had previously made a number of sensible observations about microwave exposure, including this one made on September 6, 1971, in reply to a letter from the Department of Labor:

> Protective aspects of the present microwave regulations are questionable under specific circumstances. . . . When two or more Target Tracking Radars, or two or more Ground Control Approach Radars,

or a combination of the two types, meet the distance requirement for personnel safety from the propagating antenna but are closely aligned or spaced and operating simultaneously, then the power density exceeds safe levels. This condition triggers an incident, near and at coincidence, an especially harmful incident to personnel who have had many years of actual work in the vicinity of microwave transmissions. I am one of such persons and I have been associated with such conditions.

The high power levels of radiation that can occur at or near the convergence of two or more microwave beams are precisely why the microwave radiation hazard is so acute for thousands of Navy shipboard personnel, and why it may well have been acute for the unborn children of the 16,000-odd student helicopter pilots at Fort Rucker, who spent their days flying at low altitudes from one radar beam to another and riding converging radar beams right down to ground level as they made practice landings. Moreover, at the Tobyhanna Army Depot, Montgomery was exposed time and again to radiation from AN/TPN-18 and AN/FPN-40 radar sets, the same Ground Controlled Approach Radars whose emanations saturated the skies around Fort Rucker during the late sixties and early seventies. There were at least nineteen of these, though the Army subsequently tried to lead the FDA to believe there was only one.

As might be expected, the military-industrial complex studiously ignored the Montgomery case. Since the cause of Montgomery's blindness and deafness could not be conclusively proved, his afflictions were easily consigned to the realm of chance. But what if other radar technicians should exhibit similar problems after occupational exposure to microwave radiation? Obviously, the military-industrial complex would then need another tactic. In this light, let us examine the case of Ronald P. Karras, a forty-four-year-old radar repairman from Skokie, Illinois.

From 1959 through 1972, Karras was employed by the Department of the Army's National Guard to maintain, repair, and operate fire-control radars at Nike Ajax and Nike Hercules antiaircraft missile sites that had been set up to protect Chicago, Milwaukee, and Gary from enemy attack. During these thirteen years, Karras and some twenty fellow repairmen were required to climb into the radomes in order to align and adjust the beams of several types of radar sets, including high-power acquisition radars (HIPAR). While they did so, the radar systems continued to operate. A number of things suggest that this practice resulted in heavy exposure to radiation for Karras and his colleagues.

First, birds that flew into the radomes often dropped dead. Second, the belt buckles worn by Karras and some of the other repairmen got hot while they were aligning the radar beams. (Indeed, on one occasion Karras's clothes, which happened to be stained with hydraulic oil, began to smolder while he was making adjustments on the radar at the Nike site in Homewood, Illinois.) Third, on several occasions, Karras was treated for burns on his eyelids, his legs, and his scrotum after working on the Nike radar.

Not surprisingly, during the 1970s Karras began to experience serious illness as a result of such exposure. Some of his afflictions bear a striking similarity to those suffered by Montgomery. For example, Karras is deaf and he is going blind. He has pain in his eyes. He bleeds from both eyes, as well as from the ears, gums, and gastrointestinal tract—systemic hemorrhaging similar to that suffered by victims of atomic radiation. Karras's heartbeat is irregular and he has chest pain. In addition, he suffers from incapacitating polyarthritis that is also thought to be related to his years of microwave exposure.

According to Karras, one of his former supervisors is losing his hearing. Moreover, three of his fellow workers—all of whom were in their late thirties—have recently died within nine months of each other of heart attacks. For his part, Karras has claimed total disability compensation from the government as a result of work-related injuries. In addition, he brought suit for damages in 1974 against the General Electric Company and the Western Electric Company—manufacturers of radar sets for the Nike Hercules system—alleging that the two corporations were careless and negligent for failing to properly install and place the radars, and for failing to warn him that radio-frequency energy emitted from the sets would injure him.

In order to answer the interrogatories filed by Karras's lawyers, General Electric and Western Electric requested that the Army Missile Command (MICOM) at Redstone Arsenal, in Huntsville, Alabama, declassify certain confidential information about the radars Karras had worked on. On May 2, 1977, however, Arnold M.

Kohn, attorney adviser of the Army's Adversary Proceedings Division, told GE that the Missile Materiel Readiness Command (MIR-COM) could not declassify the information on the grounds that it was "of a nature for which conclusions can be drawn that would suggest for the enemy tactics most likely to defeat the Nike Hercules system."

If this were the case, one wonders why the information was not classified secret or top-secret to begin with. Or, for that matter, why the fire-control radar sets used by Karras and his co-workers during the 1960s are now being sold as surplus on the open market. In any case, on June 15, 1977, Karras's lawyer wrote Kohn a letter that read in part as follows:

> It would appear that the Defendants have leaned on your office in support of their objections to production of relevant materials, even on publicized information that has appeared in magazines and other lay publications. We believe that it is in the joint interest of Mr. Karras and the U.S. Government to disclose all matters that may relate to the issues in this suit.

The Army's claim that no information can be given out about Karras's exposure to microwave radiation because of national security is patently false. Indeed, it constitutes a gross misuse of national security by the Army. If the Army really believed that information about Karras's radiation exposure should be classified, it would surely have classified the radiation protection survey that was conducted by the Environmental Hygiene Agency in October 1969 at the Nike Hercules radar site in Homewood, Illinois, where Karras's clothes caught fire. The agency's survey report, which is dated December 5, 1969, describes five different radars at the Homewood site. The abstract of the report begins as follows:

> This report concerns the microwave and X-ray hazards associated with the Nike Hercules radar system, including the HIPAR located at Site C-50, Homewood, Illinois. Potentially hazardous microwave and X-radiation levels were encountered at various locations at this site (for example, microwave radiation of a potentially hazardous power density level could be unnecessarily directed toward the residential area.) The areas where these potentially hazardous microwave and X-ray levels exist were outlined in paragraph 4.

Paragraph 4 of the report clearly states that during certain operations the Missile Tracking Radar (MTR) and the Target Tracking Radar (TTR) at Site C-50 will radiate power densities greater than ten milliwatts per square centimeter beyond the fence of the military compound. Paragraph 3 says that "the area surrounding this site is highly congested with private homes."

Thus does the Army use national security as a stonewalling tactic designed to thwart what appear to be the legitimate claims of an injured worker and the judicial system of our constitutional democracy. And thus does the Army's own report put the lie to the military's often-repeated claim that radar poses no hazard to the civilian population.

17

Some Poor
TV Reception

The military–electronics industry complex routinely claims that the radar technicians and microwave-oven repairmen who suffered injuries were exposed to microwaves and radio-frequency radiation long before the hazards were fully understood and protective work practices were instituted, and that such injuries would not be incurred today. It is clear, however, that these claims are worthless, for ignorance about the hazards posed by microwaves is as profound as it ever was.

Take, for example, an incident that occurred in September 1976 at the Distant Early Warning (DEW) Line radar station at Oliktok, Alaska, some fifty miles east of Point Barrow, and about the same distance west of Prudhoe Bay, where the Alaska pipeline begins. Three civilians—a young woman and a young man doing wildlife research for the University of Alaska, and a consulting electronics engineer—had gone there to conduct an experiment in which radio-transmitter collars were fastened to wolves in order to monitor the animals' whereabouts and study their habits.

While the engineer remained at the radar station, the man and woman took a small boat loaded with supplies seven miles out into the Beaufort Sea to Pingok Island, where they made camp. On the return trip, high seas drenched the walkie-talkie radio they were carrying, which made communication with the electronics engineer on shore impossible. Concerned about the safety of his companions, the engineer received permission from the civilian manager of the radar station to climb a two-hundred-foot communications tower to see if he could reestablish radio contact with them. When he reached the top of the tower, the engineer was still unable to make contact because the radio in the boat was soaked. He then began to descend the stairway inside the steel-frame tower, pausing at every landing to try to contact his friends in the boat. On one of these landings, he came level with the sweeping beam of the giant over-the-horizon radar antenna housed inside a spherical radome, a few hundred feet away. At that point, his walkie-talkie went crazy with static.

Shortly after he reached the ground, the engineer was joined by his companions, who took him out to Pingok Island. There, some twelve hours later, he suddenly became faint and dizzy and took to his bed, where he experienced such severe heart fibrillations that his companions thought he was going to die. He remained in bed for the better part of the next four days, during which time he experienced dizziness, headache, and chest pain. When the engineer, who was in his late thirties, and who had no prior history of heart trouble, felt well enough to return to the mainland, he went to Point Barrow and made a report of the incident to officials of the Naval Arctic Research Laboratory there. Since that time, he has continued to experience severe heartbeat irregularities, and in the spring of 1977 he was hospitalized for extensive tests, which showed that the electrical conduction system regulating his heartbeat was not functioning properly.

A second example of the ignorance that persists about the hazards of microwaves and radio-frequency radiation is the situation that existed at the Weinbrenner shoe plant, in Antigo, Wisconsin, during 1974 and 1975. In 1974, the firm began using a 440-volt, 27.12 megahertz radio-frequency machine manufactured by Sealomatic, a division of Solidyne, Inc., to bond precut plastic to canvas uppers on Tretorn running shoes. The women workers who took turns operating the Sealomatic Plastic Sealer machine sat about three feet in front of the radiating head, and used their hands to position the shoes and material for sealing on a metal table. When the machine was first installed, the residents of Antigo began complaining of poor TV reception, trouble soon determined to be caused by radiation from the Sealomatic. The company's solution was to build a lead-lined enclosure around the machine and its operator. The TV reception in Antigo returned to normal. However, one of the operators of the Sealomatic began to experience what she later described to Richard E. Ginnold, assistant professor of Labor Education at the University of Wisconsin's Extension School for Workers, as an "aching and tingling in the arm closest to the machine"; a "feeling like bones were aching in her cheek"; and "fingertips turning blue up to the first joint."

When the woman complained, she was transferred to another job, and other workers took her place. A second woman, who operated the Sealomatic for two months before quitting the plant, told Ginnold that after two weeks on the machine she "began losing a lot of hair"; that the arm nearest the machine got red and itchy; and that she experienced headaches and blurred vision. A third woman who operated the machine from November 1974 to May 1976 experienced blurred vision and watering eyes during this time; she also got blotches under her skin; and felt "burning and tingling sensations" when she placed her hands on the machine turntable.

In December 1974, the Boot and Shoe Workers Union filed a complaint with the Occupational Safety and Health Administration about the situation at Weinbrenner. However, when a hygienist from the Occupational Safety and Health Administration's field office in Milwaukee arrived to inspect the Sealomatic operation, it turned out that OSHA did not have equipment that could measure emanations from such a machine. As a result, the administration issued no citation to the company, and did not even bother to give any explanation to the complaining union. However, the Weinbrenner Company replaced the lead-lined enclosure with copper mesh shielding.

During the early winter of 1975, OSHA asked the National Institute for Occupational Safety and Health (NIOSH) to send someone to measure the radiation levels in the Weinbrenner plant. The request was turned down for lack of travel funds. On February 19, 1975,

Ginnold wrote a letter to John Stender, then Assistant Secretary of Labor for OSHA, outlining the problem:

> I am writing because I am very concerned that on this important health situation OSHA does not have the capability to independently carry out enforcement and that . . . a sister agency is allowing travel budgets to stand in the way of response to a union complaint. Of course, another important issue is the vagueness and impracticality of the present OSHA radiation code which prescribes no preventive measures or work practices for different radiation operations and sets up an impossible method of detecting violations.

Ginnold was obviously describing a pure case of Catch-22. The Sealomatic operated at a frequency of 27.12 megahertz and OSHA microwave and radio-frequency personnel exposure standards were not readily applicable to frequencies between 10 and 300 megahertz. Stender finally got around to replying on March 14, telling Ginnold that "the microwave radiation at Weinbrenner was beyond our capability to measure," and that "it is the duty of the employer to determine the safety of the microwave operation and to correct any overexposures."

This, too, was pure Catch-22 for if OSHA didn't know how much radiation constituted an overexposure, couldn't measure the radiation in any case, and had no standard to apply even if it could have measured the radiation, how was the employer to deal with the problem?

Meanwhile, on February 24, Wordie H. Parr, of NIOSH, visited the Weinbrenner plant. There he made electric and magnetic field strength measurements of the Sealomatic machine, and found that the electric field strengths of the radiation emanating from it were up to twice as high as those recommended as safe by the American National Standards Institute (ANSI), and that the magnetic field strengths were up to twelve times the recommended level.

While on the same trip, Parr visited a number of other plants in Wisconsin and in Illinois. He found that in twelve radio-frequency generating devices the electric field strengths of all of them exceeded the ANSI recommended standard, as did the magnetic fields of ten of the devices. In his official report, Parr noted mildly that "there would appear to be a potential hazard associated with the radio-frequency radiation emitted by some of the units surveyed."

In October 1975, Parr and his colleagues presented a paper at the Boulder conference, pointing out that most commercial microwave and radio-frequency measuring devices cannot measure magnetic fields, and are only calibrated to measure power density in terms of milliwatts per square centimeter. (Since power density is not readily measureable at frequencies below about forty megahertz—forty million cycles per second—this meant that a large family of radio-frequency devices such as the Sealomatic, could not be accurately monitored.) Parr and his colleagues also pointed out that "almost all radio-frequency personnel exposure measurements must be performed within one meter of the radio-frequency source where the operators are located," and that "since present Federal standards do not specify exposure limits in terms of field strengths, compliance with Federal standards cannot be determined."

Following Parr's survey of the Weinbrenner plant, the union let the matter drop. On December 28, 1976, Ginnold described the existing situation at the factory in a letter to Sheldon Samuels, director of Occupational Health, Safety, and Environment for the AFL-CIO's Industrial Union Department:

"I am not too concerned with the Weinbrenner plant at this time except as an example of how little control OSHA has over the expanding use of microwave and radio-frequency equipment. In fact, because of worker complaints the Weinbrenner people have tried hard to eliminate the use of this machine. However, according to Dr. Parr of NIOSH, the use of radio-frequency sealing is expanding like wildfire in industries such as wood, shoe and other areas. One Wisconsin chemical company uses induction heating to produce chemical reactions, and the electromagnetic fields are so strong in the plant that no metal objects can be taken in. Many foundries are now using induction heating for their furnaces. Thus, we have a situation where many thousands of workers are being exposed to non-ionizing radiation with considerable evidence that there are serious hazards involved. Yet there is no enforceable OSHA standard under 1910.97 and administratively OSHA has failed to use the general duty clause or machine-guarding requirements or any other provisions to deal with the problem.

But there is more to the story. On January 16, 1976, almost a year earlier, Professor Ohm Gandhi, of the Department of Electrical Engineering at the University of Utah, had written to NIOSH (Parr's

agency), reporting the results of some recent power absorption studies he had conducted for the Army. As acting director of the Division
of Biomedical and Behavioral Science, Parr had found Gandhi's
study important enough to bring to the attention of the chief of
NIOSH's Physical Agents Effects Branch, and to arrange for Professor Gandhi to present it in person at NIOSH. In terms of the exposures that may have been undergone by the women at Weinbrenner,
Gandhi's findings were ominous indeed. He had said in his letter that
"at frequencies on the order of 25 to 26 megahertz the whole body
power deposition in an adult human subjected to ten-milliwatt-per-
square-centimeter incident plane waves may be 490 watts or more,"
and that "this is a truly large amount of absorption when one realizes
that there are hot spots in the distribution of distributed power."

On January 7, 1977, Samuels relayed Ginnold's concern of a month
before about occupational exposure to radio-frequency radiation to
Dr. Finklea, the director of NIOSH. He suggested that the institute
convene a task force to study the problem. On March 1, Samuels
received a reply from Vernon Rose, which indicated that either he
and Finklea had not been told about Gandhi's data, or that they had
decided to ignore it. One paragraph of Rose's letter read as follows:

> In regard to the published literature on radio-frequency–microwave
> bioeffects, many of the "effects" are difficult to assess due to their
> subjective and often transitory reversible nature. Some "effects" may
> not be fully realized as resulting from occupational exposure because
> of the widespread general population exposure from low level electro-
> magnetic "pollution" of the environment. Also, one must be careful
> to place into proper perspective short-term reversible biological
> "effects," and differentiate them from far more serious "hazards" to
> man. In other words, not every "effect" is of equal hazard. In fact,
> many important applications of radio-frequency and microwave radia-
> tion exist, such as diathermy and certain types of tumor therapy.
> The Ginnold report of a potential radio-frequency problem is of
> great concern to us for this reason, and will be given very careful
> study.

It is not known what sense Samuels was able to make out of this
analysis of the knotty problems posed by radio-frequency and microwave radiation, let alone where Rose ever acquired the expertise
to place into "proper perspective" the biological "effects" of radiation in relation to human "hazards." This, however, is the same Rose

who maintained a proper perspective concerning the brain tumor situation at Philco-Ford and the abnormalities of the skin and genitalia experienced by the microwave-oven repairman he had studied. Caution on the part of anyone at NIOSH should come as no surprise, however. Consider the institute's "aggressive study" of the TACAN workers, and the fact that in spite of Professor Gandhi's alarming findings, NIOSH does not intend to put radio-frequency and microwave radiation on its criteria-documents priorities list until fiscal year 1980–81. Perhaps NIOSH's priorities will be shuffled if the rising levels of radio-frequency radiation cause widespread poor TV reception.

Meanwhile, as other countries such as Sweden tighten microwave standards, the American legal tangle thickens.* So many claims for radiation injuries are now being filed by federal employees in the United States that the Department of Labor has established a special claims branch to process these cases. Furthermore, while essential priorities are being deferred and the cover-up continues, the general population of the nation continues to be widely exposed to radio-frequency and microwave radiation through low-level electromagnetic pollution of the environment.

---

*Worker Protection Authority in Sweden has issued radio-frequency protection standards twice as strict as the ANSI recommended guides, and required that Swedish workers be informed by their employers about the health risks involved.

18

The "Golf Ball"

The lackadaisical, business-as-usual approach to the microwave problem on the part of government health agencies has, of course, given the military–electronics industry complex a free hand to manufacture, sell, install, and operate the millions upon millions of radiating devices that create the climate of electromagnetic pollution in which we live. One such device was the U.S. Air Force Air Defense Command's, AN/FPS-45 spacetrack radar—a giant rotating antenna housed in a 140-foot-in-diameter, snow-white geodesic dome made of interlocking hexagonal pieces. The antenna, which sat beside Borton's Landing Road, in Moorestown, New Jersey, within a few hundred yards of the New Jersey Turnpike, was promptly and aptly dubbed the "golf ball" by turnpike travelers who used it as a landmark for Exit 4.

Built by RCA in 1959 at a cost of thirty million dollars, this huge facility was the prototype for similar radar installations in the Ballistic Missile Early Warning System (BMEWS). Others were constructed during the early 1960s in Scotland, Alaska, and Greenland (where the domes were needed to protect the antennas from high winds and cold weather) in order to provide fifteen-minute notice of Soviet missile attack against the North American continent and Western Europe.

During the next fifteen years, the radar inside the "golf ball" was used for a variety of purposes. It tracked all kinds of space activity, including Russian Vostok satellites and U.S. Tyro weather satellites. In 1961, when the planet Venus came closest to earth, it was able to bounce signals off Venus in order to measure the distance between the earth and the sun. In 1962, it tracked six tiny needles that had been placed in orbit two thousand miles above the earth, in order to study the feasibility of satellite communications. During the eclipse of 1963, it studied the effect of sun spots on radio transmissions. And in 1964, it was able to locate 329 pieces of junk in space, mostly refuse from American space flights.

In 1969, the "golf ball" radar was shut down by the Air Force, which deemed it obsolete. During 1970 and 1971, however, the facility underwent "electronic modification," and in January 1972, the Air Force announced that it had been reactivated as part of the Sea-Launched Ballistic Missile Detection and Warning System (SLBM). On January 5, the *Burlington County Times* carried a story by Stephen Makler, which read:

> Robert Kavula's stereo system has a case of the "blahs" and an RCA engineer named Mr. Springle says it is all tied up with U.S. Air Force security but he will not explain why.
>
> Kavula, of 26 Tennyson Lane, Willingboro, said he began last October to notice an annoying, low-pitched buzz that affected both the FM radio and phonograph output of his system.
>
> "It sounds like blah, blah," he described. Three times Kavula brought his set into a repair shop to be checked out. He was given a bill for $25 and told that there was nothing wrong with the system. Then, while passing the USAF Spacetrack radar facility on Borton's Landing Road, Moorestown, often called the "golf ball," Kavula noticed the same interference on his FM car radio.
>
> While in the Navy in 1965 on the island of Shemya in the North Pacific, he had experienced similar difficulties from the missile radar system on the island. Kavula became sure that radar was again the cause.

He contacted an RCA engineer named Springle who told him, "It very well could be."

Kavula was not satisfied, however, with Springle's reply about when the situation might be corrected. "I got the definite impression that they would be in no hurry. You know—'We'll get around to it!' "

When asked yesterday, Springle, who would not give his first name, said, "We are investigating to see what can be done. In some cases interference is caused by power lines or various things. We have retained a subcontractor to do some work on this."

Springle requested that nothing of what he said be released because of U.S. Air Force security. He would "explain no further."

The "golf ball" is ostensibly a radar facility for tracking objects in space—nose cones, satellites, payloads, and other effluvia. It was the protoype for the stations of the Distant Early Warning System.

Kavula, a pilot with Trans World Airlines, has had some engineering training and believes that the problem affecting him and several other families in the Twin Hills area is caused by a "radar leak." The particular configuration of the land in Twin Hills, he thinks, is the reason it is limited to that area.

"They could deaden it (the interference) with a lead deflector," Kavula claimed.

He has gathered a petition with the names, so far, of about a dozen upset stereo listeners nearby and said he hopes that public pressure will persuade RCA or the Air Force to quickly rectify the situation.

On January 7, Makler wrote a second story, "RADAR UNIT GETS BLAME FOR STATIC." He quoted Michael S. Terpilak, a radiation consultant for the Environmental Protection Agency, as saying that a survey of the "golf ball" would be conducted the following week. "We have to get the appropriate instrumentation," Terpilak said. "Then we have to determine the wattage of the emissions, their frequency, the distance from populated areas, and the size of the population involved." Makler also reported that since his first article Kavula had received dozens of calls from residents suffering stereo interference, and that all but three of them came from Twin Hills Park, which is two miles north of the radar. Makler then wrote about Kavula's subsequent experience in a passage that was vintage Kafka.

Kavula then contacted the regional office of the Federal Communications Commission in Philadelphia. An official named Wilson told him that Springle "would be doing something about it, correcting it by coming into individual homes."

The airline pilot does not believe this is the correct way to settle things. "Rather than having people complain and going to every house," he said, "they ought to correct it out at the site."

Three days later, the *Camden Courier-Post* ran a story by Douglas Campbell, who saw things in a different light. The piece began as follows:

> Folks in the vicinity of the United States Air Force's space-tracking station on Borton's Landing Road may be trying to boot the wrong ball.
>
> Interference with various electrical appliances goes back several years. But, according to a spokesman for RCA, which set up the facility for the Air Force, the radar unit has been operating for only a couple of weeks.
>
> There appears, then, the possibility that some of the interference is coming from other sources—perhaps one of a number of radio and television towers in the rolling, rural area.

Campbell's theory of where the radiation might be coming from depended upon the truth of RCA's story that the newly modified radar inside the "golf ball" had not been subjected to the months of testing and calibration that would normally precede official operation. Anyone who continued to read Campbell's story, however, would have come upon the following passage.

> The curve of a side of the radar unit—known as the "golf ball"— is visible through the living room window of the Beauchamp home on Hartford Road, Mount Laurel. John Beauchamp, his wife, Gail, and their children, Cheri, 12, John III, 10, and Wendy, 9, live three-tenths of a mile from the ball.
>
> When Mrs. Beauchamp flips the switch on the family organ for little John to practice, there's a low fluttering sound in the foot-level speaker. In a matter of seconds, the palpitation has increased in volume, enough to quake the chest of a person sitting beside it.
>
> "I had to cancel the organ lesson entirely because you just can't play it," said Mrs. Beauchamp. "That upsets me and my son, who was doing quite well with his lessons."
>
> The Beauchamps suspect the golf ball radar is the cause of their organ problems. They believe similar sounds that emanate from the record player, portable radios and tape recorder are caused by the same source.

"Probably the organ is the worst offender," commented the mother, whose children agreed they first noticed the problem six months ago. But the radio interference is an irritation, even if, as she claims, the volume there is lower. "You're lucky if you can find three hours a week when it's not present."

On January 18 John Himmelein wrote a story in the *Burlington County Times,* which described the efforts of Kavula and other Twin Hills residents to alert the Mayor of Willingboro to the situation. At a Township Council meeting, Kavula said he had been informed by officials of the FDA's Bureau of Radiological Health that they were not sure what effect the "golf ball's" radiation would have on electronic devices. Kavula then told the meeting that a woman who had driven past the radar "heard a loud noise in her hearing aid," and that afterward "the hearing aid lost the fidelity it formerly had."

On the next day, Himmelein wrote a story that contained an attempt by the bureau to clarify its position on electronic interference. It began as follows:

> Cardiac "pacemakers" can be affected by radio frequency microwaves such as those emitted by the Moorestown radar "golf ball," a spokesman for the Federal Bureau of Radiological Health said today.
>
> The spokesman said it is doubtful that a motorist passing the Borton Road Air Force facility on the New Jersey Turnpike or Route 295 would be affected, but that there was no guarantee.
>
> The spokesman also said, however, that other more common emitters of such waves could also affect the pacemakers, some car ignitions and soldering irons, to name two.

Car ignitions and soldering irons notwithstanding, the Air Force apparently knew what was causing the interference, as the last part of Himmelein's article clearly shows.

> An Air Force statement released yesterday explained why home owners were receiving the interference, but also indicated the expense of correcting the problem would have to be borne by the individual residents.
>
> "Although the Air Force cannot properly accept the responsibility for eliminating the interference since our radar operates precisely in the frequency band assigned to it by the appropriate authorities, it is the Air Force's policy to do all within our means to

assist those who live near our installations in eliminating the interference."

"To do all within our means" so far has meant distributing a book
entitled "Suppression of High Power Radar Signals in Home Entertainment Equipment," as well as visiting affected residents.

On January 20, Adele Ross, of the *Courier-Post* wrote a story that
appeared beneath the headline "U.S. SAYS AIR FORCE GOLF BALL
NOT DANGEROUS TO PACEMAKERS." According to the story, four
governmental agencies—the EPA, the FDA, the Air Force, and the
New Jersey Department of Environmental Protection—concurred
that the radiation levels measured in the Twin Hills section of Willingboro amounted to only one hundredth of a millionth of a watt,
and, therefore, could not possibly be harmful to human health. What
really happened was that the three civilian agencies concurred with
the results of an Air Force radiation survey that had been made on
January 12. They did so because they lacked equipment to measure
the radiation. By some curious omission, a joint press release put out
by the Air Force and the three agencies failed to say that on Hartford
Road, where the Beauchamps lived, the Air Force had measured a
power density of 1.06 milliwatts per square centimeter—an unusually
high level for a residential area.

On January 28, Mayor Paul W. Krane announced a Willingboro
Township Council meeting to give the Air Force a chance to air
"their side of the story." An account of what went on at the meeting
was carried by the *Burlington County Times,* on February 3. The last
part of the article read as follows:

> The problem, as reported by residents and demonstrated by the Air
> Force last night, is that "side lobe" or stray radar rays are transmitted
> toward the Willingboro homes.
>
> While four government agencies have reported the emissions are no
> danger to human or environmental health, they do cause a low buzz-
> ing sound in some sound producing equipment such as television,
> stereos, tape recorders, and intercoms.
>
> The sound can be heard in the affected units approximately every
> 35 seconds as the radar scans the Atlantic Ocean, an Air Force spokes-
> man reported.

Another account of the meeting appeared on February 4 in the
Courier-Post. The final section of this story shed some new light on
the "golf ball's" emanations:

Twin Hills resident Owen Gearhart said he had lost three radio-controlled model airplanes because of the interference from the Moorestown station.

Gearhart, president of the Burlington County Radio Control Club, said he flies his planes in a field at Elbow Lane and Burlington–Mount Holly Road, Burlington Township, and on three occasions they were taken out of his control by another signal and crashed erratically.

He said in each case they were at a height of 50 to 80 feet, which is said to be the range affected by the Moorestown signal.

The Air Force promised to send out test equipment to investigate Gearhart's complaint.

With that, believe it or not, the whole story dropped out of sight. Indeed, the story not only disappeared from the newspapers, but was apparently put out of the minds of the residents of Twin Hills and Willingboro. They may well have thought there was nothing they could do anyway. More than three years passed. Then, on November 21, 1975, the *Courier-Post* published the following piece of nostalgia, entitled "FORE! AND THERE GOES THE GOLF BALL":

It's been despised by a few, revered by most and known to everyone who has driven the New Jersey Turnpike.

And now it will only be a memory.

The "Golf Ball," the giant U.S. Air Force radar installation here, is going to that great 19th hole in the sky.

The U.S. Air Force is tearing it down.

The 15-story globe, built by RCA during the days of the Cold War to track missiles, is now scientifically obsolete in the days of Detente.

The demise of the radar station will be hailed by Willingboro residents, who complained that it botched their TV and radio reception and spirited away radio-controlled model airplanes.

But to most South Jersey residents and travelers, the loss of the radar station is the loss of a familiar landmark.

A few months later, on March 7, 1976, the *Burlington County Times* noted the progress of the demolition in a piece that appeared beneath the headline "TECHNOLOGY DRIVES 'GOLF BALL' OUT." "The military is nearly finished dismantling the space tracking installation, an operation which began several months ago," the story read. "Much of the web of steel that makes up the actual tracking device has been removed. All that remains is the 15-story white sphere which earned the installation its nickname."

Today, nothing is left of that scene, not even the "golf ball" itself. However, in the 1975 draft proposal of the Department of Defense's Tri-Service Electromagnetic Radiation Bioeffects Research Program, the following paragraph appears under a section entitled "Specific Systems Impact":

> The AN/FPS-85 spacetrack radar is a fully operational phased array system which operates in a frequency range of 450 megahertz with a peak power of 32 million watts. Current systems modifications to include a SLBM (Submarine Launched Ballistic Missile) detection mode require additional electromagnetic hazards analysis. Electromagnetic data from this system is of utmost importance to two subsequent surveillance radar developments (details are classified).

As it happens, certain details about phased array radar systems—first developed at Raytheon under Martin Schilling, technical director of Germany's V-2 rocket research center at Peenemünde during World War II, and until recently Vice-President of Research and Development for the company—have now been declassified. Moreover, information about them has been made available for publication. For example, in the March-April 1977 issue of *Electronic Warfare,* the Cobra Dane phased array radar was described in a section that provided an incidental yet fascinating corroboration of Robert Kavula's initial suspicions concerning the "golf ball":

> Cobra Dane is an early warning station beginning operation in Alaska's Aleutian Islands. The conventional dish antenna system it replaces on Shemya Island is limited to tracking a single object at a time. Cobra Dane can simultaneously follow 300 missiles in the air and 200 objects in space. The manufacturer, Raytheon, has also been awarded two contracts for detection of submarine-launched ballistic missiles from as far away as 3,000 miles. One $46.6 million system will be installed at Otis Air Force Base in Massachusetts, and a second at Beale Air Force Base, in California. Cobra Dane uses 34,768 sensors on 96 antenna plates. A CDC computer coordinates signal transmission and processing. The solid-state radar was developed under a $52.4 million contract. Another $26 million was awarded Raytheon for operational testing through January.

This statement has ominous implications. The two contracts for detection of submarine-launched ballistic missiles refer to PAVE PAWS (Precision Acquisition of Vehicle Entry Phased Array Warning System) radars. The one at Otis Air Force Base, in Falmouth, Massachusetts, will be housed in a gigantic poured-concrete structure 115 feet tall, which is now under construction. No one knows the extent of the health hazard posed by this immensely powerful radar for the residents of Cape Cod. Nor does anyone know whether other phased array radars such as Cobra Dane and the AN/FPS-85 are safe. Indeed, in a 1975 report that will be examined in detail in the next chapter, the military has admitted that it has no data on the long-term, chronic biological effects of any of these radar systems.

As for the SLBM detection mode of the AN/FPS-85 that requires "additional hazards analysis," that will undoubtedly remain in the murky realm of classified information for some time to come. However, one can put two and two together by remembering that whatever modifications were performed in 1971 on the detection mode of the radar inside the "golf ball," they surely had to include raising the power level and a change in the angle of the antenna. In other words, in order to detect missiles as they might emerge from the surface of the Atlantic Ocean, the giant dish antenna that had previously been angled toward space had to be tilted forward and aimed toward the sea. Lying between the sea and this immensely powerful, continually sweeping, radiating antenna was the same thing that lay between an SLBM radar at Laredo, Texas, and the Gulf of Mexico. And the same thing that will lie between the sea and the PAVE PAWS now being installed on Cape Cod—thousands upon thousands of square miles and everyone and everything alive upon them.

One should keep in mind that the giant microwave antenna inside the "golf ball"—a device that alone irradiated much of New Jersey —as well as the enormously powerful PAVE PAWS radars now being placed on Cape Cod and in California, are merely three of thousands upon thousands of radars and other radiating devices in the military's vast arsenal of electronic weaponry. To this total add the thousands of radars and radio-frequency transmitters that have been installed at every airport, in airplanes, on ships, and in pleasure craft. Add the increasing number of police radars that can be seen beside the nation's highways. Add the thousands of radio and television transmitters that are located on towers and buildings across the country, and the communications and surveillance satellites that are beaming microwave radiation back to earth from outer space. Then add the hundreds of microwave telephone and television-signal relay towers that crisscross the land. Continue by adding four or five million microwave ovens, all of which leak some radiation and which, indeed, are allowed by law to leak up to five milliwatts per square centimeter—five hundred times the Russian standard. Include the thousands of microwave and radio-frequency induction heating devices now in use in industry all over the United States. Add fifteen million or so Citizen's Band radio transmitters, whose antennas can broadcast radio-frequency radiation far in excess of the ten-milliwatt standard, as well as thousands upon thousands of extremely powerful radio transmitters in police, fire, and emergency mobile units, which can give off hundreds of milliwatts per square centimeter. Then add several million walkie-talkie radios—the kind carried by cops and kids—which can transmit radiation far in excess of the standard in regions close to their antennas. Tack on thousands upon thousands of cathode-ray-tube video display units (VDTs)—the kind used by newspapers, banks, airlines, libraries, and insurance companies—which are also suspected of leaking harmful radiation. Don't forget all the microwave burglar alarm systems and automatic garage-door openers, or, for that matter, electronic games and remote-control transmitters for model airplanes. Include the electrosurgical devices—electronic knives that are used for cutting into tissue and for stopping blood flow—which can be found in virtually every hospital operating room in the nation, which typically emit radiation levels of about one hundred milliwatts per square centimeter, and which not only pose potential health hazards but can also interfere with other electrical medical devices such as patient monitoring and life-support equipment. And, finally, just to top off the list, consider the complex electric fields that are generated in the vicinity of high-voltage overhead power lines.

No wonder that in some urban areas the radiation background created by these myriad radiating sources and devices is estimated to be at least one hundred million times as great as the natural radio-frequency radiation background provided by the sun. No wonder that as far back as 1971 the Electromagnetic Radiation Management Advisory Council of the President's Office of Telecommunications Policy warned that "power levels in and around American cities, airports, military installations and tracking centers, ships and pleasure craft, industry and homes may already be biologically significant" and that the population at risk "may well be the entire population." No wonder, considering the very real possibility that the health consequences of microwave radiation may be cumulative, that the council also warned that "the consequences of undervaluing or misjudging the biological effects of long-term, low-level exposure could become a critical problem for the public health, especially if genetic effects are involved."

It should be abundantly clear by now that, in spite of the denials and claims to the contrary that flow from the military–electronics industry complex, the microwave and radio-frequency radiation problem is not a limited threat. Indeed, the microwave radiation problem affects virtually every man, woman, and child in the land. In fact, the microwave problem is nothing more or less than the zapping of America.

19

The Money Trail

In order to follow the Department of Defense microwave cover-up it might now be worthwhile to delve into a new Tri-Service Electromagnetic Radiation Bioeffects Research Program, which was instituted in the Spring of 1975. On April 25, 1975, the Assistant Director for Environmental and Life Sciences of the Office of the Director of Defense Research and Engineering requested that he be furnished with an executive summary of the Tri-Service draft proposed research plan; on June 11, such a summary was duly forwarded to him under the signatures of the members of the Tri-Service Electromagnetic Advisory Panel: Captain Tyler, of the Navy; Colonel William R. Godden, of the Air Force; Lieutenant Colonel Edwin N. Dodd, Jr., of the Army; and Lieutenant Colonel Andrew P. Blasco, of the Armed Forces Radiobiology Research Institute, located in Bethesda, Maryland. Both the executive summary and the proposed research plan make interesting reading.

The summary started out by saying something practically everybody knows by now—that the "Department of Defense is the nation's largest user of non-ionizing electromagnetic radiation (EMR) devices including a wide variety of reconnaissance, surveillance, and communications systems in air, sea, and ground operations." A few sentences later, the report went on:

> The principal objective of the EMR research program is to maximize personnel safety while minimizing operational constraints. In these austere times, where it is mandatory that all military organizations "do more with less," the Department of Defense cannot afford a program that would "avert all risks" on a short term basis. Rather, the program is being organized to apply a practical "level of effort" to achieve answers to logical questions in a priority sequence. While proceeding in this manner, it is recognized that many isolated reports of so-called "low level bioeffects" will not be addressed nor, therefore, resolved in the near future. On the other hand, the program will provide the best available collective data base of EMR bioeffects to make timely and appropriate decisions in support of specific DOD systems operations. This means, in effect, that through this program each service can provide the best guidance available at any point in time to prepare and/or defend everything from environmental impact statements to detailed operating procedures concerning any of their EMR emitters.

Translated, the DOD proposal called for research not to find the truth, but to "defend" itself against other research which might point an accusing finger at electromagnetic emitters such as the PAVE PAWS radar being installed on Cape Cod and in California. Four advantages of the DOD's particular brand of research were listed in the next paragraph:

> The principal advantages of this coordinated research program are (1) To avoid any unnecessary duplicative efforts, (2) To maximize use of EMR research manpower and facilities, (3) To focus collective competence to resolve the more difficult priority problems in the shortest time, (4) To maintain a united position concerning EMR exposure standards that encroach on, or would tend to unnecessarily constrain DOD operations.

On page 2 of the executive summary there was a paragraph that shed light on the need for this "united position," as well as the kind of "coordination" that lay behind it. In order to understand this paragraph, however, one should first read a paragraph entitled "Summary," which appeared in the draft proposed research plan:

> Unless the Services develop and support a coordinated EMR bio-effects research program, the DOD will be confronted with continuing pressure from other Federal Agencies to issue more restrictive EMR occupational and environmental protection standards. This research program must provide biophysical data delineating the threshold for deleterious effects so that rationale and scientific arguments can be used to evaluate current standards and recommend more appropriate standards if indicated. DOD can expect attempts to promulgate an environmental standard of one milliwatt per square centimeter or the adoption of a one milliwatt per square centimeter occupational standard with a corollary environmental standard of one-tenth of a milliwatt per square centimeter within the next two to five years. These standards will significantly restrict the military use of EMR in a peacetime environment and require the procurement of substantial real estate around ground-based EMR emitters to provide buffer zones.

Returning to page 2 of the executive summary, one learns what amount of real estate the military had in mind. The classified ECAC report mentioned in the initial sentence of the following paragraph refers to a survey of electromagnetic radiation emitters capable of producing power densities of ten milliwatts per square centimeter or more at a distance of 100 meters. The survey was conducted by the Department of Defense's Electromagnetic Compatibility Analysis Center during 1974 and 1975.

> The ECAC report (classified) was completed. The report illustrates the importance of DOD studies to include a wide range of frequencies, and confirms the major impact on DOD operations if the national EMR exposure standard were reduced from ten milliwatts per square centimeter to one milliwatt per square centimeter. Specifically it would require the Air Force to control an additional 318,000 acres, the Army to control an additional 12,000 acres, and the Navy to control an additional 168,000 acres.

There is a maxim to the effect that when one wishes to uncover a cover-up one should follow the money trail. In this case, the money trail is quite literally on land. To be precise, it is on *498,000 acres* of land. One can only guess at how much money it might cost for the Department of Defense to acquire and, therefore, "control" that much land. Twenty billion dollars? Thirty billion? Fifty? Here, is a money trail indeed and a motive for the cover-up of health hazards posed by microwave radiation.

Many of these 498,000 acres, needless to say, have people on them, including members of Congress, who are thus far conveniently ignorant about this incredible situation.

Of course, this is merely the on-land part of the problem. The implications of a reduction of the ten-milliwatt standard for the sea-going Navy would be the cessation of naval operations as they are conducted today. For the phased array fire-control radars now used by the Navy are known to irradiate a large portion of any ship on which they have been installed with power levels that exceed ten milliwatts per square centimeter. (Proof of this can be found in the Naval Ship Engineering Center's December 1976 report of power density levels that were measured on the U.S.S. *Virginia* in October of that year by the RCA Service Company, in Hyattsville, Maryland.) Indeed, if the ten-milliwatt standard were to be lowered to one milliwatt (and enforced), the yellow hazard lines that now define shipboard areas where microwave radiation levels are deemed dangerous would in some cases have to be painted hundreds of yards out to sea. No doubt the Navy would dearly love to forget Military Handbook 238, issued in August 1973, for on page 18 of that document can be found the following paragraph:

Non-thermal effects. Much of the early work in the field of biological hazards concluded that the only significant biological effect of EMR was thermal response. In recent years, however, many distinctly non-thermal effects have been documented, some of which have been shown to be dependent on peak powers whose average value is not great enough to produce heating. Frequency dependence, with no heating, has also characterized many of the observed effects. While the full significance of these effects to human hazard has not been established, the fact that they occur at average power levels considered to be negligible suggests that, at the least, an awareness of their existence should be assumed. Some recorded non-thermal effects are listed:

(1) Minor changes in human blood properties upon exposure to EM energy of proper frequency and intensity.

(2) Auditory response. Certain people can hear a buzz when exposed to microwave radiation. The sensation of sound is probably not the microwave frequency but response to the pulse repetition frequency.

(3) Abnormalities of the chromosome structure occurring upon exposure have been detected.

(4) Movement, orientation and polarization of protein molecules in pulsed radio-frequency fields.

(5) Unexplained response of man to radar. Epigastric distress, emotional upsets, and nausea may occasionally occur at as low as five to ten milliwatts per square centimeter and are most commonly associated with the frequency range from 8×10^3 to 12×10^3 megahertz.

Returning to the executive summary and the draft research plan from which it was drawn, we pursue the question of who knew what and when. On page 3 of the summary, there is a paragraph beneath the heading "Problems," which contains a double-think explanation of the thousandfold difference between the U.S. and Russian exposure standards. It reads:

> To more realistically define existing safe levels to reflect frequency effects, one must also consider the different philosophies in the Eastern vs. Western approaches. Warsaw Pact countries' safety criteria appear to reflect exposure levels such that biologic changes are not observed; this philosophy obtains even if the alternation is nondetrimental from a tissue injury point of view. The Western view accepts a level of exposure which may result in noninjurious biologic change such as the change associated with normal thermoregulatory mechanisms, but which is lower than the level producing a demonstrable thermal detrimental effect. Hence, the safety standards can differ by as much as three (3) orders of magnitude.

A few sentences later, the authors of the executive summary dropped the pretense of comparative philosophy and displayed some of the firmness that so often characterizes the military mind at work. They wrote:

> "It is of the utmost priority in the DOD program to "take a stand" on EMR exposure standards, i.e., to apply the best collective judgment to set appropriate standards at any point in time and yet to remain flexible to change these standards in accordance with the best available evidence as it is developed.

Switching to page 4 of the draft research plan, one finds the military's "taking a stand" under the heading "NATO Standardization Agreements":

STANAG 2345 which has been circulated for comment to NATO members proposed a one milliwatt per square centimeter power density limit to demark where personnel radiation control procedures are initiated. While there is no time limit on personnel exposure in areas containing one to ten milliwatts per square centimeter of EMR, the establishment of controlled access at one milliwatt per square centimeter in essence sets a general population exposure limit of less than one milliwatt. Several member nations have agreed with the proposed STANAG and urged ratification. The U.S. has rejected this proposal stating that a change from the present U.S. standard is unwarranted. Adoption of a lower standard will be continually pressed by some NATO countries until adequate bioeffects research studies have been conducted.

Whatever the authors of the 1975 research plan intended the word "adequate" to mean, it seems doubtful that they would have used it to describe the kind of microwave studies that were called for by Professor Czerski, who spoke at a European conference held that same year, and whose comments were reported in the following detail in ESN–29–12, a report issued and distributed on December 31, 1975, by the Office of Naval Research Branch Office, in London:

The speaker, Czerski, made an impassioned plea for more investigative efforts on microwave effects on nervous and hematopoietic systems and on genetic and chromosome aberrations. In view of the increasing use of high-power electromagnetic devices, this plea carries a degree of urgency. The interdisciplinary cooperation of biologists, biophysicists, physiologists, electronic engineers and medical research workers appears imperative.

Czerski pointed out that primary interactions of microwaves with living systems cannot be explained solely by electromagnetic theory in terms of the conversion of the absorbed energy into kinetic energy of molecules; quantum mechanical effects come into play in complex subcellular structures. Besides frequency, the type of modulation, and the duration and the repetition period of irradiation all have bearing on the total microwave biological effect. Because of the absence of well-documented epidemiological studies, the authors expressed doubt on the relatively high (compared to USSR and Poland) safe-exposure limit (ten milliwatts per square centimeter) recommended in the U.S.

A page or two later, the Office of Naval Research report goes on to describe "Lecture Series Number 78 on Radiation Hazards," sponsored by the NATO Advisory Group for Aerospace Research and Development (AGARD) in the autumn of 1975. It was not surprising, of course, that Professor Czerski—a Pole and, therefore, a Warsaw Pact national—was not invited to participate in this lecture series. After all, the series was designed to "adequately" inform our NATO allies of the potential microwave hazard problem. On the other hand, it should come as no surprise that the director of the lecture series was none other than Professor Sol M. Michaelson, of the University of Rochester's Department of Radiation Biology and Biophysics. Professor Michaelson had appeared before Congress on behalf of the Association of Home Appliance Manufacturers—a trade organization representing the makers of microwave ovens—and had also conducted microwave research for the United States Navy. For example, during 1973, 1974, and 1975, Professor Michaelson received funds from the Navy's Bureau of Medicine and Surgery to study the neuroendocrine aspects of microwave exposure in rats and dogs, in order to assist with "hazard evaluation and standard setting." In fiscal year 1974, Michaelson received $90,000 for such research; in 1975, $115,000; and in 1976, the planned allocation for his work was listed on the Tri-Service project résumé as $120,000.

Other than finding thermal effects, it is not known what results the professor obtained from his experiments. They are still in progress. It is known, however, that Michaelson's program contact at the Navy has been Captain Tyler, who monitors practically all of the Navy-funded research on microwave effects. Tyler is, of course, one of the authors of the 1975 research plan that calls for resistance to any demands by NATO nations for a lower microwave exposure standard. It is also known that when he lectured in Oslo in the autumn of 1975, Professor Michaelson told his listeners that he was unconvinced by most of the experimental evidence linking microwave radiation with a direct effect upon the central nervous system; that one could not conclude that the mechanism of interaction was nonthermal just because the average body temperature had not changed; and that an argument about the mechanism must take second place to a determination whether or not there were any real low-average-power effects to begin with.

Professor Michaelson, whose colleagues occasionally josh him about his devotion to the thermal theory, should feel free to express his scientific opinions wherever and whenever he can. Should Michaelson's opinions, however, not be considered in light of the expressed determination of the authors of the 1975 research program to resist all pressure from NATO to lower the ten-milliwatt standard—a determination that, in effect, included "taking a stand" against any admission that nonthermal hazards might exist?

If the reader has not yet tired of observing Catch-22 as played by the Navy, he or she is invited to return to the 1975 Tri-Service Research Plan. It contains much evidence that the military's firm support of the thermal theory and the ten-milliwatt standard flew in the face of dangers the military knew about. For example, the authors of the plan cited work in France and the United States that demonstrated that neural activity is stimulated in animals exposed to either microwaves or very-high-frequency radio waves. "This activity occurs at the same frequency as the pulse repetition of the EMR, and may persist for a few hours after the termination of the irradiation," they wrote. "The average power is below that considered safe for prolonged exposure in this country."

Next, there was a description of Allan Frey's work, showing that low power, pulsed microwave radiation produces changes in the central nervous system. "Significant increases in the permeability across the blood-brain barrier were reported for exposure to two milliwatts per square centimeter pulsed microwave radiation," the report stated.

The rest of the research plan reads in similar fashion. The authors state that extra-low-frequency electric fields, which are modulated at from six to twenty hertz, produce a progressive increase in the calcium efflux in the brains of animals—a fact that has a bearing on Project Seafarer—and they go on to admit that "this effect is independent of any ongoing metabolic processes in the brain."

They speak of changes that occur in the thalamic region of the brain when test animals are exposed to microwave radiation at the ten-milliwatt level, and they report that "chronic exposure for periods up to 30 days appears to cause a more severe deterioration of the neurons." They also take note of the fact that Polish scientists have found that "repeated irradiations at five to seven milliwatts per square centimeter daily for 3–4 months indicated functional and biochemical disturbances as well as morphologic changes in the CNS [central nervous system]."

As for alteration of behavior, the 1975 research plan cites studies demonstrating "sizeable decrements in the performance of trained animals following exposure to microwave irradiation at and below the ten-milliwatt level," and says that "pulsed radiation, similar to that used in many military radar systems, was used in this study." Further, the plan states that "some investigators have found that as the psychological task is made more complex the intensity of EMR required to alter behavior decreases." And "if the tasks are made more complex, approaching those required in a military operation, the thresholds for microwave effect may well decrease."

Moving on to ocular effects, the authors declare "virtually all litigation resulting from EMR exposure includes ocular damage as an effect of such exposure." Then, in a breathtaking bureaucratic sweep, they first complain about the lack of information on ocular effects; second, they note that "Zaret has maintained that numerous cases of EMR-induced cataracts have occurred and were the result of chronic EMR exposure to low levels of radiation"; and, third, they go on to call for "a long-term study of animals receiving chronic exposures to low power densities of radiation." This amounts to a brazen about-face. After all, one of the authors of this research plan was the ubiquitous Captain Tyler, who, back in 1971, was instrumental in cancelling Navy funds for Zaret's study of chronic microwave exposure in primates. And why did Captain Tyler and others suddenly want to conduct such a study? The answer lies in the next sentence. "This work must be done soon," they declare, "since cases of litigation involving purported ocular damage appear to be increasing and scientific data to resolve the question is lacking."

Let us flip back now to page 5 of the research plan. There, beneath the heading "Claims and Lawsuits for Service Connected Disabilities," one can find a passage about ocular damage that provides another off-shoot of the money trail. It also indicates how cynical the military can be when it comes to dealing with its own people and provides an explanation for the military effort to discredit Dr. Zaret for nearly a decade:

In recent years, the possibility of delayed cataract formation as a result of exposure to radar has received extensive publicity and appears to be a significant cause for concern among veteran groups. Veterans have filed claims alleging that cataracts and other lenticular defects are the result of chronic exposure to low level (one to ten milliwatts per square centimeter) EMR while in the service. Several claims have been settled and involved payments in excess of $100,000. It is expected that the number of claims will increase in the future, based on informal information from the FAA, and that settlement will favor the plaintiff until studies are accomplished that disprove this EMR effect.

Studies to *disprove* that microwave radiation causes cataracts? That last sentence deserves rereading. It not only serves to corroborate the Federal Aviation Administration's deep involvement in the microwave cover-up, but also to describe just what kind of "studies" the authors of the report had in mind. Informal information? That's one way of putting it. A trifle euphemistic, though. Why not just come right out and say long-suppressed information about a secret study which shows the incidence of cataracts in the eyes of airline pilots to be significantly higher than expected?

Thus there is apprehension in high military, governmental, and industrial circles about the effects of electronic systems. But what is the extent of this hardware? A complete listing of the systems would both boggle the mind with its length and stagger the imagination with the military's penchant for code names and acronyms. However, a quick and arbitrary rundown of only a few of the Pentagon's latest gadgets will give some idea of the investment our country has made in electronic warfare.

• ABRES—the Air Force's Advanced Ballistic Re-entry System.

• AEGIS—the Navy's advanced shipboard weapons system developed by RCA, which integrates phased array radars with missile-launch and missile-guidance systems, in order to engage multiple air and surface targets.

• ALCOR—"A" stands for the Advanced Research Projects Agency, "L" stands for the Massachusetts Institute of Technology's Lincoln Laboratory, "COR" stands for Coherent Observable Radar, and the whole is a huge radar installed on Kwajalein Island in the Pacific to observe reentry vehicles.

• ALTAIR—another Kwajalein instrument; ARPA's Long-range Tracking and Instrument Radar, a 150-foot-in-diameter dish antenna that is used for midtrajectory testing of missile systems.

• AWACS—Airborne Warning and Control System; a unique airborne, rotating phased array antenna system which transmits a high-power pulsed microwave signal that enables its users to view an entire battlefield. AWACS will be housed in modified Boeing 707 airliners—each plane and radar system costing about $170 million—and in spite of strong congressional opposition, the Carter Administration and Boeing are hoping to sell them to Iran and a number of NATO nations.

• COBRA AMBER, COBRA ANGEL, COBRA BALL, COBRA DANE—the multi-beam phased array radar that has been installed in the Aleutians and elsewhere.

• COBRA JUDY—a shipboard phased array designed to track Soviet reentry vehicles at low altitudes.

• COBRA MIST and COBRA TALON—the latter is a ballistic missile tracking radar designed to observe Chinese ICBMs launched over the Pacific Ocean.

• COMPASS COPE—a remotely piloted reconnaissance drone developed by Boeing and Teledyne Ryan. The COMPASS series includes COMPASS COUNTER, COMPASS DART, COMPASS DAWN, COMPASS SAIL, and COMPASS TIE.

• CONELRAD—Control of Electromagnetic Radiation; not a hardware system but a national operational plan to minimize the use of electromagnetic radiation in the United States in the event of hostile attack.

• DIXIE CUP, a ballistic missile penetration decoy developed by Philco-Ford, which is shaped like a reentry vehicle and which radiates electronic jamming signals that will enable our ICBM's to enter the earth's atmosphere undetected.

• HARM—the Navy's Hypervelocity Anti-Radiation Missile, designed to knock out enemy surface-to-air missile guiding radars.

• PAVE PAWS—the Air Force Phased Array Warning System already described.

• PAVE PENNEY, PAVE SPIKE and PAVE TACK—other microwave and laser systems for Precision Acquisition of Vehicle Entry.

• SADRAM—Seek and Destroy Radar Assisted Mission; a technique developed by the Westinghouse people for locking airborne fire-control radar on to a hostile ground-based radar.

• SEPAK—Suspension of Expendable Penetration Aids by Kite.

This partial list is intended merely to give some idea of the vast and complex Department of Defense arsenal of electronic weaponry. However, in order to understand how vast and complex the department's biological problems are, one should return to the 1975 Tri-Service Bioeffects Research Program and the executive summary of it. For example, at the bottom of page 5 of the summary, beneath the heading "Data Gaps," is the following paragraph:

> There are essentially no data on the effects of Phased Array Radars such as the Army SAFEGUARD PAR, Navy PHOENIX system and the Air Force FPS–85, COBRA DANE, and PAVE PAWS systems. The latter system is funding biological effects research on this new evolving system. Lastly, there are no comprehensive long-term chronic effects data for major system frequencies and this area, due to its complexity, cost and long duration, is proposed for a Tri-Service cooperative program.

As might be expected, the proposed research plan goes into these "data gaps" at some additional length. For example, the first part of a section entitled "Specific Systems Impact" reads as follows:

> In addition to the many conventional EMR emitters which this program will support, several unique (one-of-a-kind) DOD systems have major program impact. Systems such as ELF, CONUS OTH-B Radar, the AN/FPS–85, PAVE PAWS, AWACS, and SAFE-GUARD PAR are of special concern because: (1) they serve or will serve high priority communications and aircraft and missile surveillance functions vital to national defense, (2) their physical size and/or high power propagation results in high power densities over large areas thus requiring formal submission of environmental impact statements, (3) operations personnel will be exposed to relatively high power densities (compared to previous systems operations) in so-called "near-field" zones where the E- and H-field energy transfer to man is not well understood, and (4) they operate over diverse frequency ranges posing unique questions concerning man's bio-response.

The authors of the 1975 research plan go on to say that the CONUS Over-The-Horizon Backscatter (OTH-B) radars, to be installed in Maine and in the Pacific Northwest, will operate in the

frequency range of from three to thirty megahertz, and are so powerful that they are expected to produce power densities of ten milliwatts per square centimeter or more at a distance of 2,200 feet from
the antenna. The report also reveals that as far back as 1974, studies
were conducted at the School of Aerospace Medicine at Brooks Air
Force Base, in Texas, which suggested that a safe level of exposure
to this radar might be fifty milliwatts per square centimeter. The
number is convenient since these radars (theoretically at least) could
not be allowed to go into operation otherwise. The following paragraph from the executive summary describes how the Air Force
research was used to persuade Maine residents that the OTH-B was
safe.

> The contractor (General Electric) has been selected to develop the
> prototype system (cost $40 million). The Air Force has performed
> EMR bioeffects studies for the OTH-B for several years and provided
> major inputs for preparation of Environmental Impact Statement
> (EIS), siting criteria, and operational procedures used during the pub-
> lic hearing at the sites in Maine.

In January 1977, *Aerospace Daily* announced that because of performance problems the OTH-B radar program was in trouble, and
that the construction of the prototype, near Moscow, Maine, would
be delayed. Whatever its performance problems, there is another
good reason for delaying construction of the OTH-B radar in Maine
—a reason not even hinted at by the Air Force. Early in 1976,
Professor Gandhi's studies showed that at frequencies of twenty-five
to twenty-six megahertz (which lie within the frequency range of the
OTH-B and which can penetrate deeply into tissue) the whole body
power deposition in an adult human subjected to ten milliwatts per
square centimeter—the power density expected to occur 2,200 feet
from the OTH-B antenna—may be 490 watts or more. Gandhi described this as "a truly large amount of absorption."

Later in their report, the authors of the research plan address the
troublesome problem of how to assess the health hazards posed by
the new phased array radars even as they are being installed and put
into operation:

> High powered phased array systems such as the AN/FPS-85, an
> operational spacetrack radar currently modified for an SLBM mis-

sion, the Cobra Dane system nearing operational status, and the Pave Paws/Seek Sail systems in initial development stages, pose new questions concerning personnel exposures. These systems are physically large, energize thousands of operational elements, are electronically steered at high search rates, and operate at a frequency range having a maximum whole body energy transfer to man and for which little bioeffects data exists. . . . Additional experimental protocols will be developed using inputs and subsequent program direction will be coordinated with the Pave Paws/Seek Sail SPO. Field measurements will be performed at the FPS–85 site to obtain a more meaningful understanding of personnel exposure profiles.

This is another way of saying that, in addition to rodents, human beings will be used to assess the health hazards posed by exposure to the radiation emanating from the FPS-85, Cobra Dane, and PAVE PAWS radars. Let us now examine how this prospect has been foisted upon the residents of Cape Cod, who will soon be exposed to radiation emanating from the Raytheon PAVE PAWS now under construction at Otis Air Force Base, in Barnstable County. In March 1976, the Air Force Systems Command at Hanscom Air Force Base, near Boston, issued an Environmental Assessment for the PAVE PAWS system, which said that there would be no serious adverse environmental or biological effects from the radar. In addition, the Air Force assured officials of the towns surrounding the proposed radar site that PAVE PAWS would bring jobs and income to Cape Cod, which has a high rate of unemployment. What the Air Force did not tell these officials, and what it conveniently omitted from the assessment, was the fact that eight months earlier the authors of the Tri-Service Bioeffects Research Program (who included Colonel Godden of the Air Force) had admitted that there were essentially no data on the biological effects of phased array radars such as PAVE PAWS.

Bearing this admission in mind, the Environmental Assessment makes for some rather interesting and informative reading. PAVE PAWS is a six-story, 105-foot-high edifice measuring 100 feet by 150 feet at the base. When completed, the two angled facades of the structure that look out over Cape Cod toward the Atlantic will contain 3600 radiating elements in phased array. The main beam emanating from PAVE PAWS will be a combination of all of these radiating elements; it will scan 240 degrees; it will be aimed 3 degrees above the horizon; and it will be powerful enough to detect submarine-launched ballistic missiles at a distance of more than 2500 nautical miles.

According to the Air Force, PAVE PAWS has a frequency of between 425 and 450 megahertz. It will operate at a peak power of 700 kilowatts and at an average power of 140 kilowatts. Forty percent of its radiating power will be used for detecting SLBMs; sixty percent will be used for target tracking and space object identification. The assessment says that a fenced-off radiation hazard zone with a radius of 1000 feet will surround the installation and "prevent personnel and wildlife from entering the biological hazard zone." It also says that, at a distance of 3000 feet, the main beam of the radar will generate a power density of ten milliwatts per square centimeter, but that the average power density will be much less because the radar is constantly scanning.

Without knowing more about the characteristics of the beam and the manner in which PAVE PAWS will be operated, it is not possible to estimate how much radiation will be present at ground level 3000 feet from the radar, or at a distance of 3500 feet, where there is a mile-long stretch of the Mid-Cape Highway. Nor is it possible to estimate how much radiation will be present at ground level in the towns of Sandwich and Sagamore, which are situated about a mile to the north, or in Hyannisport, which is about fourteen miles to the southeast. There are, however, instruments that will measure this.

As is often the case with such reports, the authors of the Environmental Assessment choose to be optimistic about the safety of PAVE PAWS. They also manage to be somewhat contradictory. On page 44, they say that "objects in the air such as birds or aircraft will not receive enough radiation for a sufficient period of time to be considered harmful, due to the sporadic nature of the beam," and that "aircraft with metal skin offers additional shielding to the passengers." Later, they include as an appendix an earlier survey stating that "it would be necessary to restrict non-metallic aircraft with passengers having cardiac pacemakers from flying closer than 1.7 miles to the site." Nowhere in the assessment do they suggest how this restriction is to be accomplished. Nor do they consider the possibility that passengers in metallic aircraft may be sitting next to windows.

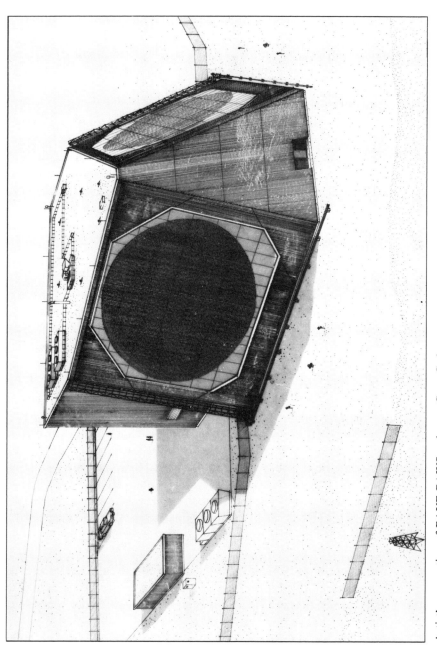

Artist's conception of PAVE PAWS radar on Cape Cod. COURTESY OF U.S. AIR FORCE

The authors of the assessment are preoccupied with the well-being of birds. (Apparently the Air Force wishes to avoid alarming the Audubon Society.) On page 24, they say that "birds will continue to use the forested area surrounding the radar installation, and very likely will fly through the biological hazard zone," but that "since the radar beam will not dwell at any spot for more than a fraction of a second, the possibility of an energy accumulation sufficient to cause tissue damage in wildlife is slight." Later, they include the preliminary draft of a 1975 report which says that "birds may fly into the direct beam of the radar," but that "the danger to birds is thought to be minimal except at close range." A few sentences later, the report says that birds are so tolerant of the phased array radar at Eglin Air Force Base in Florida, that "they can sit on the radar face without any noticeable harmful effects."

This last bit of reassurance is not only gratuitous but downright misleading. For one thing, the observation clearly has little biological significance unless the Air Force has performed follow-up studies of such birds. Also, since the face of any phased array radar consists of many radiating elements, it is entirely possible that a bird could sit on one of them and be irradiated only by a very low power density emanating from that single element. But how would the same bird fare if it were to fly in front of the radar at the point where the radiations of all of the operational elements are combined to form a main beam so powerful that it is dangerous out to thousands of feet? The answer is, of course, poorly.

Still later in their report, the authors return to the subject of birds, citing some laboratory studies performed in the late sixties, which showed that in certain test situations birds will try to avoid microwave radiation. They then say, "according to this evidence, our judgment is that . . . migrating birds will avoid the radar proposed at Otis Air Force Base and therefore the radar should not pose any threat to avian species."

Returning to page 44 of the assessment, one learns that, in accordance with the ANSI standard, officials at the Air Force School of Aerospace Medicine at Brooks Air Force Base, in Texas, have determined that a radiation power density of ten milliwatts per square centimeter can be withstood for six minutes without adverse biological effects, and that a power density of sixty milliwatts per square centimeter can be withstood for one minute with no harmful effects.

The assessment then says, "these effects are not cumulative," which, of course, is nothing more than wishful thinking on the part of the Air Force.

If the town fathers of Sandwich, Sagamore, Bourne, Barnstable, Falmouth, Hyannis, and Mashpee had taken the trouble to read and to study the Air Force Environmental Assessment, they might have entertained sufficient doubts about the safety of PAVE PAWS to call for public hearings. This, in turn, would have compelled the Air Force to issue a formal environmental impact statement and, perhaps, to tell the world just how it knows for sure that the effects of microwave radiation are not cumulative. Instead, at the invitation of the Air Force, the town fathers attended a meeting where they were told, in effect, that PAVE PAWS would be a good thing for Cape Cod and the country. Some citizens of Yuba County, California, were not so gullible. In the summer of 1977, they filed suit in United States District Court in Sacramento to halt construction of the PAVE PAWS at Beale Air Force Base, charging that the Air Force violated the National Environmental Policy Act by failing to file an environmental impact statement.

On June 11, 1975, Captain Tyler, Colonel Godden, Lieutenant Colonel Dodd, and Lieutenant Colonel Blasco sent the executive summary of the Tri-Service Electromagnetic Radiation Research Plan to the Assistant Director for Environmental and Life Sciences of the Office of the Director of Defense Research and Engineering (DR&E), within the DOD. At that time, the director of DR&E was Dr. Malcolm R. Currie, often described as the Pentagon's top scientist. (Dr. Currie would later be reprimanded and fined by the Department of Defense when it came to light that he had accepted a trip to Bimini in an aircraft belonging to the Rockwell International Corporation, whose Condor air-to-surface missile system he was supposed to evaluate and either approve or reject for production.) Dr. Currie is no longer at the Pentagon. He has, as the *New York Sunday Times* put it, "rejoined the Hughes Aircraft Company, for which he was instrumental in getting contracts while in Government service." The newspaper went on to point out that Dr. Currie's employment history is legal and not unusual. "Policy-making circles in many Federal agencies, and in the Defense Department especially, are largely populated by business executives in midcareer," the

Times account continued. "The phenomenon is commonly called the revolving door; a common charge is that the practice involves inherent conflict of interest."

There is hardly anything new about the revolving-door syndrome. Or, for that matter, about the military–electronics industry complex. It is part of the same complex with the same modus operandi—the business-as-usual-trade-off—that President Eisenhower warned the nation about in 1959. The phrase, so often used, deserves new definition. What, for example, in addition to the Department of Defense, does the military-industrial complex actually consist of? To begin with, it encompasses a significant portion of the entire private enterprise system. However, one can get some idea of its dimensions by glancing over the Department of Defense's annual list of top-ranking defense contractors. In fiscal year 1976, the first dozen firms were, in order: McDonnell Douglas Corporation, Lockheed Aircraft Corporation, Northrup Corporation, General Electric, United Technologies, Boeing, General Dynamics, Grumman, Litton Industries, Rockwell International, Hughes Aircraft, and Raytheon. As for the Pentagon's top dozen research and development contractors, they were: Rockwell International, with $606 million in R & D contracts; Lockheed Missile & Space Company, with $599 million; General Dynamics, with $446 million; and then Boeing, General Electric, McDonnell Douglas, Hughes Aircraft, Raytheon, RCA, TRW, Northrup, and Westinghouse, in that order.

Strange as it may seem at first glance, Johns Hopkins University ranked fifty-fifth, and the Massachusetts Institute of Technology ranked sixtieth in the list of the top hundred defense contractors. What are these institutions doing on such a list? The answer is that, together with the Aerospace Corporation, the Mitre Corporation, and the Rand Corporation, the Pentagon has designated the Applied Physics Laboratory at Johns Hopkins and MIT's Lincoln Laboratory as Federal Research Contract Centers. It has given the same designation to the Center for Naval Analyses at the University of Rochester and to the Applied Research Laboratory of Pennsylvania State University. Thus has the military-industrial complex grown to include not only most of the nation's leading corporations, but some of its most respected institutions of learning as well.

Apparently, very few members of Congress paid much attention to Eisenhower's chilling prophecy about the military-industrial complex, and those who did listen have apparently forgotten it and gone about their business as usual. For a lesson in the fine congressional art of rubber-stamp, one has only to browse through the House and Senate Defense Appropriations Committee hearings for research and development for fiscal year 1977. (The House subcommittee was chaired by Representative George M. Mahon, of Texas, and the Senate committee by Senator John L. McClellan, of Arkansas.) Particularly interesting is the testimony given before these committees in February and March 1976 by Dr. Currie and by Dr. George H. Helmeier, director of the Defense Advanced Research Projects Agency. Not once was either of these top Pentagon officials (or, for that matter, any of the dozens of other witnesses from the Department of Defense) asked a single question by any member of Congress about the possible health hazards posed by the military's vast electronic arsenal. (Indeed, the only time the subject was even mentioned was on March 30, when Senator Gaylord Nelson, of Wisconsin, appeared before McClellan's committee to object to the Navy's proceeding with Project Seafarer until its biological and environmental impact could be determined.)

Thanks to this dumbfounding deference to the Department of Defense, the military was given a free hand to continue its cover-up of the health hazards posed by microwave radiation to the general population. The Congress—supposed protector of the people—in this whole affair resembles a hooded bird tethered to the wrist of a falconer. Every once in a while, the bird flaps its wings; occasionally it is unhooded; and every so often it is allowed to fly off and snare a pigeon. Most of the time, however, the bird is content to roost quietly upon the falconer's wrist. The falconer—the military-industrial complex that Eisenhower warned the nation about nearly twenty years ago—has by this time largely tamed the Congress, and he is a falconer who now bids fair to rule the land.

20

Some Further Unraveling

As is so often the case with such documents, the executive summary of the draft proposed research plan that was forwarded through channels on June 11, 1975, by Captain Tyler, Colonel Godden, Lieutenant Colonel Dodd, and Lieutenant Colonel Blasco, of the Tri-Service Electromagnetic Radiation Advisory Panel, was as interesting for what it omitted as for what it included. For example, the summary contained not a single word about the biological effects of electromagnetic pulse (EMP), which had been under development since the early 1970s as a super-secret weapon. As it happens, however, EMP was discussed several times in the proposed research plan from which the summary was drawn. The first reference provides a review of the EMP situation as it was left in Chapter 12:

> In February 1974, DOL [Department of Labor] requested information on the need to develop and promulgate an occupational health standard for Electromagnetic Pulse (EMP). This action was in response to a petition submitted by the Boeing Company, an Air Force

contractor assessing the vulnerability of weapon systems to EMP. Data from Air Force and AFRRI [Armed Forces Radiobiology Research Institute] research studies and some epidemiological data indicated no evidence to date that EMP exposures have resulted in adverse effects. This information was forwarded to DOL with a strong recommendation to not propose an EMP health standard. DOL has indicated they will reject the Boeing petition and not propose an EMP standard at this time. A personal injury claim (alleged EMP and laser effects) for $890,000 filed by a Boeing employee against the Air Force is expected to publicize the EMP question again and pressure DOL to reconsider the development of an EMP health standard.

The second time EMP was mentioned in the research plan occurred in the next-to-last line of a table describing the operating characteristics of special military electromagnetic radiation transmitters. (The last line described a highly classified directed-energy weapons system known as HEP, which stands for High Energy Pulse.) Toward the end of the summary, EMP was discussed again, but this time in a fashion both bizarre and ambiguous. "Another specialized area with high visibility within DOD that must be studied is that of possible biological effects subsequent to exposures to Electromagnetic Pulse (EMP)," the authors of the plan declared. "This is a unique situation involving multiple frequency bursts of very narrow pulse widths with rapid rise times. EMP is used to simulate the effect of nuclear weapons on existing electromagnetic system components and determine if there are deleterious effects on man."

Deleterious effects on man? Of nuclear weapons? Surely not what the authors had in mind. No, indeed, for this was only a draft proposal of the research plan and the grammar needed to be straightened out. The authors intended to say that EMP was being used to simulate the possibly deleterious effects on man of the brief but immense surges of radio-frequency and microwave radiation—sometimes called radio flash—which accompany nuclear explosions. But why simulate the deleterious effects of that, since, as everybody knows by now—especially the citizens of Hiroshima and Nagasaki —it is the radioactive fallout from any nuclear explosion which has such a devastating effect upon human health and life?

The answer to this question provides the answer to many questions. It explains why the authors of the research plan declared that "the effect of prolonged and repeated exposure to HEP must be investigated," even though no mention of either electromagnetic pulse or high-energy pulse was made in the executive summary forwarded to Dr. Currie's office. (Currie, of course, knew all about them since the Defense Advanced Research Projects Agency, the Navy, and the Air Force had for more than three years been hard at work developing them for special weapons systems.) It may well explain the motive behind the Soviet irradiation of the American Embassy in Moscow. It could possibly explain the murder of three American electronics technicians in the streets of Teheran in the summer of 1976. It certainly explains much of the feverish satellite activity going on in space, as well as some of the dire predictions being made that the Soviet Union is on its way to achieving a lead in space warfare techniques. It undoubtedly explains the deep reluctance of Congress, in typical see-no-evil-hear-no-evil fashion, to become involved in the whole microwave affair. It particularly explains why the Navy became deeply enmeshed in electromagnetic pulse research during the early 1970s. Indeed, it marks the beginning of the final unraveling of the microwave mystery and the cover-up behind it.

As the reader knows, EMP was first used in the 1960s to determine the effects of the electric fields accompanying nuclear explosions on the warheads and guidance-and-control systems of the nation's thousand-odd Minuteman intercontinental ballistic missiles in underground silos. Air Force Regulation 161–42, issued on November 7, 1975, contains the following description of EMP and these early tests:

> Nuclear explosions generally produce a short, intense electromagnetic pulse (EMP) which, depending on the altitude, can radiate over many hundreds of miles. This pulse is produced by a flow of Compton electrons generated in the atmosphere as the front of gamma rays from the burst interacts with air molecules. Because of the very short rise time [ten billionths of a second] and large amplitudes of the EMP, large voltages and currents can be induced in conductors exposed to the electromagnetic fields. It was found in the early phases of nuclear weapons testing that cables and electronic test equipment could be upset or damaged by the energy contained in the EMP; hence EMP represents a threat to communications systems, missile guidance devices, computers, etc.
>
> The understanding of EMP, its interaction with weapons systems

and the prevention of damage, has, therefore, been a matter of great importance and concern in national defense. The restrictions on atmospheric testing have made it necessary to construct simulators of an electromagnetic environment relatable to that produced by this type explosion for the empirical investigation of military hardware, ranging from small electronic components to large missiles, airplanes, and ships.

Some of the information contained in Air Force Regulation 161–42 has been expanded upon in *EMP Radiation & Protective Techniques,* published in 1976 by John Wiley, New York, and written by L.W. Ricketts, a senior staff scientist at the Magnavox Company, of Fort Wayne, Indiana; by J. E. Bridges, a senior engineering adviser at the ITT Research Institute, in Chicago; and by J. Miletta, of the Harry Diamond Laboratory, in Washington, D.C. In a fascinating opening chapter, much of which they acknowledged was taken from the Defense Nuclear Agency's *EMP Awareness Course Notes,* the authors wrote as follows:

> The fundamental mechanism of EMP generation involves an energy transformation process. Essentially, a small fraction of the nuclear energy is transformed by several intermediary steps into energy in the radio-frequency electromagnetic spectrum. The first step in the conversion is the release of gamma rays during a nuclear detonation. Next, the gamma rays interact with the atmosphere or other materials to produce electrons and positive ions. This separation of charge translates some of the energy of the gamma rays into energy associated with moving charges and electromagnetic fields. The region where the gamma rays interact with the atmosphere is called the *source region.* The flow of electrons in this source region constitutes a current that can radiate electromagnetic energy, provided that some asymmetry in the current flow exists.

The authors then contrast the electromagnetic pulse radiating from near-surface or lower atmospheric nuclear bursts—those that might occur anywhere from ground level to an altitude of twenty kilometers above earth—with EMP radiating from exoatmospheric or high-altitude nuclear explosions—those occurring fifty kilometers or more above the surface of the earth:

> In a near-surface burst, the hemispherically shaped source region is typically several miles in diameter. The asymmetrical shape of the

source region causes potentially degrading EMP fields to be radiated a few tens of miles beyond the burst point. The dense atmosphere near the earth's surface restricts the range of the gamma rays and limits the size of the source region. The extent of the source region coincides roughly with that of the region where most of the other severe prompt nuclear weapon effects occur. Thus, in an atmospheric burst, the EMP always occurs with these other prompt effects.

On the other hand, if the weapon is detonated outside the atmosphere, the gamma rays can travel many hundreds of miles before encountering an air molecule. In addition, because the air is so thin, a significant fraction of the gamma rays can penetrate well into the atmosphere. A high-yield weapon under these circumstances can create a source region over 1000 miles in diameter and about 12 miles thick, having a lower limit at about 60,000 ft. in altitude. The presence of the earth's magnetic field in this source region causes the asymmetrical current flow that efficiently converts the electromagnetic energy in the source region into a radiated downward-traveling EMP wave.

The writers went on to point out that "the large size of the source region of exoatmospheric bursts causes high-level EMP to be radiated downward over a large fraction of the earth's surface." A figure map illustrated just how large a fraction, showing that high-level EMP from a nuclear explosion occurring 50 miles above the Iowa-Nebraska-South Dakota border would irradiate an area whose circumference would extend through Saskatchewan, Manitoba, Ontario, Ohio, Louisiana, Texas, Utah, and Montana; and that a nuclear bomb detonated 120 miles above this spot would send a powerful electromagnetic pulse upon the entire North American continent. "Of significance is the great range of severe EMP exposure," they wrote.

> Of almost equal impact is the fact that this EMP *is not accompanied to a noticeable degree by other prompt nuclear weapon effects.* Thus systems, both civilian and military, that would not normally be expected to be targets or near-likely targets for nuclear bombs can experience severe EMP exposure from nuclear attacks on distant targets. This severe EMP exposure can burn out sensitive electronic and electrical components associated with large antennas or exposed conductors such as power lines. The EMP can also introduce massive disruption into digital processing or control circuits, often without permanent degradation effects. Thus the effects of EMP from a high-altitude nuclear burst must be considered for all electrical and elec-

tronic systems. If the systems are important, suitable countermeasures or hardening must be employed.

Small wonder that in 1968 the Department of Defense became concerned about the effect of electromagnetic pulse upon the nation's billions of dollars worth of electronic weapons systems, and undertook to build EMP test facilities in a number of localities across the land.*The Air Force has operated EMP simulators at Kirtland Air Force Base, near Albuquerque, for at least ten years, and has recently completed work on Project Trestle, a large ramp-and-platform facility at Kirtland, which will be used to test the electronic systems of aircraft for their ability to withstand EMP. The Army maintains an EMP testing facility at its Mobility Research and Development Center at Fort Belvoir, Virginia, and another at the Harry Diamond Laboratory in Woodbridge, Virginia.

The Navy's Electromagnetic Pulse Radiation Environment Simulator for Ships (EMPRESS)—located on the Patuxent River at Solomons, Maryland, and designed and constructed by the ITT Research Institute, in 1972—employs an electromagnetic pulser capable of putting out two and a half million volts. EMPRESS is used not only to irradiate ships, but also missiles and airplanes. EMP simulators for studying biological effects are maintained at the Navy Weapons Laboratory at Dahlgren, Virginia, and at the Armed Forces Radiobiology Research Institute, in Bethesda, Maryland. Other EMP facilities are operated by Martin-Marietta at Orlando, Florida; by ITT at Crystal Lake, Illinois; and by the University of Denver at Cherry Creek, Colorado.

Considering the massive disruption caused by electromagnetic pulse in electronic systems, the Department of Defense soon became interested in the possibility that the pulses being used to simulate secondary effects of nuclear explosions might themselves become potent weapons. From then on the Defense Advanced Research Projects Agency, the Air Force, and the Navy plunged into development of a number of so-called directed-energy weapons systems—the phrase applies to high-energy pulse weapons, charged-particle beam devices, and high-energy lasers—with the Navy taking the lead since

---

*An additional reason for this concern was undoubtedly the fact that shortly after lift-off, on November 14, 1969, some important electronic equipment on Apollo 12 was put out of commission when the spacecraft was struck by lightning.

EMP had raised serious doubts about the survivability of the Minuteman missiles in their underground silos.

In order to understand the nature of directed-energy weapons systems, as well as some of the problems inherent in their development, one must go back to a symposium on the Biomedical Aspects of Non-Ionizing Radiation, held on July 10, 1973, at the Naval Weapons Laboratory, in Dahlgren, Virginia, and attended by nearly 150 people. Some of the attendees, by now familiar to readers of this book, were Colonel Appleton, of Walter Reed Army Hospital; Dr. Alfred Bruner, of the Lovelace Foundation; Janet Healer of the President's Office of Telecommunications Policy; Professor Michaelson, of the University of Rochester; Dr. Osepchuck, of the Raytheon Corporation; Dr. Pollack, of the Electromagnetic Radiation Management Advisory Council; Professor Schwan, of the University of Pennsylvania; Dr. Sharp, of the Walter Reed Army Institute of Research; and three members of the Tri-Service Electromagnetic Radiation Advisory Panel—Colonel Godden, Lieutenant Colonel Dodd, and Captain Tyler.

As things turned out, the opening address of the symposium was delivered by Captain Tyler, who, after a passing mention of EMP, declared that scientists at the Naval Weapons Laboratory had a unique opportunity "to do basic research along with the hardware development," so that "when such systems are introduced into the fleet for operational use, we can at the same time provide the fleet with information on how they can best utilize the system and also provide adequate protection and safety for their personnel." Captain Tyler was followed by Professor Schwan, who spoke in defense of the ten-milliwatt standard, and he was followed by Professor Michaelson, who assured the audience that "as of now it appears that the major, if not the only effect of microwaves is due to thermal conversion." Professor Michaelson was followed by Dr. Dietrich E. Beischer, a German scientist during World War II, who proceeded to describe some now-discontinued experiments he had been conducting since March 1970 on human volunteers, who were being irradiated with low-intensity electromagnetic energy, including extra-low-frequency radio waves and microwaves, at the Naval Aerospace Research Laboratory, in Pensacola, Florida, in order to determine why the Soviet safe level of exposure limit was one thousand times less than our own. "By far the most important and unique advantage of the approach presented in this report is that the exquisitely complex and dynamic nature of the living human organism is automatically taken into account in the proper perspective," Dr. Beischer declared. "Direct measurement of the reflection and transmission of microwave energy by human subjects will provide information concerning the interaction of man in a microwave environment that can be obtained in no other way."

But it was none of these men who provided the high point of the symposium at Dahlgren; that distinction was taken hands down by Dr. M. F. Rose, of the Naval Weapons Laboratory, who chose to speak about high-power pulse transmitters. Dr. Rose began by telling his audience that a group of transmitting devices had been developed which were different from the ordinary radio-frequency generators they were accustomed to use in their laboratory experiments. "It is primarily these that I want to talk about," Dr. Rose continued. "These devices represent the state-of-the-art in attainable power levels. They are primarily short-pulse, high power transmitters and, as you will see, they cover a rather large portion of the frequency spectrum."

After observing that the new transmitters "provide the means for some very interesting biological experiments," Dr. Rose went on to describe how they worked in some detail:

> You are all familiar with the normal devices that are used to generate radiofrequency—triodes, the klystrons, magnetrons and so forth. I do not want to deal with any of these except to perhaps summarize some of their performance characteristics toward the end of this paper. There are new devices, as I have mentioned, which generate power levels far in excess of those generated by conventional transmitters. Some of these are extensions of the techniques employed when radio was in its infancy. These LC [coil-condenser] oscillators give you rather large powers. Development of these Hertzian generators was essentially stopped when the vacuum tube was invented. But now an increase in the use of extreme power devices for such things as upper atmosphere mapping, electromagnetic testing, and short pulse radar have brought these devices out of hiding and into the research labs where significant R & D is being done to improve them for several applications. We are interested in the whole electromagnetic spectrum, because we find we produce pulses over a wide frequency range.

Concomitant with the production of high power is also high voltage, with the resultant danger from pure electrical shock. The second class of rather novel RF sources is the beam plasma devices, invented by NRL [Naval Research Laboratory].

The sweep of history and the scope of science contained in these observations by Dr. Rose were nothing short of breathtaking. In the first sentence, he covered all the major radio-frequency generating devices developed during the seventy-odd years that had passed since Lee De Forest invented the triode. Then, jumping all the way back to 1888, he announced that the new high-power pulse transmitters were similar to the original spark gap device that had been used by Heinrich Hertz to produce and detect the first man-made electromagnetic radiation. From there, Dr. Rose proceeded to give some vague but nontheless ominous hints about the uses to which these newly rediscovered, high-power pulsing devices might be put. And, finally—shades of Nikola Tesla, the electronic wizard who, in 1934, at the age of seventy-eight, claimed he knew how to invent a death beam capable of destroying enemy airplanes at a distance of 250 miles—Dr. Rose mentioned "a second class of rather novel RF sources"—beam plasma devices being developed at the Naval Research Laboratory, in Washington, D.C.—by which he meant nothing more or less than ship-mounted, high-energy pulse, charged-particle electron beam weapons capable of knocking aircraft from the sky, and of neutralizing incoming missile warheads at incredible distances.

It seems likely that some of Dr. Rose's listeners may have had neither the technological nor the military background to appreciate the implications of what he had told them, or, for that matter, of what he was about to tell them. It seems highly unlikely, however, that this could be said of the vast bulk of his audience, for they included representatives from the Office of the Chief of Naval Operations; the Naval Research Laboratory; the Naval Weapons Laboratory, the Naval Ordnance Laboratory; the Naval Space Surveillance System; the Naval Weapons Center; the Naval Air Systems Command; the Defense Nuclear Agency; the Nuclear Weapons Effects Laboratory; and the Central Intelligence Agency. At any rate, Dr. Rose proceeded to show his audience some slides, and to present them with an analogy of what the future radio-frequency environment on shipboard might be like:

> Just to illustrate something which I am sure you are aware of, take a look at the first figure. It is a friend to a lot of you in the Navy. She is the U.S.S. *Enterprise.* There are nearly a hundred radiators located on the island structure. There's any number of others in the aircraft that are normally aboard and there are whip antenna on the side and in the forward sections. In that relatively small area you might have as many as 200 radiating systems. Biological tests to date have helped to establish safety standards aboard ships. But the laboratory researcher who is making the next generation devices that will perhaps be in this environment may not have nearly enough safety standards to serve him. For example, researchers are probing the upper limits of RF power production for a given set of conditions. Figure 2 illustrates a calculation of what these limits are. Electric field strength in volts per centimeter is plotted as a function of altitude. At standard temperature and pressure, the breakdown strength of air is a function of pulse length. For extremely short pulses, the breakdown strength is greater than 100,000 volts per centimeter which is equivalent to roughly 10 million volts per meter. Experience dictates field strengths in practical structures to be near 3 million volts per meter.

As Dr. Hirsch had stated at the Lovelace Foundation's EMP conference in 1970, three million volts per meter was equivalent to the electric field accompanying a lightning stroke. When one considers that even as Dr. Rose was speaking, the Department of Labor was wrestling with the problem of what to do about the Boeing Company's petition requesting promulgation of an EMP exposure standard—a petition the Boeing people had filed because they were worried about an Air Force proposal to raise the EMP exposure level to a mere 50,000 volts per meter—one begins to comprehend the true extent of the electromagnetic radiation cover-up that was underway in the early seventies. One also begins to understand what went on at a meeting of the American National Standards Institute's (ANSI) C-95.4 subcommittee held in Boulder, Colorado, just one month before the symposium at Dahlgren. The C-95.4 subcommittee had been established by the institute to recommend safe levels for human exposure to electromagnetic radiation; it was being sponsored by the Navy and the Institute of Electrical and Electronics Engineers, Inc.; and it had been asked by the Department of Labor for advice on what to do about the Boeing petition. In order to respond to the department's request, the subcommittee formed a four-man working group to look into the EMP problem. Its members included Gerald Karches, of NIOSH; Dr. James W. Frazier, of the Air Force's School of Aerospace Medicine; Dr. Franz Bartl, director of occupational medicine at Boeing; and Professor Michaelson. These gentlemen agreed that the ten-milliwatt standard was not applicable to EMP; that the available data was too limited to set a meaningful EMP standard; that no acute effects had been observed in animals or humans exposed to EMP; and that no chronic effects had been noted. They then recommended that chronic occupational exposure levels for EMP should be maintained at ten thousand volts per meter for a continuous forty-hour work week; that acute exposure levels on an infrequent basis should not exceed fifty thousand volts per meter; and that the general public should not be subjected to chronic exposures of more than one thousand volts per meter, or to acute exposures of more than five thousand volts per meter.

In light of the fact that these were his recommendations at Boulder on June 5, one can only imagine what must have gone through Professor Michaelson's head at Dahlgren, on July 10, when he heard Dr. Rose suggest that EMP field strengths could soon be expected to reach three million volts per meter. For that matter, one can only imagine what thoughts occurred to the other people attending the Dahlgren symposium, who had also been present at the Boulder meeting. They, it turned out, included Captain Tyler, who, on August 4, 1972, had suggested that if EMP standards "must be set now, then try for as high a level as possible," for the simple reason that "if adverse effects are determined in the future, it is far easier to further lower the standards than to relax them." Other people who attended both meetings were H. Mark Grove and Dr. Joseph C. Sharp, of the Walter Reed Army Institute of Research; Arthur A. Riggs, of the Army Environmental Hygiene Agency; Lieutenant Raymond L. Chaput, of the Navy's Bureau of Medicine and Surgery; Earl B. Massengill, of the Naval Air Systems Command; Dr. Osepchuk, of Raytheon; and William W. Mumford, of the Electromagnetic Radiation Management Advisory Council, who, in October 1972, advised the chairman of the C-95.4 subcommittee in writing that "in view of the fact that Dr. Heller and his colleagues have observed chromosomal aberrations and genetic mutations at peak pulse voltage gradients of 300 volts per centimeter [30,000 volts per meter], we should probably suspect any gradients approaching this value as being potentially hazardous."

Whatever all these gentlemen may have thought about electrical field strengths of three million volts per meter, they soon had other things to think about, for Dr. Rose went on to give a description of high-power transmitters, which amounted to a blueprint for understanding how the new directed-energy weapons systems would work. He described Hertzian generators that were capable of producing pulses of fifty million watts of power. He described Marx generators capable of producing a high-voltage, short-pulse electron beam with so much energy—several millions of electron volts—that it traveled close to the speed of light, producing microwave radiation at several frequencies simultaneously, as well as intense bursts of X-rays. He also described the travitron—a cylindrical-waveguide generating device equipped with a series of spark switches, and designed to combine the power of a series of spark discharges into a single electromagnetic pulse—which could, in fact, become the very heart of a directed-energy weapons system. And then, after passing quickly over the EMP simulators used to test the electronic systems of Minuteman missiles, Dr. Rose ended his talk with a brief comment concerning the possible health implications of the new weapons. "In summary, I have described two classes of experimental radiators which produce high power levels," he said. "Because of the nature of these devices and the fact that they are experimental, personnel working near them could be exposed to power levels and pulse shapes for which biological studies have not been made."

Concerning the biological effects of EMP, the people who attended the Dahlgren symposium heard three investigators from the Armed Forces Radiobiology Research Institute—Dr. S. J. Baum, Lieutenant Commander Wesley D. Skidmore, and Captain Merlin E. Ekstrom—describe an experiment they had conducted, which produced no changes in bone-marrow cells, chromosome structure, or lymphocytes in rodents that had been exposed to electromagnetic pulses with a peak electric field intensity of 447,000 volts per meter. The three men also found that exposure to EMP fields did not induce the onset of leukemia in a strain of mice that were known to spontaneously develop the disease when they were between six and twelve months old. Their reason for conducting this experiment was "to determine whether exposure of personnel to an EMP field could trigger the onset of leukemia, particularly in leukemia-prone individuals"—a motive obviously triggered by the onset of leukemia in Boeing employees and other people who had been exposed to EMP at the missile sites in Montana. As for their conclusions, the three scientists from the Radiobiology Research Institute said that "it is difficult to predict from the present data whether exposure to EMP could increase the incidence of malignancies in personnel working in an electromagnetic field," and that "this must await further studies during the second half of life of the experimental rodents."

The cancers that had developed in the Boeing employees had already been taken care of by no less an office of authority than the President's Office of Telecommunications Policy. This had occurred on March 14, 1973, in a letter sent to Silvio Patti, chief of the Electronic and Electrical Branch of the Department of Labor's Occupational Safety and Health Administration, by W. Dean, Jr., who identified himself as Assistant Director for Frequency Management of the O.T.P. Dean's letter read:

> It has come to my attention that you are considering the need for a protection guide on Electromagnetic Pulse (the simulation of pulses accompanying nuclear detonations in the atmosphere). As you may know, this Office has responsibility for management of the radio spectrum on behalf of the Federal Government. We are advised in this capacity by the Interdepartment Radio Advisory Committee (IRAC).
>
> It is our view that at this time there is not sufficient evidence to justify establishing an EMP standard. This conclusion is concurred in by the IRAC. A summary of the more detailed views of the Side Effects Working Group of the IRAC Technical Subcommittee is contained in the Attachment.

The attachment, it turned out, was an interesting document. In the fourth paragraph, for example, the members of the Side Effects Working Group wrote:

> The evidence at hand indicates a substantial margin of safety for EMP generators in existence, or currently under design considerations, if the suggested criteria and procedures are followed. The margin, in fact, may be too conservative since there is little concrete evidence which suggests effects or damage to biological systems fol-

lowing repeated exposures to levels considerably above the proposed guideline. The caveat in interpretation of available data are: (1) in the Air Force's report of work done at both the Lovelace Foundation and the Boeing Company; and (2) the observation that three Boeing employees who have been exposed to simulated EMP's have developed abnormal cellular proliferations. In the first instance, there is mention of increases of bilirubin and uric acid ("gout" in the Boeing report). In the second, one case each of lymphatic leukemia, myeloid leukemia, and skin carcinoma have been diagnosed. To date there has been no cause-and-effect relationship demonstrated in any of these observations and "best judgment" of officials associated with these observations or cases minimizes the possibility of a relationship.

It is not clear just who the "officials" associated with these "observations" were, let alone how or on what basis they arrived at their "best judgment" that the "caveat" in the studies conducted by the Lovelace Foundation and the Boeing Company could be dismissed. However, it is known who the thirty-five members of the Side Effects Working Group of the Interdepartment Radio Advisory Committee were. (The IRAC was established in 1922 and it is made up of radio frequency management representatives of principal government agencies engaged in use of the frequency spectrum, who now serve as advisors to the President's Office of Telecommunications Policy.) They included John Villforth, director of the FDA's Bureau of Radiological Health, and Dr. Sharp, of the Walter Reed Army Institute of Research, as well as people from the Naval Weapons Laboratory at Dahlgren; from the Naval Ship Engineering Center at Hyattsville, Maryland; and from the Naval Research Laboratory, in Arlington, Virginia, where work was proceeding at a feverish pace to perfect a traveling-wave accelerator for use in directed-energy weapons systems. The Navy was also represented by Stephen Caine, of the Naval Electronics Systems Command, who also happened to be Secretary of the American National Standards Institute's C-95 Committee on Radio-Frequency Hazards, and who had written a letter on August 17, 1972, advising Sava I. Sherr, director of the Standards Office of the Institute of Electrical and Electronics Engineers, Inc., that if EMP standards "must be set now, it is recommended that they be set as high as possible," so that "if adverse effects are determined in the future, it will be far easier to lower the standards than to relax them."

Caine's advice to Sherr on August 17 was, of course, practically word for word the advice that had been given to Caine's committee on August 4 by Captain Tyler. And, as things turned out, it just so happened that the Secretary of the Side Effects Working Group was none other than Captain Tyler. Moreover, a fellow member of the working group was none other than Colonel Dodd (then a major), who would soon become Captain Tyler's colleague on the Tri-Service Electromagnetic Radiation Advisory Panel. But for sheer coincidence—indeed, the last link in this ring-around-the-rosy—one only needs to know that still another member of the Side Effects Working Group was none other than Silvio Patti, of the Department of Labor, who had received the letter from W. Dean, of the Office of Telecommunications Policy, advising him that in the OTP's view there was not enough evidence to justify establishing an EMP standard, and informing him that this conclusion was concurred in by the Interdepartment Radio Advisory Committee's Side Effects Working Group, of which—to complete a round of resounding redundancy—Patti happened to be a member.

21

A New Game of Gap

It will be no surprise to the reader to learn that since the Dahlgren symposium almost no information concerning the biological effects of EMP has been made public. Indeed, for more than four years, the entire subject of electromagnetic pulse has been muted at microwave conferences and all but banished from scientific literature. As for EMP studies being conducted at the Naval Weapons Laboratory at Dahlgren, nothing more was heard of them, except for one brief description in the OTP's 1974 projects résumé. That was of a study just begun of the effects of EMP on the blood chemistry and sleeping time of the Dutch rabbit.

Meanwhile, down at the Naval Aerospace Laboratory, in Pensacola, Dr. Beischer was still at work on human volunteers. His experiments had begun in March 1970 and were not scheduled to be completed until June 1978, but they seemed to be producing results, judging from the OTP's 1974 projects résumé, which said that "exposure of naval personnel to microwave radiation is an acute problem," and that "even low doses are likely to reduce the efficiency of personnel in vital duty positions." Indeed, not long after these findings were indicated, Beischer's studies were discontinued.

Putting this all together, one sees that the biological effects of microwave radiation and electromagnetic pulse were being scrutinized at a snail's pace at Dahlgren, while intense activity went on elsewhere in the Department of Defense to develop microwaves, EMP, and other high-energy pulses (HEP) for use in directed-energy weapons systems. The military objective of this charade was simple: it bought time for the Department of Defense to develop and present as a *fait accompli*—even an absolute necessity—to the Congress and the American people an arsenal of directed-energy weapons. At the same time, DOD could claim to have carefully studied the biological effects of microwaves, EMP, and HEP during this period and to have found none that could be considered hazardous to human health.

In order to convince Congress and the people that directed-energy weapons are essential to the national security, the Department of Defense has found it necessary to invent "directed-energy gap"—a new version of the old game of "bomber gap" and "missile gap." The Department now claims that the Soviet Union is far ahead in the race to develop directed-energy weapons, and that since this technological lead threatens our capability to launch a retaliatory strike, it threatens the very life of our nation. The game is, of course, designed to fool the Soviets as much as the Congress and the American people, and it is played by leaking information to various segments of the press over a period of time.

Regarding directed-energy weapons, these leaks began back in the autumn of 1975, when considerable publicity was given to reports that the Soviets had used high-energy lasers to "blind" the infrared sensors of U.S. Air Force early warning satellites. An article that appeared in the January–February 1976 issue of *Electronic Warfare* speculated that the Soviets might have accomplished this feat with a land-based, long-range infrared laser. It went on to quote one analyst as saying that "the USSR has the capability of rendering warning satellites temporarily useless, which 'necessarily invalidates the existent SALT edifice.' "

Since the summer of 1976, there has been a steady stream of stories about (and denials of) various Soviet breakthroughs in space weaponry. The August 2, 1976 edition of *Aviation Week &*

Space Technology announced that the effects of pulsed laser radiation on solar cells would be investigated by TRW under a $213,000 contract awarded by the Air Force Propulsion Laboratory. The magazine went on to say that the Defense Department "has denied that anomalies detected by a U.S. early warning satellite last fall were caused by Soviet lasers, but the incident has spurred investigation into the consequences of laser radiation on spacecraft solar cells and sensors."

On September 3, *Science* published an article by Deborah Shapley, who said that after a four-year hiatus the Soviet Union had resumed the testing of "killer" satellites which could threaten vital U.S. reconnaissance, military, and navigational satellites. According to Shapley, this development posed a serious problem for the nation's space policy makers. "If the United States adopts a more active military stance, a number of programs, most of them highly classified, could receive a boost," she wrote. "An example is the $27 million high-energy laser research sponsored by the Advanced Research Projects Agency (ARPA), which in recent years has been redirected toward outer space applications—largely against other satellites ('but we're not building a satellite to put laser weapons in space,' protests one ARPA official)."

Scarcely had this protest been published than the October–November 1976 issue of *Microwave Systems News* hit the stands with an article by its Pentagon correspondent, John Rhea. Rhea wrote that "George H. Heilmeier, director of Defense Advanced Research Projects Agency (DARPA), which oversees the entire HEL [high-energy laser] effort, has left no doubt that the program is oriented toward lasers in space." Indeed, Rhea quoted Heilmeier as telling Congress that "we are requesting funds to continue to develop both chemical and visible laser technology for space applications." Rhea went on to point out that an antiballistic missile system in space had first been suggested and studied during the early 1960s and that development of such a system had now become possible because of new laser and space technology, and because "the Air Force also will have a platform for a space-based ABM system in the reusable Space Shuttle being developed jointly with NASA." After describing Deputy Defense Secretary William Clement's warning that "the Soviet Union could be developing orbiting laser weapons capable of knocking out U.S. ICBMs at launch," Rhea wrote:

The fact that top U.S. officials are attributing this capability to the Soviets is a subtle way of warning them that the U.S. is developing a capability itself, in the opinion of Peter Schwartz, a policy analyst at Stanford Research Institute (home of the top secret Jason Committee that is reviewing the HEL and directed energy programs). The Soviets have nothing comparable to the Space Shuttle and therefore would have to use other, less efficient means to orbit an ABM system.

The Soviets do have a strong high energy laser program, and Dr. Malcolm Currie, director of defense research and engineering, has warned that "they are leading us in some areas" during Congressional testimony.

During the autumn of 1976, high-energy lasers appeared to be much on Dr. Currie's mind. In October, he outlined the government's HEL program at a secret meeting in San Diego, which was reported to have been attended by representatives from many of the top-ranking firms in the military-industrial complex. (In August 1975, *Aviation Week* had listed the nation's leading high-energy laser firms as United Technologies Corporation, Hughes Aircraft, Avco Everett Research Laboratory, TRW Systems, Northrup, and Rockwell's Rocketdyne Division.) On November 10, 1976, Dr. Currie spoke about high-energy lasers at the Institute of Electrical and Electronics Engineers' International Pulsed Power Conference, in Lubbock, Texas. The United States, he said, would not be able to assess the weapons potential of HEL devices until the end of the decade. And on November 18, Dr. Currie was the featured speaker at a classified conference that was held at the Air Force Academy, in Colorado Springs, and attended by eight hundred representatives from major aerospace contractors. Also in attendence were personnel from the Air Force Special Weapons Laboratory, the Army Missile Command, the Naval Research Laboratory, the Naval Sea Systems Command, MIT's Lincoln Laboratory, the Advanced Research Projects Agency, the Central Intelligence Agency, and the National Security Agency.

On November 24, the *New York Times* published a story by John W. Finney, which said that "the Defense Department has been watching with growing concern a long-term Soviet program to develop hunter-killer satellites for destroying other satellites, a step that some Pentagon Officials fear could extend warfare into space." Finney went on to say that the Defense Department not only denied reports that the Soviets had used laser beams to blind an American satellite in the autumn of 1975, but attributed the problems to the fact that "the infrared sensors on the satellite had detected large fires along a Soviet gas pipeline rather than deliberate interference." According to Finney, the State Department had also denied the reports. The spokesman who issued the denial was Robert Funseth, who, during the spring and summer, had issued a series of denials about the effects of the Soviet irradiation of the American Embassy in Moscow. "I have looked into the allegations and no U.S. satellite has been damaged," Funseth declared. "There has been no interference."

On January 17, 1977, *Aerospace Daily* announced that the Jason Committee had reported favorably on the Chair Heritage study program for using a ship-mounted high-energy particle accelerator to neutralize incoming enemy missile warheads. On February 4, Dr. Currie submitted the annual defense research report to Congress, declaring that "we must also be concerned with Soviet activities in the area of directed-energy weapons." According to an *Aerospace Daily* article on February 4, directed-energy weapons are "similar to high-energy laser weapons except that they use nuclear particles, also traveling at the speed of light, as is the case with lasers." On the same day, the *New York Times* ran a piece by David Binder, who described American intelligence officials as saying that "both the Soviet Union and the United States were trying to develop high-energy beams of charged sub-atomic particles that would destroy incoming nuclear missiles," and that "the Soviet particle-beam program was comparable in size to the huge Manhattan Project." The last part of Binder's article read as follows:

> Lasers, as distinct from particle beams, are highly concentrated and organized beams of light particles called photons.
>
> The particle-beam concept involves the acceleration of charged particles—electrons or protons—and the aiming of a stream of them at a target. Aiming particle beams is performed by precisely tuned electromagnets, but is difficult at great distances. Particles can be produced by splitting the hydrogen bomb, for example.
>
> In the case of nuclear warheads, the idea would be to melt the plutonium explosive with the beam, neutralizing it before it could be detonated over a target. To accomplish this from a ground base, however, would require "boring holes in the atmosphere so the beam can go through," Mr. Garwin [Richard L. Garwin, a former scientific

consultant to the Defense Department and now with the IBM Research Center, in Yorktown Heights, N.Y.] said.

He remarked that the "heaviness" of the atmosphere scatters and weakens particle beams. To make the beams effective would require heating a portion of the atmosphere, perhaps with a laser beam, before using the weapon, he said.

In the case of ballistic missiles, Mr. Garwin continued, it is conceivable to put particle-beam accelerators in orbiting satellites, which could be targeted on a missile in its booster stage after it leaves the atmosphere.

However, Mr. Garwin said a satellite-based beam would have to contend with the earth's magnetic field, which would deflect particles from an intended target. "The problems tend to vitiate the possibility," he said.

Mr. Garwin said that theoretical studies had also investigated the use of neutral hydrogen atoms to form weapon beams based on satellites, thereby avoiding the magnetic-field problem. But he said small amounts of gas distributed in the thin upper atmosphere would neutralize the hydrogen atom beam.

On February 15, the *New York Times* published an article by Drew Middleton, who wrote that "space defense has assumed a high priority in Air Force research as a result of experiments in the Soviet Union," and that "Rockwell International, for example, has completed a study on satellite maneuvering to escape hunter-killer satellites." On the very next day, Middleton wrote a story that began:

> The "death ray" is still in the realm of science fiction, but lasers powerful enough to inflict significant damage are moving toward the arsenals of the Soviet Union and the United States.
>
> Dr. Kumar Patel, inventor of the high-energy carbon monoxide laser, said recently that, with current technology, his laser had the potential size, efficiency and power to be packaged into a transport aircraft from which it could knock other aircraft from the sky "at long distances."
>
> This statement focused attention on the Defense Department's laser-weapons development group at Kirtland Air Force Base in Albuquerque, N.M. Known by the code name "Eighth Card," the base is run by the Defense Advanced Research Projects Agency (DARPA).

All of this speculation and counterspeculation came to a head in the spring of 1977. For months a fierce debate over whether the Soviets had developed a charged-particle beam weapon had raged within the Department of Defense, the CIA, and the Air Force. In the April 22 issue of *Science,* Nicholas Wade quoted retired Major General George J. Keegan, former head of Air Force Intelligence, as warning the American Security Council that the Soviet Union was "twenty years ahead of the United States in its development of a technology which they believe will soon neutralize the ballistic missile weapon as a threat to the Soviet Union." After noting that General Keegan has "a reputation as a worst-case analyst," Wade got down to specifics about the particle beam weapon. "Physicists who work at particle accelerators know that if the beam is discharged into a brick, the brick will absorb the energy and explode," he wrote. "In accelerators, however, the beams are propagated in a vacuum. Firing a beam through the atmosphere is a different proposition. But should it be feasible, a beam might deliver more energy than would a laser, say, on an incoming missile during the few seconds it was within range."

Later in his article, Wade returned to the question of whether a particle beam weapon was practical:

> As to the technical feasibility of using particle beams as weapons, none of several physicists consulted said the concept was possible but none dismissed it out of hand. "It doesn't violate the second law of thermodynamics," observed a scientist knowledgeable about military interest in the particle beam concept. "Just getting the beam to propagate over the long distances has been thought of as the principal difficulty. You have high-current beams of relativistic particles. No matter how you slice it this means very large powers. Also the design of a suitable accelerator is rather problematical."

In assessing Keegan's warning about the Soviet technological lead, Wade went on to quote a West Coast physicist as saying that "in principle it could be considered possible but even if it were, I would seriously question if it would be worth doing," and giving as his reason the opinion that "you would need radar systems and a very large accelerator and I doubt if it would be cheaper than a conventional ABM system." Wade then quoted an East Coast physicist as saying that homing missiles provided a more effective ABM system than particle beams. He concluded his article by observing that "Keegan has his own reasons for believing the Russians have found a way to use particle beams as weapons, but the view of at least some physicists seems to be that particle beams are most useful inside accelerators."

Wade's assessment of the particle beam situation did not go unchallenged for long. On May 2, *Aviation Week & Space Technology* published a highly detailed 7,000-word article by its military editor, Clarence A. Robinson, Jr., who said that the Soviet Union was not only developing a charged-particle beam device "designed to destroy U.S. intercontinental and submarine-launched ballistic missile nuclear warheads," but that a fusion-pulsed magnetohydrodynamic generator (which is a nuclear explosive device) to provide power for the particle beam weapon had been tested in an underground chamber beneath the desert near Azgir in Kazakhstan, not far from the Caspian Sea. According to Robinson's account, the Soviets were also deploying large over-the-horizon radars in northern Russia to detect and track U.S. ICBM reentry vehicles, and were preparing to test a spaceborne hydrogen fluoride high-energy laser designed to destroy American satellites. Robinson went on to say that "because of a controversy within the U.S. intelligence community, the details of Soviet directed energy weapons had not been made available to the President or to the National Security Council."

Much of the rest of Robinson's article was devoted to an analysis of a four-or-five-year running battle between General Keegan and the Air Force Intelligence people, on the one hand, and the CIA, the Defense Intelligence Agency, and a number of leading high-energy physicists at the Energy Research and Development Administration's Lawrence Livermore Laboratory, on the other. At issue was whether the Soviets had the technological capability to develop a particle beam weapon, and especially the capability to produce the necessary levels of energy for such a weapon, which were estimated to be between one and one hundred billion electron volts. Also at issue was whether the Soviets were actually engaged in testing a particle beam weapon at the Semipalatinsk nuclear test area in Central Asia—an installation that Air Force Intelligence people refer to as PNUT (an acronym for Possible Nuclear Underground Test) and that the C.I.A. identifies as URD-3, which stands for Unidentified Research and Development Facility Number Three.

According to Robinson, Keegan's dour hypotheses were rejected by the members of a munitions panel of the Air Force's Science Advisory Board. After a three-day meeting at the Livermore Laboratory, they were supposed to have discounted any possibility that the Soviets could have developed the technology for nuclear explosion generation, power storage, power transmission, and collective acceleration—all of which would be necessary for the production of a particle-beam weapon. Robinson quoted one official as explaining that "the bottom line was that the panel said there is no way to control or stabilize such a beam if a weapon is produced," and that "the net result is that evidence about possible beam weapons development was rejected."

After describing Keegan's efforts to prove that the Soviets did, indeed, have the multiple technological capabilities to produce a particle beam weapon, Robinson revealed that in 1975 the general had disclosed his findings to William Colby, then head of the CIA, and that Colby had convened the CIA's Nuclear Intelligence Panel to consider them. According to Robinson, the panel was unable to accept the Air Force's conclusions about either the Soviet technological capabilities, or the nature of the tests that were being conducted at Azgir and Semipalatinsk. "The major argument now raging within the intelligence community is whether the facility at Semipalatinsk is experimental in nature and whether it will require a major effort by the USSR over many years to build more such facilities to use for weapons purposes," Robinson continued.

Some members of the scientific community had raised objections that charged-particle weapons were impractical because the beams would have to be propagated and bent, in order to intercept incoming warheads in reentry vehicles. Robinson quoted an Air Force official as saying that "all that is needed is for Soviet long-range precision radars now deployed in violation of the ABM agreement to detect avenues or windows for re-entry vehicle trajectories against targets in the USSR," and that "by airing rapidly pulsed proton beams into these windows, ICBMs and SLBMs could be quickly saturated and destroyed." The official went on to tell Robinson that "with this method, many acquisition and tracking problems could be overcome," and that "by using the window concept to scatter the beam over a wide area through which warheads must transit, it is believed that not many beam weapons would be required to protect the USSR from a U.S. retaliatory strike."

According to Robinson's article, the United States had attempted to develop a charged-particle beam weapon during the early 1970s under an ARPA-funded project code-named "Seesaw," but the project was abandoned several years ago. Later in his piece, he described the testimony given to the House Armed Services Research and Development Subcommitee by John L. Allen, Deputy Director of Defense Research and Engineering. Allen spoke as follows:

> Science fiction writers have been fascinated with the concept of a directed-energy weapon that beams energy directly to a target, obviating the need for bombs, missiles or projectiles. A weapon of this type now appears not only to be possible, but we may even have a choice of the beams that can be used . . . electrons or other fundamental particles.
>
> These beams travel at or near the speed of light so that the delivery time is negligible, an attractive attribute for a weapon. The beams can also be moved rapidly from one target to the next. Thus, for defense against nearly simultaneous multiple attackers, directed-energy weapons are appealing.

Adding that high-energy lasers were the most advanced of the directed-energy devices, Allen explained that it had been known for about a decade that the generation and propagation of damaging levels of energy might be feasible. "However, the technical problems forseen were formidable," he told the subcommittee. "High power is needed for useful lethal ranges. The achievement of such high power requires a strong foundation of basic knowledge of the physics and chemistry of highly excited gases, coupled with, in some systems, sophisticated high-volume, high-velocity gas flow technology. The flow rates involved in gas dynamic high-energy lasers are like those from a jet engine. The physical size is also comparable to a jet engine."

According to Allen, the Defense Advanced Research Projects Agency "is looking at the possible applications of lasers in space defense with emphasis on chemical lasers." He then explained the problems of directed-energy weapons:

> Particle beams—beams of electrons, for example—are not directly affected by the weather and may provide longer ranges than high-energy lasers in adverse weather. However, they have other problems. Charged-particle beams have a tendency to be unstable. They also are deflected by magnetic fields, so pointing and tracking uncertainties exist. If these problems can be solved, a viable weapon could result. We believe that charged-particle weapons might, in some applications,

present a useful alternative or complement to the high-energy laser for giving us "zero-time-of-flight" weapons. We are pursuing projects at an exploratory level.

Toward the end of his article, Robinson said that the Navy was continuing exploratory development of beam weapons in its Chair Heritage program, and that the Navy planned to move the program into an advanced development phase in fiscal year 1979. Robinson indicated that the Navy was believed to be working with an auto-resonant accelerator, which has the potential for generating extremely intense beams of ions whose power can be measured in billions of electron volts. According to Robinson, the auto-resonant accelerator combines the basic concepts of traveling wave and collective acceleration, and operates by converting electron beam energy to ion energy. He then listed a number of installations where test accelerators were under development, including the Naval Research Laboratory at Dahlgren, Virginia. Robinson ended his article by quoting a senior U.S. official:

> "It does seem that the Soviets have taken a very different course which may eventually prove most U.S. planners and analysts to be wrong. If this proof comes early enough, it may then be too late for our research and development establishment to catch up on what may finally be agreed to be a very long Soviet lead in this field of strategic defense.

As might be expected, Robinson's disturbing article was quickly seized upon by newspapers across the country. Typical of these follow-up pieces was a story that ran in the *New York Times* on May 3, which stated that "in large part the article and accompanying editorial reflected the controversial views of Maj. Gen. George Keegan, recently retired chief of Air Force intelligence, who has maintained for years that the Russians were developing a charged-particle beam weapon and were attaining superiority in all other weapons systems." Indeed, the *Times* devoted nearly a quarter of its story to a series of hard and soft denials issued by Pentagon officials, who said that a Soviet particle-beam breakthrough "is considered remote"; that Robinson's article was "highly speculative"; but that "there is a possibility this is happening," because "there's no question they're working on something."

Other reaction to Robinson's article was similarly ambiguous. On

May 17 the *Washington Post* ran a story which said that "knocking down an enemy plane with a beam of light or destroying an incoming missile with a manmade lightning bolt are concepts being explored at the Pentagon," but that "Pentagon scientists stressed at a briefing yesterday, neither a light beam nor a lightning bolt weapon is close at hand in the United States or the Soviet Union." On the same day, the *Washington Star,* whose reporter presumably covered the same briefing, ran a story stating that "the United States expects to begin building a prototype of a laser beam weapon—the first American death ray directed-energy military device—about 1981 and might have usable laser weapons by the late 1980s." The story in the *Star* went on to say that "a more potent and more controversial type of directed-energy weapon using charged particle beams (CPB) is less certain to be realized by current research and therefore is further off"; that "CPB weapons of atomic or subatomic particles can deliver more power on a target than lasers, which direct strong, narrow beams of light to destroy by heat"; and that "beams of charged electrons or protons can produce more energy in whatever they hit, burning up a target."

On May 21, John H. Douglas and Dietrick E. Thomsen wrote a critique of Robinson's article in *Science News,* which quoted President Carter as saying at a press conference on May 3 that there was no evidence that the Soviets had achieved any major breakthrough in directed-energy weapons. "I think that is, first of all, a report that is based on some inaccuracies," the President said. "Secondly, the assessment of the report in the aviation magazine has been exaggerated."

Regarding the practicality of using a particle beam weapon against incoming missiles, Douglas and Thomsen said that "the task is about like trying to shoot a bullet coming toward you on a foggy day while your gun hand is shaking and the wind is blowing." They went on to point out that in order to deflect a charged-particle beam an enemy would merely have to explode a nuclear device above the atmosphere just before launching his ICBMs.

The *Science News* article debunking the charged-particle weapons concept was followed by another article written by Nicholas Wade, which appeared in *Science* on May 27. "The affair of the charged particle beam, the death-ray weapon with which the Soviets will allegedly soon be able to neutralize an American strategic missile attack, has been the sensation of the week in Washington," Wade began. "Congressmen have received secret briefings, the CIA has been moved to issue one of its infrequent statements, and there has even been a presidential assurance that the nation is not in jeopardy."

Thus was the new game of gap played in 1976 and 1977 in newspapers and magazines all across the country. By and large, the writers and publications were being used as unwitting mouthpieces for a catch-up campaign orchestrated by Department of Defense officials who strummed the news media as if it were a guitar. The trouble with all of it—meaning virtually all of the articles that had been published about directed-energy weapons during this two-year span—was that they amounted to little more than a series of phony alarms and phony denials. These were designed not only to drum up public apprehension—and, therefore, congressional support—for a directed-energy weapons program that had been in full bloom since the early 1970s, but also to fool the Russians about the true nature of this program. In order to accomplish this deception, the Department of Defense has not only played directed-energy gap, but also an elaborate game of hide-and-seek with the Congress. In this game, Congress closes its eyes, counts to twenty (over a period of, say, five or six years), and opens them, to be presented not only with the necessity for a new weapons system, but, magically, the system itself.

To satisfy oneself that such has been the case with directed-energy weapons, one might return to the Dahlgren symposium of July 1973, and listen to Dr. M. F. Rose describe Figure 8—a diagram of an accelerator devised by the Naval Research Laboratory people during the early part of 1972. Here is what Dr. Rose said:

> Figure Eight is a schematic of a radio-frequency source being researched by Naval Research Laboratory. A Marx-generator is discharged through a pulse former to produce a relativistic electron beam. This beam interacts with a magnetic field in the drift space producing microwave radiation at several different frequencies simultaneously. There is also a rather intense burst of X-rays. This source produces radio-frequency in the microwave region of the spectrum. Power levels in the 30 to 50 megawatt range are produced at a number of frequencies for each pulse.

Now contrast Dr. Rose's description of Figure 8 with the description and diagram of the Navy's supposedly experimental auto-resonant accelerator as described by Clarence Robinson in *Aviation Week* nearly four years later. Here is what Robinson wrote:

> The name auto-resonant accelerator is derived from the process involved—the novel feature is that as the cyclotron eigenmode [electron wave configuration] delivers energy to the accelerated ions, it automatically extracts energy from the relativistic electron beams. Power is thus automatically fed from the relativistic beam to the resonant ions. To provide the accelerating medium, the electron beam is propagated in a vacuum over a distance of several meters. The relativistic beam is the accelerating medium and is used to accelerate protons to high energies.

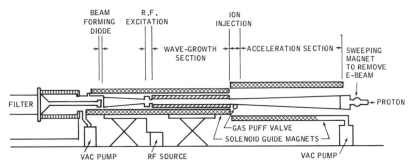

CREDIT: AVIATION WEEK & SPACE TECHNOLOGY

At top is the diagram of the experimental auto-resonant accelerator that appeared in *Aviation Week & Space Technology* on May 2, 1977. Below is the diagram of the electron beam accelerator shown at the Naval Weapons Laboratory, in Dahlgren, Virginia, on July 10, 1973.

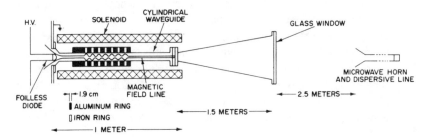

Most physicists would have a hard time making much sense out of this paragraph, let alone understanding what the right-hand portion of the diagram shown in *Aviation Week* is supposed to signify. However, if one blocks out the right half of the diagram in *Aviation Week* and compares it with the Figure 8 described by Dr. Rose four years previously, one suddenly gains a new perspective. Indeed, the two accelerators appear to be closely related, except that the newer auto-resonant accelerator undoubtedly emits a giant high-power microwave pulse of purer frequency, one that can be aimed and propagated with considerable efficiency either in space or through the atmosphere. Robinson, of course, was led to believe that the energy radiating from the so-called auto-resonant accelerator is in the form of charged particles that have the potential to burn through metal and to destroy nuclear warheads. What seems far more likely, however, is that the radiating energy is not a charged-particle beam but a powerful microwave pulse. Because such a pulse can be beamed and transmitted over long distances through the atmosphere, and because it can disrupt the guidance systems of incoming missiles, it provides a far more efficient directed-energy weapon than a charged-particle beam, which can only be propagated through the atmosphere with great difficulty.

Thus, all the talk about death rays and charged-particle beams has been little more than an elaborate smokescreen designed to hide the fact that the United States is developing a directed-energy weapon that uses a high-power microwave pulse.

So much for the directed-energy weapons gap.

22

Seafarer

Clemenceau once said that war was too serious a matter to be entrusted to the military, and certainly the public health is. While no one should question that it may be necessary for the Department of Defense to dissemble when it comes to developing secret weapons, no one should assume that the department will at the same time undertake scientific research designed to protect Americans from microwave damage. In order to protect their health and well-being, the citizens of a constitutional democracy obviously have either to be informed, or to inform themselves about health hazards, for only when the people are informed about the hazards can they insist that protective measures be taken. This has been true of DDT, asbestos, vinyl chloride, aerosol propellants, and a host of other harmful substances and toxic chemicals, and it is equally true, of course, of an insidious, tissue-penetrating agent such as electromagnetic radiation.

A case in point is the U.S. Navy's Project Seafarer, which stands for Surface ELF Antenna For Addressing Remotely-deployed Receivers. Project Seafarer, formerly known as Project Sanguine, is the scheme that would bury a gigantic, three-to-four-thousand-square-mile underground radio antenna system, costing $315 million, three to six feet below ground in the Upper Peninsula of Michigan, in order to permeate the biosphere with extremely-low-frequency (ELF) radio waves. Because they can penetrate sea water they would enable the Navy to communicate with deeply submerged nuclear submarines. As far back as 1963, the Navy satisfied itself that an ELF system would work by using a 109-mile-long antenna in the Appalachian Mountains, radiating half a watt of ELF power, to send a message to a submerged submarine 2,500 miles away. In 1971, the Navy used a thirty-mile, prototype ELF antenna system buried in the nonconducting rock strata of the Laurentian Shield, at Clam Lake, in northern Wisconsin, to send a message to a submerged submarine several thousand miles away, using less than a watt of radiated power. Unlike EMP and the directed-energy weapons, of course, the Navy could not possibly bury an ELF system and keep it secret. Thus, Project Sanguine/Seafarer eventually came under public scrutiny.

When it was learned that electrical conductors such as fences, power lines, and telephone lines running parallel to an ELF antenna could have sufficient voltage induced in them to cause operational interference and to pose a possible hazard to people and animals, it was only natural that environmental groups should mount opposition to the test facility at Clam Lake. At first, the Navy tried to counter such opposition by claiming that there were no harmful biological effects caused by extremely-low-frequency radio waves. However, in 1972 and 1973, one of Dr. Beischer's now-discontinued ELF experiments on human subjects down at the Naval Aerospace Medicine Research Laboratory, in Pensacola, produced rises in blood-serum triglycerides in nine out of ten volunteers; and another study of eleven men exposed to ELF showed a significant decline in their ability to perform simple addition. The results of both these studies were suppressed by the Navy for two years. The Navy has since announced that rises in triglycerides have not been observed in monkeys irradiated with ELF.

In 1974, the Office of Telecommunications Policy's bio-effects projects resumé described a behavioral experiment performed on monkeys at the University of California at Los Angeles, which showed that "at very low voltage levels (ten volts per meter) there was evidence that seven hertz electric fields resulted in shorter interresponse times and reduced variability of responding." Another study described in the 1974 resumé showed that "pigeons may be deflected toward an energized antenna and may orient faster in the presence of ELF fields." Still another study was conducted in the summer of 1973 by researchers at Northern Illinois University, in order to determine if the normal migration of Ringbilled Gull chicks would be affected by the Navy's ELF antenna at Clam Lake. The progress report of this study read as follows:

> About 391 trials were conducted at the buried antenna site while the east-west antenna was energized and the north-south buried [antenna] was turned off. Under these conditions all but two of the test groups showed statistically significant mean headings. Thus increasing the distance between the test subject and the energized antenna may reduce the effect. Therefore, birds flying over the facility should be exposed to significantly lower magnetic fields than we used for experimentation. It is possible, however, that the fields estimated to occur at even 1000 feet above the operating system may be sufficient to cause disorientation of juvenile Ringbilled Gulls. It is suspected, however, that the adaptability of the avian orientation system and the ability of adult birds to use multiple cues during migrational orientation will result in bird migration being unimpeded by the presence of Sanguine.

Not surprisingly, as word of such results got out, opposition to Project Sanguine/Seafarer continued to grow, and in 1974 local citizens defeated an effort by the Navy to locate an ELF system in Texas. Then, in 1975, Governor William G. Milliken, of Michigan, invited the Navy to consider putting its ELF system in the Upper Peninsula, not far from the original Clam Lake test facility in Wisconsin. Determined opposition to this proposal was mounted by environmental groups, and during the spring of 1976, the residents of the Upper Peninsula voted down Project Seafarer by a margin that exceeded three to one.

Meanwhile, blockaded by public opposition to Seafarer in three states, the Navy asked the National Academy of Science to undertake an "independent and objective evaluation" of the biological and environmental effects of ELF, and the Academy's National Research Council organized a fifteen-man multidisciplinary Committee on

Biosphere Effects of Extremely Low Frequency Radiation, which held its first meeting on February 11, 1976. As it turned out, three of the committee's fifteen members, including Professor Michaelson, either held or had held Navy contracts for studying the biological effects of microwave radiation, and two others—Professor Schwan and George M. Wilkening, director of Environmental Health and Safety at the Bell Laboratories, in Murray Hill, New Jersey—had been staunch defenders of the ten-milliwatt standard for many years. As might be expected, an organization called People Against Sanguine/Seafarer, which had objected to the make-up of the National Academy's committee from the outset, was quick to criticize a preliminary statement on Seafarer that was released by the academy during the first week of 1977:

> Although it recognizes the existence of numerous biological effects, the statement fails to relate these effects to human health or animal behavior. For example, the statement does not attempt to evaluate experiments associating magnetic fields with elevated serum triglycerides and mental dysfunction in humans. It also ignores experimental evidence leading to the recommendation that Seafarer should not be placed in the route or nesting areas of migratory birds. The NAS statement provides only unsubstantiated opinions which do not adequately respond to the serious concerns of Upper Peninsula residents.

The spokesman for the group added that "it should be obvious to the governor that waiting for still another ambiguous report from the NAS will neither contribute to public understanding nor alter public opposition to Project Seafarer." Three months later, there was evidence that the Governor may already have seen some political writing on the wall, for on March 28, 1977, the *Washington Post* ran the following story:

> Republican Gov. William G. Milliken of Michigan is hopping mad at President Carter and Defense Secretary Harold Brown for going back on what he considered a firm promise not to wire the state for a doomsday communications system if he objected. He objects, fiercely, to Project Seafarer, a grid system for communicating with nuclear submarines that was kicked out of Wisconsin and Texas for all sorts of reasons. The White House says "the President won't get involved in this at all until the Secretary of Defense has made his

recommendation." The furious Milliken says that's not at all what Carter said during the campaign. Maybe the grid project could be tied in with a couple of water projects.

Meanwhile, on March 15, Secretary of the Navy W. Graham Clayton, Jr., had written to Governor Milliken, informing him that Project Seafarer "has an extremely high priority because of its direct contribution toward the safety and effectiveness of our strategic submarines." Secretary Clayton enclosed a memorandum written by Admiral J. L. Holloway III, Chief of Naval Operations, who declared that "the need for Seafarer is real and urgent," and that "there are no adequate alternatives for communicating with our submarines without their having to put an antenna near the surface, and run the danger of detection." On April 12, the Navy upped the tempo of its pro-Seafarer campaign by releasing a barrage of pro-Seafarer statements from Admiral Holloway, former President Gerald Ford, and Deputy Secretary of Defense C. W. Duncan, Jr., who, presumably, would not have gone out on a limb for Seafarer unless he had permission from Secretary of Defense Harold Brown, who, in turn, must surely have checked the matter with President Carter. On May 10, the Senate Armed Services Committee fell into predictable line in the face of this mounting pressure, and recommended the authorization of $20.1 million of the $23.7 million requested by the administration for Seafarer. (The House Armed Services Committee had previously deleted the entire sum from the budget, and recommended using an alternative system that would contact submerged submarines with a laser ray beamed from space by a satellite.) On May 26, Secretary Clayton sent a letter to Station WLUC-TV, in Marquette, stating that "Governor Milliken has never been given the right to 'veto' the building of Seafarer in Michigan," and that "it is unlikely that Congress would or could grant to the Governor of a state the right to decide on an issue of national security to the United States."

To no one's surprise, when the House and Senate Armed Services Committees met in the early part of June to resolve their differences over Seafarer, it was decided that the project should go forward as scheduled. And when the National Academy of Science's report was issued in August, it stated that, except for possible shock hazards, the likelihood of serious adverse biological effects from ELF was very small.

No matter what Secretary of Defense Brown and President Carter have decided behind the scenes about the future of Seafarer in Michigan, the Navy is in any case determined to install an ELF antenna system that will enable it to communicate with deeply submerged nuclear submarines. As alternatives to a buried ELF system, TRW has proposed using an 850-mile-long power line extending from Los Angeles to Oregon as a giant antenna; the Boeing Company has proposed the deployment of a 20-mile-long trailing ELF antenna from a 747 aircraft; and the Naval Research Laboratory has come up with a scheme to suspend a giant ELF antenna from balloons. Which, as usual, leaves it squarely up to the American people to inform themselves of the potential hazards of ELF, and, like the residents of Wisconsin, Texas, and Michigan, to decide whether to oppose on their own a project that would permeate the entire biosphere with extremely-low-frequency radio waves.

23

Some
Loose Ends

Needless to say, the American people have not had the opportunity to oppose numerous other schemes and devices resulting in the proliferation of microwave and radio-frequency radiation. The reason is that information about them has been highly classified (and thus suppressed) for reasons of national security. In no case, perhaps, has this been more true than in the case of electromagnetic pulse, which has not only been the object of strict security regulations, but also of the largest cover-up of all. As a result, virtually no one in the general public has been able to learn much about the biological effects of electromagnetic pulse—let alone voice objection to it. The one exception to this would, of course, be the unsuspecting people exposed to EMP at the missile sites in Montana, who have filed for Workmen's Compensation, or made claims for damages against the Air Force.

This calls to mind once again the prophetic and totally unheeded warning that was given in the summer of 1972 by Leo Birenbaum, who, when asked to write his thoughts about a proposed EMP standard, had the courage to call for more research and to stand alone amidst a scientific community coopted by military considerations.

For better or worse, however, EMP and other forms of electromagnetic radiation may well provide a valuable, though hard, lesson for a society that seems not only uncertain of how to assess the biological consequences of its own technological capabilities, but far too quick to classify them for supposed reasons of national security before it has even begun to determine what their biological consequences may be. Surely, if the questions that should have been asked about the various applications of electromagnetic radiation continue to go unasked about future applications, this nation will one day be faced with a public health disaster of monumental and perhaps irreversible proportions. In fact, since nobody knows the extent to which microwave radiation may pose a carcinogenic and genetic hazard, we could be approaching that day already.

Meanwhile, since EMP and other microwave and electromagnetic radiation applications remain under tight security wrap, one can only continue to speculate about their uses and the biological consequences that may result. In this way, however, one can sometimes tie up loose ends. Take, for example, the murder of three American employees of the Rockwell International Corporation, who were ambushed and killed in a minibus while driving through the streets of Teheran, on August 28, 1976. The official explanation for the killings, as given in the Iranian newspapers, was that they were the work of Islamic Moslem terrorists. However, according to an article written by Bob Woodward for the *Washington Post,* on January 2, 1977, the Shah of Iran told Richard Hallock, a retired Army colonel representing Secretary of Defense James Schlesinger, that the Soviets were behind the murders. On the same day, Hallock was told it was the Russians by Richard M. Helms. Then Ambassador to Iran, Helms had formerly been director of the CIA.

Almost thirty thousand Americans live and work in Iran these days. The murder of American technicians by Soviet agents in Iran or anywhere else in the world is a thing of great rarity. Thus, one naturally wonders about the motive for such a deed, which obviously reflected extreme displeasure. There has, for example, been no trouble reported over the presence of Raytheon Service Company employees in Iran. Judging from a company poem—"From backgrounds that are as diverse as can be/These nowaday nomads continue to roam/From Shemya, Alaska, to the Caspian Sea/All continents are theirs, all cities their home"—these technicians have probably set up a phased array radar in Iran, in order to look into Russia across the Caspian. Reading on in Woodward's article, one learned that the three Rockwell International employees were "working on a secret project of truly Buck Rogers proportions called IBEX." IBEX is a highly sophisticated and automated, $500-million signal intelligence collection system that was being installed on the border between Iran and the Soviet Union. One also learned that fifteen employees of the CIA in Iran, who were operating under cover as the United States Advisory Team, had drawn up the plans for IBEX, and that the CIA had, in fact, for many years operated secret monitoring posts on the Soviet-Iranian border. None of this, of course, explained the assassination of the three Rockwell technicians by Soviet agents. It did indicate, however, that IBEX was most probably not the kind of communications-monitoring equipment which has been deployed and operated in many countries around the world by the National Security Agency. What, then, does IBEX monitor? Why did it provoke the Soviets to murder three civilian technicians? And why was this deed almost totally ignored by the Administration in Washington?

Unfortunately, Woodward was not able to answer these questions. His article dealt mainly with corrupt practices and illegal payoffs in the Pentagon's Iranian arms sale program. Toward the end of the piece, however, he described the IBEX system as complicated and unworkable, and said that one Pentagon official, who was familiar with the equipment, had called it "garbage." This was one of the few false notes in an otherwise excellent exposé. Indeed, it had all the earmarks of a phony disclaimer.

To begin with, in fiscal year 1976, Rockwell International was the Pentagon's top-ranking research and development contractor with $606 million in R & D contracts alone; it was also the tenth-ranking defense contractor in terms of overall contract dollars; and it had received awards of more than $10 million from NASA. Why, then, should Rockwell, of all firms, try to peddle a defective electronics system? Why would the Shah of Iran pay millions of dollars for a piece of "garbage"? And, finally, if IBEX *were* "garbage," why would the Soviets be so upset about its installation as to risk an international incident by killing three Americans?

Any answers to these questions must, of course, be speculative. It is possible, however, that IBEX was not a piece of junk but rather a complex surveillance system designed to intercept signals given off at the moment of launch by Soviet hunter-killer satellites, or by ABM satellites carrying directed-energy weapons. Such a surveillance system could trigger off a directed-energy response of our own, perhaps in the form of a vast electromagnetic pulse sent down from space upon the Soviet homeland.

With regard to the possibility of total space warfare it is well to remember a number of interlocking developments:

(1) Rockwell International had recently completed a study for the Air Force on maneuvering techniques that would enable American satellites to escape from Soviet hunter-killer satellites.

(2) In 1976, at a symposium co-sponsored by the National Academy of Science's Naval Studies Board and the Office of Naval Research, William H. Pickering, a former director of NASA's Jet Propulsion Laboratory, said that satellites and precision-guided weapons "will dominate the design of the next-generation Navy."

(3) During 1976 the Advanced Space Program at the Air Force's Space and Missile Systems Organization (SAMSO), in Los Angeles, began development of a satellite-attack warning system (SAWS), and also began to explore the possibility of launching small satellites from missiles or high-flying aircraft, in order to escape detection by the Soviets.

(4) Also during 1976, the Advanced Research Projects Agency financed a study by the Air Force's Rome Air Development Center, in Rome, New York, of the effectiveness of spaceborne radar surveillance systems.

(5) Concurrently, SAMSO sponsored similar studies by Grumman Aerospace, Hughes Aircraft, TRW, and Raytheon.

(6) In November 1976, the Soviets sent half a dozen satellites into orbit whose mission puzzled Western observers, and in December they launched three satellites—Cosmos 881, 882, and 885—which were believed to be involved in satellite intercept-and-destroy tests.

(7) In February 1977 the Air Force held a briefing for the electronics and aerospace industries concerning the Department of Defense's rapidly expanding $100-million-a-year space defense program. The program is highlighted by devices that protect military satellites

from attack by hunter-killer satellites. Some space surveillance satellites are outfitted with infrared sensors designed to keep track of all Soviet satellites.

Because space is now accessible, it seems obvious that the directed-energy weapons now under development will be deployed in space. Such a combination raises the possibility that NASA's space shuttle program, its space power-generator programs, and some of the sixteen satellites it put into orbit in 1976 for the avowed purposes of communications, weather observation, and scientific study may be the celestial counterparts of the CIA's Glomar-Explorer.

In any case, whatever the CIA and Rockwell International were up to in Iran during 1975 and 1976, it was certainly enough to make the Soviets risk confrontation with the United States. This brings us full circle to the loosest end of the microwave cover-up—the motive for the sharply increased Soviet irradiation of the American Embassy in Moscow during 1975.

At its simplest, this was another crude sign of displeasure that occurred at the same time that IBEX was being installed. However, it has continued for more than two years, and has provoked from Washington no more than an ambiguous "protest." For example, on May 31, 1977, William Beecher, of the *Boston Globe,* wrote that "the Carter Administration has quietly but firmly urged the Soviet Union to stop bombarding the American Embassy in Moscow with microwaves." According to Beecher, the message was carried to Moscow in March by Secretary of State Cyrus Vance. "The Russians were told this is one of an array of serious issues that lie between us," one senior official told Beecher. "We're not threatening anybody, but they know we don't take it lightly." As for how lightly the Russians were taking it, one simply needed to continue reading Beecher, who went on to say that while the Russians had told Vance they would "take note" of his protest, "they considered the problem a figment of American imagination," and insisted that "microwave levels around the embassy were no different than anywhere else in Moscow." Beecher then went on to write a stunning personal account of his own experiences at the embassy earlier in May. It read as follows:

> But this reporter, in four out of eight interviews at different times in the embassy on Tchaikovsky Street, experienced a weird combination of sensations—sweating, dry mouth, sudden loss of concentration,

forgetfulness and general unease. On the four other occasions absolutely none of these symptoms occurred.

I was prepared to write off the first occurrence, during my first visit on May 3, as springing from the fact that I was slightly weary from travel, that the office had a busted air conditioner, and that having written in Washington about the microwaves, I might, subconsciously, have expected strange sensations and then experienced them psychosomatically.

But when it happened on three other occasions, when I was rested, where air conditioning was functioning, and after interviews in other embassy offices and having no strange effects, I can't help but suspect that microwaves might have been involved. Some American diplomats thoroughly agreed, but were loath to have such sentiments attributed to them.

At this point, one must ask: What is going on here?

The Soviets may well be irradiating the American Embassy in Moscow in retaliation for what they consider either the threat or the fact of unwarranted irradiation of their population by powerful electromagnetic devices that now encircle them and look down upon them from outer space. Perhaps, as a warning, the Soviets have chosen to irradiate the only population of Americans they can hold electronically captive. It would be an effective means of demonstrating to the United States, which has for twenty years denied that adverse biological effects accompany low-level microwave radiation, that it is as wrong about the hazards of such radiation as it was about the hazards of low-level X-rays. The Soviets have possibly irradiated Americans in Moscow in order to demonstrate, first to Dr. Kissinger and now to Mr. Vance, that they have developed an electromagnetic pulse weapon of their own. Would not the flabby response of the American government to the irradiation of its Moscow Embassy be better explained in this fashion than by the implausible excuses advanced by the Department of State?

All these things are conjectural and speculative. They are also possible and logical. Indeed, anything becomes possible when the institutions of a constitutional democracy are held in thrall by the kind of massive threat that has been posed to the United States since the Soviet Union stunned the nation—first by developing the hydrogen bomb and then by sending up Sputnik. The logic flows from a connection—the cancer connection. Three cases of leukemia and two cases of other cancer among a handful of people exposed to EMP at the missile sites in Montana. Sixteen breast cancers, several known cases of leukemia, and a high incidence of blood disorders among people living and working at the American Embassy in Moscow, who, according to Zbigniew Brzezinski, the national security adviser to President Carter, are suffering the highest rate of cancer in the world.

The cancer connection between the EMP testing in Montana and the Soviet irradiation of the Moscow Embassy will no doubt be denied and assailed. Studies and surveys will surely be undertaken to prove or disprove it, just as studies were made over the years to prove and disprove the carcinogenicity of asbestos, DDT, vinyl chloride, and other cancer-producing substances. No amount of affirmation or denial of the cancer connection will be of much use until independent studies—studies not financed by the State Department or the military—are conducted. In other words, if we allow scientific inquiry to replace stonewalling, time will reveal the truth.

24

The Mind-Control
Connection

The record thus far, regarding information about microwave and radio-frequency radiation, suggests that a lot of powerful people in this country are sufficiently caught up in considerations of national security and corporate profit so as to feel no urgency to settle the bio-hazard issues. Nor do they have much compunction about bringing economic and political pressure to bear upon anyone who might feel that urgency. As a result, the military and the electronics industry are in close cooperation over what to make public about the health effects of microwaves. Nowhere is this more clearly stated than in a report entitled "Biological Effects of Electromagnetic Radiation (Radiowaves and Microwaves)—Eurasian Communist Countries," prepared for the Defense Intelligence Agency by the Army Medical and Information Agency. This report was issued in March 1976 as a classified document; however, most of its contents—twenty-six pages to be exact—were declassified in November of that year, after Barton Reppert, of the Associated Press, wrote letters to the Pentagon requesting that it be made public under the Freedom of

Information Act, which, of course, meant that the Pentagon wanted it to become public.

After acknowledging in a summary section that microwave exposure standards in Communist countries "remain much more stringent than those of the West," the report warned, "If the more advanced nations of the West are strict in the enforcement of stringent exposure standards, there could be unfavorable effects on industrial output and military functions." This, of course, provides an excellent motive for the military and the electronics industry to be in close cooperation over what to make public about the health effects of microwaves. The DIA report goes on to present the rationale that "the Eurasian Communist countries could, on the other hand, give lip service to strict standards, but allow their military to operate without restriction and thereby gain the advantage in electronic warfare techniques and the development of anti-personnel applications."

The rest of the document is a compendium of obviously deliberate, but unintentionally comic, contradiction, misinterpretation, and omission. The first page of the summary says, for example, that "Eurasian Communist countries are actively involved in evaluation of the biological significance of radiowaves and microwaves," while the next declares: "no significant research and development has been identified that could be related to work in this field in the People's Republic of China, North Korea, and North Vietnam." Further, the entire middle section of the report, which is entitled "Biological Significance of Radiowaves and Microwaves," turns out to be little more than a general review of well-known studies conducted by scientists in the Communist countries between 1968 and 1975.

However, it is in the final paragraph of a section entitled "Trends, Conclusions, and Forecast" that the authors of the report achieve their most significant omission, for in their zeal to expose the machinations of the "Eurasian Communist investigators" they manage to avoid any mention of the fact that virtually all the work whose usurpation by the Communists they are suggesting, and whose potentially disastrous consequences they are describing, was originally conducted by Allan Frey, published in the medical literature in the United States, and financed by the Office of Naval Research. The paragraph reads:

No Eurasian Communist research activity has been identified which can be clearly or directly related to any military offensive weapons program. However, Soviet scientists are fully aware of the biological effects of low-level microwave radiation which might have offensive weapons application. Their internal sound perception research has great potential for development into a system for disorienting or disrupting the behavior patterns of military or diplomatic personnel; it could be used equally well as an interrogation tool. The Soviets have also studied the psychophysiological and metabolic changes and the alterations of brain function resulting from exposure to mixed frequencies of electromagnetic radiation. One physiological effect which has been demonstrated is heart seizure. This has been accomplished experimentally in frogs by synchronizing a pulsed ultrahigh-frequency microwave signal of low-average power density with the depolarization of the myocardium and beaming the signal at the thoracic area. A frequency probably could be found which would provide sufficient penetration of the chest wall of humans to accomplish the same effect. Another possibility is alteration of the permeability of the blood-brain barrier. This could allow neurotoxins in the blood to cross. As a result, an individual could develop severe neuropathological symptoms and either die or become seriously impaired neurologically.

No one knows to whom the authors of the next Defense Intelligence Agency report on radio waves and microwaves will attribute one of the more recent experiments conducted by Frey, let alone how dire they will imagine its consequences to be, for he has since found that pairs of caged male rats, which are accustomed to fight viciously when their tails are pinched, accept pinching of their tails with relative passivity when they are being irradiated with pulsed microwaves in the ultrahigh-frequency television range at a power density of one milliwatt per square centimeter. However, an educated guess can be made from the summary section of the 1976 report, in which the DIA specialists hint broadly of mind control. "The potential for the development of a number of anti-personnel applications is suggested by the research published in the USSR, East Europe, and the West," they write. "Sounds and possibly even words which appear to be originating intercranially can be induced by signal modulation at very low average power densities."* Later on, they predict

*The authors of the DIA report surely knew that in the spring of 1973, Dr. Sharp and some colleagues at the Walter Reed Army Institute of Research conducted an experiment in which the human brain received a message carried to it by a pulsed microwave transmission. Sitting

that the Soviets will continue to investigate the nature of internal sound perception, perceptual distortion, and other psychophysiological effects, and that "the results of these investigations could have military applications if the Soviets develop methods for disrupting or disturbing human behavior."

Thus most of the report is a kind of red herring, designed to show Americans that the Communist countries are deeply and nefariously involved with microwave technology. The real purpose behind the Pentagon's release of this threatening scenario is not known, unless it would be to suggest that microwave radiation might be used as a mind-control weapons system, but that only the communists would be inhuman enough to do it.

There is, however, a small portion of the DIA report which remains classified. It clearly indicates that efforts to develop microwave radiation as an antipersonnel weapon have been underway in the United States for some years. Take, for example, the following paragraph:

> A study published in 1972 by the U.S. Army Mobility Equipment Research and Development Center, titled "Analysis of Microwaves for Barrier Warfare" examines the plausibility of using radio-frequency energy in barrier-counterbarrier warfare. It discusses both anti-personnel and anti-materiel effects for lethal and non-lethal applications for meeting the barrier requirements of delay, immobilization, and increased target exposure. The report concludes that:
>
> a. It is possible to field a truck-portable microwave barrier system that will completely immobilize personnel in the open with present-day technology and equipment.
>
> b. There is a strong potential for a microwave system that would be capable of delaying or immobilizing personnel in vehicles.
>
> c. With present technology no method could be identified for a microwave system to destroy the type of armored materiel common to tanks.

A bit later in their report, the DIA specialists indicated how these microwave weapons might accomplish the immobilization of people:

---

in an anechoic chamber—a room with absorbent walls designed to prevent microwave reflection—Dr. Sharp was able to recognize spoken words that were modulated by an audiogram —a graphic representation of the sound waves that humans can hear—and that were then sent into the chamber at a microwave frequency of about two gigahertz.

The immediate danger from microwave barrier weapons is burns. The U.S. Army Medical Research Laboratory at Fort Knox, Kentucky, has conducted tests on burns with microwaves. They have produced third-degree burns on human skin with twenty watts per square centimeter in two seconds, with frequencies of approximately three Gigahertz. The study also points out that a microwave barrier can be set up with existing state-of-the-art technology and off-the-shelf hardware. Considering the Soviet expertise in the area of electromagnetic energy, which is probably very close to, if not on a par with that of the U.S., the possibility must be accepted that they too have investigated microwave energy for barrier warfare and that they are also concerned with the biological effects of this type of radiation. Close monitoring of their research efforts on burns and burn therapy may possibly reveal Soviet efforts to develop countermeasures against microwave barrier warfare.

One scarcely knows how to react to this passage. First, barrier warfare sounds like a euphemism for crowd control. Second, the fact that a microwave beam with a power density of twenty *watts* per square centimeter can produce third-degree burns on human skin should come as no surprise. A beam of twenty watts per square centimeter amounts to an electronic flamethrower. Moreover, three gigahertz (three billion hertz) happens to be a frequency that can easily penetrate the human skull and, therefore, the brain. What is behind this experiment? Who authorized it, and why? As for "burn therapy" possibly revealing "Soviet efforts to develop countermeasures," what could that possibly mean? Super Unguentine? In any case, so much for the notion that only the Russians would think of utilizing microwave radiation for antipersonnel purposes.

The suggestion in the DIA report that microwave radiation might be used as a mind-control weapons system is not new. More than ten years ago, Dr. Zaret suggested as much. As Project Pandora was in full swing, Zaret undertook to analyze the Soviet literature on microwaves for the CIA, and wrote as follows:

The primary emphasis of Soviet-bloc research on the biological effects of non-ionizing electromagnetic radiation is concerned with induced neuro-physiological or behavioral aberrations. These may be either inhibitory or excitatory; the primary locus of action may be in either the peripheral or central nervous system, and the effects may be reversible or irreversible. Super-imposed upon these three sets of variables are the concepts of thermal versus non-thermal effects, the role of continuous versus pulsed waveform, and the degree of wavelength specificity. Although the various reports appear, at first glance, to represent a confused and conflicting mass of data, a logical, orderly and meaningful pattern can be evolved in evaluating their data. The basic factors which must constantly be borne in mind are (1) that microwave radiation is electromagnetic in nature, (2) that the nervous system functions as an electronic network normally shielded or protected from spurious fields and (3) that when extraordinary electromagnetic fields are created around neural elements this can produce functional or organic neurological anomalies.

After pointing out that Soviet scientists obviously believed that pulsed microwave radiation was much more effective than continuous radiation in affecting nervous system pathways, Zaret said that the Russians defined nonthermal microwave effects as those produced by exposures that did not result in appreciable heating of irradiated tissues:

> For non-thermal irradiations, they believe that the electromagnetic field induced by the microwave environment affects the cell membrane, and this results in an increase of excitability or an increase in the level of excitation of nerve cells. With repeated or continued exposure, the increased excitability leads to a state of exhaustion of the cells of the cerebral cortex. This results in the Sechenov inhibition effect which is manifested by the elimination of positive conditioned reflexes or behavior.

Unless one assumes that Soviet research as described by Zaret ten years ago has since been ignored in the United States in favor of developing such crude devices as a twenty-watt electronic flamethrower designed to "immobilize personnel in the open," one must conclude that work on mind-control weapons systems has been going on here as well as in Russia. Indeed, there have been a number of reports to that effect. One of the most recent appeared in the *New York Times* on July 20, 1977. It said that CIA documents revealed that the agency had conducted a fourteen-year program to control human behavior with drugs, electric shock, radiation, and ultrasonics.

Another report appeared in the *National Enquirer* on June 22,

1976. It said that since 1973 the Advanced Research Projects Agency had been sponsoring a program to develop a machine that could read minds from a distance by deciphering the brain's magnetic waves. A scientist involved in the program had declared that the ultimate goal of his work was to exercise control over the brain. According to the article, scientists were studying various aspects of the problem at the Massachusetts Institute of Technology, New York University, the University of California at Los Angeles, and the National Aeronautics and Space Administration's Ames Research Center, at Moffett Field, in California. Official verification that something of the sort is going on can be gained from the following passage in a letter written on November 19, 1976, by Robert L. Gilliat, Assistant General Counsel for Manpower, Health, and Public Affairs for the Department of Defense:

> As indicated in my letter of November 12, information which I have received from the Advanced Research Projects Agency is to the effect that the so-called "brain wave" machine, which was the subject of the *National Enquirer* article . . . is *not* capable of reading brain waves of anyone other than a willing participant in the laboratory efforts to develop that particular device. Its technical limitations, I am told, do not permit any long range use. I have no reason to doubt that information.

An interesting report about behavior alteration caused by low-level electromagnetic radiation has recently been compiled by William Bise, director of the Pacific Northwest Center for the Study of Non-Ionizing Radiation, in Portland, Oregon. Bise's report, entitled "Radio-frequency Induced Interference Responses in the Human Nervous System," describes some preliminary experiments conducted with radio-frequency energy on ten human volunteers—five men and five women—between July 1975 and June 1976. According to Bise, these experiments, which were conducted without controls, showed that "biological interference responses in the human nervous system can be elicited not only by pulse-modulated but by continuous wave radio-frequency at power densities substantially below those levels that exist in a typical urban environment." Four of the male volunteers, who were subjected to irradiation by electric fields of only sixty-five to ninety microvolts per meter, experienced short-term memory impairment, followed by concentration inhibition and by irritability, and three of the women volunteers expressed apprehension and mild irritation during the course of the tests. In the final section of his report, Bise suggested that since approximately five percent of the urban population of the United States was believed to be living in an environmental power density averaged over several radio bands of about two volts per meter, his findings indicated that "a meaningful risk factor for the general population appears to exist." He then concluded, sensibly enough, that "since radio-frequency in the environment continues to increase at a phenomenal rate, there is a need for further clarifying research of radio-frequency effects on biological systems."

As for the Russians, their attempts to use microwave and radio-frequency radiation as a psychological weapon may already extend far beyond the walls of the American Embassy in Moscow. A report published in the *New York Times* on October 30, 1976, revealed that in recent months a mysterious broadband, shortwave radio signal had been broadcast intermittently from the Soviet Union. The signal was so powerful that it disrupted radio and telecommunications throughout the world. Despite complaints from other countries, from the Federal Communications Commission, and from the International Telecommunications Union, the Soviet transmissions continued.

Not surprisingly, a number of theories arose regarding the origin and meaning of these signals. According to one theory, the signals were pulsed radiation emanating from an experimental over-the-horizon radar that had been set up in the vicinity of Minsk, not far from the Polish border. The radar might be designed either to detect surface shipping and aircraft over the North Atlantic, or a ballistic missile attack over the Arctic Circle. A second theory suggested that the Soviets were studying effects upon the ionosphere caused by radiating up to two million megawatts of power in the frequency range below six megahertz. And still another theory was advanced by disciples of Nikola Tesla—that the signals were an attempt by the Russians to test Tesla's claim that significant amounts of electrical energy could be transmitted without wires by using the earth as a conductor. Tesla is said to have proved this theory during the 1930s when he installed an invention called a magnifying transmitter in northern Quebec, and used it to provide power through the ground to a laboratory a hundred miles away. Adding fuel to this particular speculation was the news that Soviet scientists had sought out and interviewed Arthur H. Matthews, of Quebec, Tesla's last known living assistant. In addition, the Director of Operations of the Canadian government's Department of Communications reported that although the strange Soviet signals originated several thousand miles east of Canada, the stations monitoring them recorded the same signals with even greater intensity coming around from the opposite direction, half an hour later.

Dr. Zaret is concerned about the Russian signal, not because of its interference with radio and telecommunications, but because of its potential hazard to human beings. He spoke about it not long ago. "This broadband signal is being pulsed at an on-off rate of ten times per second. When I analyzed the Soviet literature for Project Pandora back in the 1960s, it was very clear that such an encoding impressed onto carrier wavelengths could have a central-nervous-system effect. In the case of the present signal, I would not be surprised to find that the on-off code at a repetition rate of ten per second could have an effect on the brain's inherent alpha rhythm. So whatever purpose the Russians may have for continuing this transmission, the potential effect in human beings from altering their alpha rhythm cannot be discounted."

25

The Zapping
of America

For the past decade or so, the government has extended the presumption of innocence to low-intensity microwave radiation even as it was supposed to be encouraging an intensive investigation of the biological effects of such radiation. This situation has created a strange and often uncomfortable climate for members of the medical and scientific community who have been given government funds to study the problem. It has, for example, created a climate in which, over nearly a decade, a number of leading microwave scientists have received government research money to investigate the biological effects of low-level microwave radiation even though during this entire period they have publicly disparaged the possibility that such effects might exist. A number of wide-ranging but connected developments show how the military, the government, the electronics industry, and the scientific community operate within such a climate to influence the medical issue:

• Colonel Appleton, chief of ophthalmology service at the Walter Reed General Hospital, has found it possible to testify on behalf of a microwave-oven manufacturer in a court case involving the alleged development of microwave cataracts. He has also found it possible to write on behalf of President Ford a dubious letter of reply in November 1976 to a former Army radar technician afflicted with cataracts. The radar technician had written to the President suggesting that a commission be established to determine whether physical disabilities occur at a higher rate among people exposed to radar. Appleton, who must have forgotten about the famous case of microwave cataracts discovered by Dr. Hirsch of the Sandia Corporation back in 1951, assured the ex-serviceman that the Joint Uniform Services Committee on Microwave Ocular Effects, of which he was a member, had concluded that there was "*no* evidence to indicate that *any* human being had *ever* sustained injury to the eyes from exposure to microwave energy, regardless of how intensive the exposure may have been." He went on to say that "in all honesty and fairness, I must tell you that there is no reasonable or factual basis for assuming that you have a claim for damages from exposure to microwave energy that you should be entitled to bring against either the Veterans Administration or any of the uniformed military services." In making this statement, Appleton was apparently unaware that five former radar technicians and two air traffic controllers had by then received compensation for work-related cataracts from either the VA or the Department of Labor; also that dozens of other such cases were pending, and that since 1968, there have been at least ten diagnosed cases of cataracts among radar technicians and radar instructors working on Hawk and Nike-Hercules missile systems at the Army's Redstone Arsenal, in Huntsville, Alabama.

• For the past seven years, the only reliable vehicle of information and support for the 150-odd ex-servicemen and former air traffic controllers who are known to have developed cataracts has been an organization called Radar Victims Network. Founded by Joseph H. Towne, of North Highland, California, a former radar technician who developed cataracts after serving on EC-121 spy planes, this organization was written about extensively during the early 1970s by Jack Anderson and Les Whitten. Yet Captain Tyler, as chairman of a four-day Conference on the Biological Effects of Non-Ionizing Radiation, held by the New York Academy of Sciences in February 1974, used the opening address as an opportunity to place a label of "pure sensationalism" on the highly accurate Anderson-Whitten columns about the plight of the former radar technicians. In addition, Captain Tyler, in a 1977 meeting with a former Navy radar officer afflicted with cataracts, tried to discredit Dr. Zaret by showing the former officer a closing statement signed by two plaintiffs in a recently dismissed civil action involving eye damage allegedly sustained from exposure to microwave ovens produced by Litton Industries, Inc. The statement said: "We now believe that Dr. Zaret had no scientific basis for his claimed findings that we had microwave eye injuries and cataracts caused by exposure to leakage from a microwave oven." Tyler did not tell the officer that the case had been settled out of court to the advantage of the injured plaintiffs. And he probably did not know that a lawyer from the plaintiffs' law firm—Freeman, Friedman, Wilson, and Carney, of Newark—had subsequently given an address at a meeting of the Association of Trial Lawyers of America in which she referred to the case, saying: "I think you should also be made aware of the fact that we were advised many times during the course of this litigation that the matter could be settled if we would agree that the doctor not report his findings." Thus, the quid pro quo for the out-of-court settlement of this case was that the plaintiffs sign a statement absolving Litton and criticizing Zaret.

• In February 1977, Captain Tyler attended a Bureau of Radiological Health Symposium on the Biological Effects of Radiofrequency and Microwave Radiation, where he heard Dr. Moris L. Shore, director of the bureau's Division of Biological Effects, point out that the tenfold safety factor thought to be present when the ten-milliwatt standard was formulated had been seriously eroded by subsequent research. Tyler nevertheless wrote a letter in April 1977 to the Naval Ship Engineering Center, which had just submitted the first draft of a report on the safety of the Navy's electromagnetic systems for the Chief of Naval Materiel. The letter said: "The flat statement that electromagnetic radiation is harmful to biological organisms is very misleading. It must be changed by qualifying harmful to either 'may be' or 'we know that at high levels, i.e., greater than one hundred milliwatts per square centimeter, electromagnetic radiation can be harmful.' "

• The C-95.4 subcommittee of the American National Standards Institute, sponsored by the Navy and the Institute of Electrical and Electronics Engineers, Inc., is responsible for recommending safe levels of human exposure to non-ionizing radiation. It has reaffirmed the ten-milliwatt standard three times within the past ten years. At least thirty-five of its sixty-eight members represent the Army, the Navy, the Air Force, NASA, the microwave-oven industry, the Association of Home Appliance Manufacturers, the electronics industry, and the aerospace industry, or have conducted research on the biological effects of microwaves for one or more of these organizations. The chairman of the subcommittee is Professor Arthur W. Guy, of the Department of Rehabilitation Medicine at the University of Washington. At the Senate Commerce Committee's 1973 Oversight Hearings on the Radiation Control for Health and Safety Act, Guy sent a statement for inclusion in the Hearing Record. In his capacity as chairman of C-95.4, Guy assured the Commerce Committee that the five-milliwatt standard for microwave ovens was adequate. At the time he was engaged in a study of microwave radiation effects at oven frequencies on the eyes of rabbits and monkeys. The study was being financed by the Office of Naval Research and the Association of Home Appliance Manufacturers. Professor Guy has found it possible to testify in behalf of microwave oven manufacturers in court cases involving alleged cataract development, and to organize a workshop, sponsored by the Association of Home Appliance Manufacturers and held at the University of Washington, in order to educate lawyers and executives from microwave-oven manufacturing companies about the research he had conducted on microwave cataracts.

• Another key academic figure, the ubiquitous Professor Michaelson, has been a consultant for the Association of Home Appliance Manufacturers, and has testified on behalf of the Raytheon Corporation in a workmen's compensation hearing involving microwave cataracts. He is a member of the C-95.4 subcommittee; of the subcommittee's 1973 working group on EMP; of the 1971 ad-hoc committee that upheld the Navy's decision to terminate Dr. Zaret's research contract for studying the long-term effects of chronic microwave exposure on primates; and of the National Academy of Science's Committee on Biosphere Effects of Extremely-Low-Frequency Radiation, which has been set up to evaluate the biological effects of the Navy's proposed Seafarer communications system. In addition, Michaelson is a research scientist whose studies of the biological effects of microwaves on animals have largely been financed by the Navy. In 1975, he appeared as a witness for the Rockland Electric Company at a public hearing held in Newark by the New Jersey State Department of Utilities. At issue was whether the electric company should be allowed to install a microwave antenna tower in the town of Mahwah. Michaelson testified under oath that in his opinion there was no evidence whatsoever of any health hazard or even any biological effect from continuous exposure to microwave radiation having a power density of .85 milliwatts per square centimeter; that it made no difference to him as a medical scientist whether or not an antenna radiating that amount of energy was to be installed so that human beings might be exposed to it; that microwaves affect cells only through heating, and that a human being would feel pain before incurring cell damage from microwave radiation; that no reports of microwave-induced cataracts had been authenticated; that animal experiments showing low-level, nonthermal microwave effects on rats, which were conducted by the renowned Dr. Zinaida V. Gordon, were invalid because Dr. Gordon housed her animals in cages made out of metal that can act as an antenna; and, furthermore, that Dr. Gordon was either in error or misrepresenting the facts when she wrote in her report of these experiments that "the animals were placed in special plastic cages which are virtually transparent to all wave bands."

• The Bureau of Radiological Health is only just now getting around to proposing performance standards for the 15,000-odd microwave-diathermy devices that are used to treat some two million Americans each year. This delay is puzzling, for the bureau has known for eight years that radiation from such devices could cause cataracts. It has known for three years that pregnant women are not allowed to be occupationally exposed to microwaves in Poland, because at least five cases of birth defects have occurred as a result of microwave-diathermy treatments.

• The Occupational Safety and Health Administration lacks proper and sufficient equipment to measure radiation being emitted by thousands upon thousands of microwave and radio-frequency heating devices used in industry. It has in effect thrown up its hands over the problem, declaring that employers have "the primary responsibility for determining the level of risk to workers exposed to microwaves."

• Except for a highly suspect study—carried out by the National Academy of Sciences—that compared the health and death records of twenty thousand Korean war veterans who were exposed to radar with the records of twenty thousand veterans who were not exposed, not a single epidemiological investigation similar to the investigations undertaken in the Soviet Union and other Eastern European countries has ever been conducted in the United States.*Nevertheless, there are hundreds of thousands of civilian and military radar technicians, microwave workers, and microwave-appliance makers, as well as television, radio, and other communications personnel, who are occupationally exposed to microwave radiation.

• On June 27, 1977, the Senate Commerce Committee held oversight hearings on the Radiation Control Act. However, only one member of the committee, Senator Wendell H. Ford, of Kentucky, showed up to hear the statements given by Dr. Pollack; Captain Tyler; Major Lawrence E. Larsen, of the Walter Reed Army Institute of Research; Captain Frank H. Austin, Jr., of the Office of Defense Research and Engineering; and Guenther Baumgart, president of the Association of Home Applicance Manufacturers, who was accompanied by two colleagues. Senator Ford was so woefully ill-prepared on the subject of microwave radiation that he scarcely bothered to query Dr. Pollack's assertions that the only reason screens had been placed over the windows of the American Embassy in Moscow was to protect embassy personnel from anxiety, and that there were no physical effects attributable to the Soviet irradiation of the embassy except for a "normal anxiety state." When Senator Ford asked Captain Austin why the military had destroyed part of the Project Pandora file, he did so without seeming to have any idea that the motive might have been to remove evidence of what the real intensity of the Moscow Signal was. In addition, Senator Ford did not know enough to challenge Captain Tyler's claim that the two cases of pancreatic cancer among young TACAN workers at the Quonset Naval Air Station were unexplained chance occurrences, and that no other TACAN personnel had developed cancer. Finally, the Senator did not even know enough to question the assertion by a representative of the Association of Home Appliance Manufacturers that the only microwave ovens being recalled for repair were units whose doors had suffered serious physical damage.

• In the end, this climate has made it possible for the Soviets to

---

*The study's chance of detecting true differences in morbidity and mortality was acknowledged to be only three in five, and its findings were almost totally invalidated by the fact that fully half of the twenty thousand men who were not supposed to be exposed to radar were radarmen.

irradiate the American Embassy in Moscow with impunity, and for American warships to pull alongside Russian surveillance trawlers on the high seas, turn on their radars at full megawatt power, and "paint" the Soviet vessels with radiation. This action burns out the receivers of the trawlers' electronic listening devices and accounts for the fact that Russian sailors are seldom seen on the decks of these vessels.

A policy based on suppressing and delaying the emergence of data cannot always be adjusted to conceal the haphazard revelations that are bound to occur from time to time. This proved to be the case during the Watergate affair—most notably when a chance question revealed the existence of the presidential tapes—and it may prove to be so with the recent attempt of the State Department to assuage the anxiety of its employees in Moscow. The window screens installed at the embassy, according to the State Department, have reduced the power levels of microwave radiation there from a maximum of eighteen microwatts per square centimeter to less than one. There is, of course, good reason to believe that the State Department has been lying to its employees, and that the power levels of radiation at the embassy have been far greater than eighteen microwatts. But, the issue of the State Department's credibility to one side, this claim still places the government of the United States in the untenable position of taking measures to protect a few hundred Americans in Moscow from levels of microwave radiation to which, as it has good reason to suspect, millions upon millions of American men, women, and children are being exposed every day.

Ironically, one of the early assessments of the extent of this exposure comes from the Raytheon Company, whose wholly owned subsidiary Amana Refrigeration is the largest manufacturer of microwave ovens in the world. Back in 1973, the Raytheon research division became upset by Consumers Union's blanket "Not Recommended" edict on microwave ovens. It asked one of its microwave experts, John Osepchuk, to look into the situation and, if possible, to come up with a way of countering the adverse publicity.

Osepchuk produced a study entitled "Radiation Hazards of Television Broadcasting to the General Population and Comparison with Microwave Oven Hazards." Documenting his study from official government reports, Osepchuk found that, according to the President's Office of Telecommunications Policy, the thousand-odd television stations in the United States "are located in the centers of population and therefore are of prime concern as sources of biological hazard due to 'electromagnetic pollution.' " He then compared the total radiated power and energy of these television transmitters with the total radiated power and energy that would be put out by a million microwave ovens operating for half an hour a day, and determined that "the television broadcast industry irradiates the country and its population by a factor of more than forty thousand greater than the radiation due to microwave ovens."

Later in his study, Osepchuk quoted the Federal Communications Commission as saying that it had issued no regulations governing television-broadcast radiation, "because the health hazard from such radiations has not been defined, and because the equipment over which it has jurisdiction has tended to be constructed and operated in such a manner that significant practical radiation hazards have not been known to exist." In a section of his study headed "Estimate of Television Broadcast Radiation in U.S. Homes," however, Osepchuk revealed that there is considerable evidence that a large part of the population may be subjected to levels of television radiation as high as one microwatt per square centimeter, and that a smaller, but still large, part of the population may be exposed to several milliwatts per square centimeter—"particularly those residing or working in high-level apartments or offices in cities." Osepchuk then referred to the 1973 Office of Telecommunications Policy annual report, which states that "levels of two milliwatts per square centimeter or higher in near-by high structures" will exist in cities near television transmitters. He also disclosed that it had long been known in government circles that microwave radiation generated at television frequencies could penetrate deeply into the body and affect the central nervous system.

Osepchuk's study was never formally published or distributed by Raytheon. There is, nevertheless, much anxiety in government circles over the amount of microwave radiation in urban areas, as determined by the fact that the Environmental Protection Agency's Office of Radiation Programs has been hard at work since October of 1975 measuring the intensity of the radiation being emitted by television and radio transmitters in major cities across the United

States. Using a specially built radiation-monitoring van, the EPA people have already completed surveys in Miami, Philadelphia, New York, Chicago, Boston, Atlanta, and the metropolitan area of Washington, D.C.

In October 1976, David E. Janes and Richard A. Tell, of the EPA's Office of Radiation Programs, presented data on radio-frequency radiation levels they had measured at seventy-two different locations in Atlanta, Boston, Miami, and Philadelphia. Janes and Tell said that the FM radio band contributed the most to environmental radio-frequency exposure between 54 and 900 megahertz, and that within that range, each of the three TV-bands (there are two VHF television bands and one UHF television band) contributed about equally to environmental levels. "The maximum power density at any site summed over all bands was 2.5 microwatts per square centimeter," they wrote. "Thus no sites had a value which exceeded the Soviet occupational standard of 10 microwatts per square centimeter. However, four sites or about six per cent fell within the range of 1 to 2.5 microwatts per square centimeter so that some of the population is potentially exposed in excess of one microwatt per square centimeter, a value which has been recommended as a general population exposure standard in the USSR."

The authors of the 1976 EPA report went on to say that, according to the Bureau of Census, about five percent of the U.S. population lived within the metropolitan areas they had surveyed. "While we feel that the results reported here are a fair representation of the exposures likely to be encountered by a large fraction of the U.S. population, some care must be used in interpreting these results." They added that there could be bias in the data because of the manner in which measuring sites were selected. Later in their report, Janes and Tell said that another consideration in interpreting their results was the fact that the measurements were made with an antenna that extended no more than twenty feet or so off the ground, and thus failed to take into account exposures on all but the lowest floors of buildings. The fact that this might constitute a serious bias in the interpretation of their report was stated as follows:

> Television broadcast antennas are highly directive, with the principal axis of the main lobe of the radiation pattern directed at or slightly

below the horizon. This means that at a constant horizontal distance from the antenna field strength increases with increasing height. Calculated values have been published by Tell and Nelson (1974). In a recent study in New York City, Tell (unpublished results) found power density values of the order of 10 microwatts per square centimeter on the upper floors of tall buildings.

Janes and Tell went on to say that in unusual situations exposures could approach or exceed the recommended U.S. standard of 10 milliwatts per square centimeter. As examples, they cited the fact that power densities exceeding 10 milliwatts per square centimeter had been measured in small regions very close to walkie-talkie antennas; that a power density greater than 1 milliwatt had been measured at the base of an FM tower in Mt. Wilson, California, where a small forest of antenna towers for twenty-seven FM and TV stations serving the Los Angeles area is located; and that radiation levels exceeding 180 milliwatts per square centimeter had been measured on the tower itself. Subsequently, an article appeared in *Environmental Action* saying that the ground levels of microwave radiation measured at Mount Wilson ranged from 1 to 44 milliwatts per square centimeter, and that a level of nearly 5 milliwatts had been measured in the vicinity of the Mount Wilson Post Office, which also serves as the residence of the postmaster. One can only assume that FM towers pose a potential hazard throughout the United States. For example, in New England, electric fields corresponding to power densities of forty-five milliwatts per square centimeter have been measured on the guy wires supporting FM towers. Moreover, the dashboard lights of jeeps parked beneath such towers have been known to glow without being turned on.

In spite of the obvious constraints in the way they had made their measurements, Janes and Tell put their data in the best possible light when they reported the results of their survey at the Fourth International Congress of the International Radiation Protection Association, in Paris during April 1977. At that time, they estimated that the total population of the four metropolitan areas in which their seventy-two measuring sites were located was 8,300,000 people, and they concluded that less than one percent of these people (or fewer than 83,000) were being exposed to radiation levels exceeding the Soviet general population standard of one microwatt per square centimeter.

They did not attempt to extrapolate these figures to the entire urban population of the nation, which would have brought the estimate of people exposed to more than one microwatt to well over the one-million mark. However, in the final paragraph of their 1977 report, Janes and Tell stated the qualifier to their conclusion:

> This model for population exposure does not account for complications such as daily movements of the population within an area, exposures at heights greater than 6 meters where exposures can be higher due to non-uniform antenna radiation patterns, for any attentuation effects of typical buildings, or for times when sources are not transmitting. The results are simply the population in areas where an unobstructed measurement 6 meters above ground would result in the indicated values.

Since delivering this report, Janes and Tell have measured a broadcast radiation level of 3.5 microwatts per square centimeter at the corner of Wisconsin Avenue and Fessenden Street in Northwest Washington, D.C., and a level of 2.2 microwatts in the Westwood section of Bethesda, Maryland. Both locations are near VHF TV towers. Moreover, near an FM tower in Las Vegas, they found a level of 20 microwatts. In addition, they have measured broadcast radiation levels of nearly 66 microwatts per square centimeter on the fiftieth floor of the Sears Tower in Chicago; a level of 97 microwatts on the thirty-eighth floor of a Miami office building; and a level of more than 10 microwatts on the fifty-fourth floor of the Pan Am Building in New York.

Janes and Tell are hoping to get new equipment that will enable them to measure radiation levels in multi-story buildings more easily. In the meantime, they are still performing ninety-nine percent of their measurements with an antenna twenty feet above the ground. Their results, therefore, cannot reflect broadcast radiation exposures being experienced by unsuspecting people living or working in tall buildings adjacent to television or FM installations. They also cannot measure the area in or near the primary lobe of the antenna beam, or, worse still, in the crossover or intersection of signals from two different transmitters, which can result in very hazardous conditions.

As it happens, a perfect example of upper-story exposure was discovered by chance, early in February 1977. At the request of the New York Newspaper Guild, Dr. Parr and some co-workers from NIOSH visited the *New York Times* Building (located on Forty-

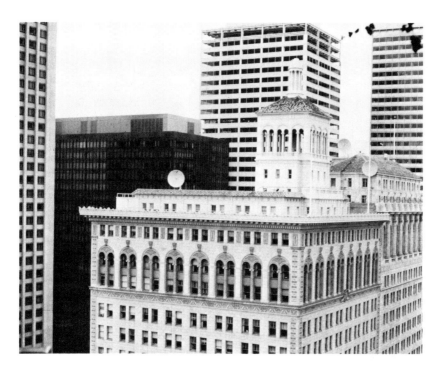

Microwave antennas seen from the revolving restaurant on top of the Hyatt Regency Hotel in downtown San Francisco. PHOTOS BY JANE RIPPETEAU

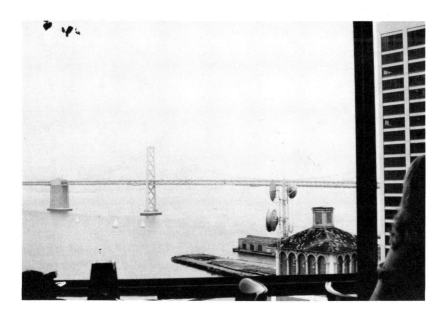

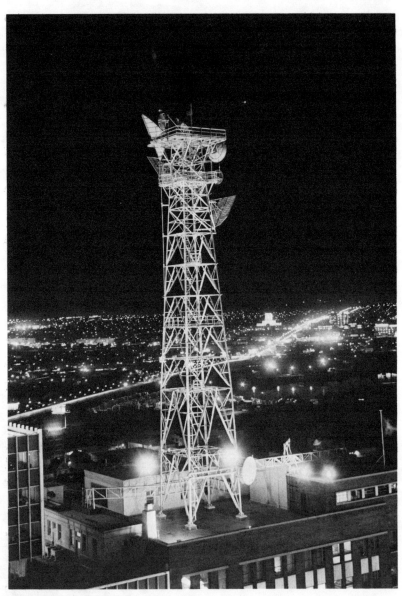

Microwave antenna tower in Vancouver, British Columbia.
PHOTO BY TED GRANT

third Street just west of Seventh Avenue) in order to determine
whether radiation was being emitted by the *Times'* video display
terminals (VDT). VDTs are now widely used at newspapers, banks,
libraries, airline offices, and insurance companies, and are suspected
by Dr. Zaret and others of leaking sufficient radiation to cause cataracts. According to Dr. Parr's report, none of the VDT units was
leaking excessive amounts of radiation—a finding that the guild has
disputed on the basis of the fact that his measuring equipment was
inadequate. However, page 7 of Dr. Parr's draft report of his survey
contains the following passage:

> In making measurements on the seventh floor, a reading of 1 mil-
> liwatt per square centimeter was obtained while measuring IBM ter-
> minals with the Narda instrument. With the terminals off, the reading
> still persisted. Because the same reading was obtained in the adjoining
> computer area, and at nearby windows, it was concluded that the
> meter was responding either to radio station WQXR located on the
> 9th floor of the *Times* Building or to signals from a nearby television
> station . . .

What might the radiation levels be, up on the ninth floor, where
WQXR is located? Or, for that matter, on the eighth, tenth, or
eleventh floor? Or in other buildings in the vicinity of the nearby
television station? Can we still believe official estimates and assurances that the general population of the United States—particularly
the urban population—is being adequately protected from potentially harmful amounts of television and radio broadcast radiation?
Few people in or out of government seem much concerned either
with the situation or the fact that it is growing worse.

A fine example of this lack of concern has been provided by the
New York Times itself. As of August 1977, the newspaper had not
seen fit to print a single word about the fact that two of its editorial
employees had developed cataracts at the ages of twenty-nine and
thirty-five, after using video display terminals for about six and
twelve months, respectively. Or about the fact that the dispute between it and the Newspaper Guild over VDTs had been placed
before an arbitrator. Nor did it cover the story of the radiation level
on the seventh floor of its own building. The *Times* did, however, run
an article on May 5, 1977, describing a new method of propagating
television signals. The new signal has been designed to eliminate

ghosts or multiple images of the sort that often plague city dwellers whose TV sets pick up signals bouncing off the faces of buildings. Alterations permitting the new signal to be broadcast are already being made in commercial and educational television transmitters at various places around the country. According to the *Times* article, if the new signals prove successful, a $100-million market in new television transmitter antennas and home roof antennas can be expected to develop over the next few years. A few lines later, the article mentioned in passing that the new system—it has, of course, been approved by the Federal Communications Commission—will require roughly double the electric power of the present system. By definition, this translates into a significant increase in the already worrisome levels of broadcast radiation that exist in cities and towns across the nation. Thus does the zapping of America proceed.

For his part, Dr. Osepchuk has been designated as the National Lecturer for 1977–1978 by the Institute of Electrical and Electronics Engineers' Microwave Theory and Techniques Society. These days he goes about delivering a talk called "Microwave Radiation Hazards in Perspective." As stated earlier, he concluded his report for Raytheon by observing that if low-level microwave radiation proved to be biologically harmful there would be a far greater hazard to the general population from television than from microwave ovens. As things turned out, he and his employers need not have worried. In spite of Consumers Union's nonrecommendation (which was reaffirmed in June 1976) and in spite of the manufacturers' having been forced to recall and repair thousands of microwave ovens that were discovered to be leaking radiation in excess of the five-milliwatt level, sales of the ovens have exceeded the most optimistic estimates of their makers. According to an article in the Sunday edition of the *New York Times,* in the spring of 1976, under the headline "MI-CROWAVE SALES SIZZLE AS THE SCARE FADES," more than eight hundred thousand microwave ovens, valued at $360 million, were sold in the United States in 1975. That year, for the first time in history, the sales of microwave ovens exceeded the sales of gas ranges.

On January 11, 1977, however, the *New York Times* ran a short piece reporting that the General Electric Company had agreed to repair without charge 36,000 microwave ovens manufactured between November 1973 and October 1975, which might be leaking radiation in excess of the five-milliwatt standard. What the *Times* failed to report was that the leakage problem in these ovens had been identified by the Bureau of Radiological Health almost a year and a half before; that the company had contested the bureau's finding at an FDA regulatory hearing; and that when the administration had upheld the bureau, GE had requested an exemption from complying with the five-milliwatt standard on the grounds that its ovens were not leaking enough to create a significant risk of injury. Nor did the *Times* report that General Electric had previously undertaken to make the necessary repairs on two other groups of ovens that were leaking radiation in excess of the standard, including repairs on 5,300 of 6,026 ovens manufactured between July and November 1973, as well as repairs on approximately 9,900 of 12,854 ovens manufactured before July 1973.

Whether microwave ovens, which are still allowed by federal regulations to leak as much as five milliwatts of radiation after purchase, are safe or not is obviously open to question. No one knows what constitutes a safe level of exposure to microwave radiation, and the average housewife cannot have the vaguest notion of how much or how little radiation her microwave oven may be leaking. The manufacturers of these appliances, for their part, continue to claim that it is safe to allow children to watch food cooking through the oven windows. Not so long ago, however, it was considered perfectly safe to allow children to study the bones of their feet in the viewing windows of flouroscope machines in shoe stores all over the country.

A year or so ago, one would have had a hard time finding anyone who believed that microwave radiation might turn out to have potent biological effects similar to those associated with X-rays and other ionizing radiation. Today, there is considerably more concern about the matter. And no one has the slightest idea what the long-term, low-level effects of microwaves will be. Of course, if microwave radiation should turn out to have irreversible biological effects, it may well be too late to do much about it. Indeed, given the mass addiction to television, and the widespread use of microwaves in all manner of communication, it seems questionable whether today's society would even want to do much about it. It is entirely possible that, regardless of how bad the situation may turn out to be, microwave radiation might pose a hazard people will choose to tolerate and continue to live with. That this possibility exists however, is hardly a reason for the public not to have been adequately informed about the potential danger posed by microwave radiation long before the radiation had proliferated to its present state of ubiquity in the urban environment, where it must now be accepted simply because submission is the only choice.

Needless to say, in order for the public to be adequately informed about any technological hazard prior to its becoming pervasive—after which, of course, people can merely cross their fingers and hope for the best—there has to be a free and enlightened scientific community, whose members are not only permitted but encouraged to think the unthinkable, if only in order to design a full range of experiments. This, of course, has not been the case with microwave radiation. Still, it is interesting to speculate about what might have happened if, instead of scorning mavericks like Zaret, laughing at pioneers like Frey, succumbing to the military's Cold War outlook, and worrying about possible misinterpretations by the press, the scientific community had undertaken to follow the Soviet lead and had seriously studied the biological effects of microwave radiation fifteen or twenty years ago, when the first disconcerting signs that something might be wrong appeared. It seems likely that at the very least such an endeavor might have prevented the government from placing itself in the position of perhaps having to install window screens for half the urban population. At best, it might have alerted the public long before now to assert its inalienable right to know, and to question the conspiracy of silence about the potential hazards of microwave radiation—a policy that the government was able to maintain for years on the very basis that the public, according to the parlance employed by military and intelligence people in matters deemed to involve security, had "no need to know." If this had been the case, it might not have been left to a handful of foreign-service officials and their wives to remind the nation that it is always eminently sensible to question government policy in any area that may affect the well-being of the people. Nor might we have found ourselves in a situation in which, for the first time in evolutionary history, we have begun to subject ourselves to levels of microwave and radio-frequency radiation that are millions of times as high as those occurring naturally in the biosphere. In doing so, we are living under an electronic sword of Damocles, for we are entirely without any idea of how such radiation may affect us, let alone of how it may affect future generations.

Epilogue

In June 1977, I went on vacation with my two children to Cape Cod, where I have spent a part of every summer for more than twenty years. While there, I read a letter to the *Provincetown Advocate* by Susan Williams, of Wellfleet, and Holly Kosikowski, of Eastham, whose husbands are stationed at the Air Force's 762nd Radar Squadron base in North Truro. This radar station, situated on a cliff 150 feet above the Atlantic Ocean, near Highland Light, on the Cape Cod National Seashore, has been in operation since the 1950s; its three spherical white radomes, approximately sixty feet in diameter, can be seen for miles around.

In their letter to the *Advocate,* the two women warned that hang-gliding from the cliffs near Highland Light—a sport that has become popular in recent years—could be extremely dangerous because "this radar complex operates on a peak power output of ten megawatts of microwave radiation." They went on to say that there was an official danger zone 800 feet in circumference around the three radomes, and they suggested that hang-glider pilots be warned to keep clear of it.

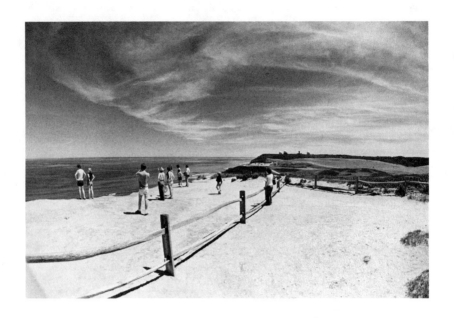

Two views of the Air Force radar station at North Truro. PHOTOS BY JIM GILBERT

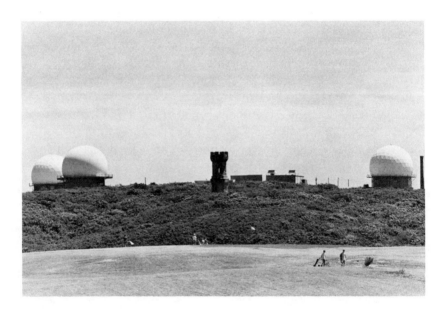

A week later, a front-page story by Gregory Katz appeared in the *Advocate* beneath the headline "TRURO RADAR COULD FRY HANG-GLIDERS." The article began:

> Powerful microwave transmissions sent out by three radar units can injure or kill hang-gliders who wander into airspace near the North Truro Air Force Station.
>
> "Under the worst combination of circumstances, a man could fry in those things," said Capt. Leland Downer, in reference to the radar units he is responsible for maintaining at the base.
>
> The radiation can cause sterility and cataracts. "A pilot could be injured by radiation without even knowing," said Lt. Col. Franklin Hall, commander of the base. "Radiation symptoms may not show for two years."

Later in the article, Colonel Hall was quoted as saying that any hang-glider pilot who sailed within 800 feet of the radar towers would be in danger. The article also said that the two most powerful radar units at the station "send out a concentrated beam that moves slowly in a vertical plane," and that Captain Downer was afraid this beam could fatally injure a pilot who was gliding through it. According to Katz, the third radar at the station "is thought to be less dangerous because it is constantly rotating and would hit a hang-glider for a very short time."

Toward the end of his article, Katz reported that an officer at the radar station had tried to prevent the Williams and Kosikowski letter from getting into print, for national-security reasons. The officer later admitted that the letter contained no classified information. Katz went on to say that hang-gliding is at present prohibited on National Seashore property adjoining the radar station but not on beaches controlled by the town of Truro. His article ended:

> Although the men in charge of the Seashore are aware of the radiation danger, nothing is presently being done to warn pilots to avoid the Air Force base. Truro Police Chief Ralph Lepore, Jr., said word of mouth was being relied upon to alert pilots to the danger. He said the government land is posted to prevent trespassing. There are no signs detailing the radiation hazard.

As it happens, in May 1974—more than a year before I began to study and write about the health hazards of microwave radiation— I bought two acres of land on Aldrich Road in North Truro, about a mile west of the radar station. In May 1977, I began to build a house on it, so the letter written by the two Air Force wives and the article by Katz were of particular interest to me. On July 1, I visited my building site on Aldrich Road with a friend who owns a microwave-detection device designed to warn motorists of police radar. Standing at ground level in a dense forest and listening on the microwave receiving set, we could hear very clearly the signal put out a mile away by the constantly rotating search radar. The search radar was irradiating the land mass that surrounds the station on three sides.

It was not, however, the search radar that concerned me as much as the two height-finder radars—the units Captain Downer had described as sending out concentrated beams that move slowly in a vertical plane. Were these units being operated so that they were also irradiating the land mass around the radar station? If so, they could be sending significant amounts of radiation into every home and school for miles around. I returned to New York City on July 5 and set about to determine whether this was the case. The information that follows is unclassified. Some of it appears in Air Force Technical Orders; some of it can be found in Military Handbook 162A; some of it can be obtained from the EPA; and much of it can be learned by talking with people who buy and sell surplus radars.

The sweep-search radar at the North Truro station is an FPS-107. It rotates 360 degrees five times a minute. It is manufactured by the Westinghouse Electric Corporation. It operates at a peak power of ten million watts (ten megawatts.) It has a duty cycle of about .0016. It has a frequency of 1.25 to 1.35 gigahertz. It has a vertical beam width of about 35 degrees, and a horizontal beam width of 1.5 degrees. Its antenna—parabolic in shape—is about fifty feet wide and twenty feet tall. From these data, it is possible to estimate that at a distance of one mile from the station, the peak pulse power density of the sweep-search radar is approximately 17.5 milliwatts per square centimeter. The average power density when the radar is rotating is about .2 microwatts per square centimeter. At eight hundred feet from the station, the peak pulse power density is approximately 770 milliwatts per square centimeter, and the average power density when the radar is rotating is about 7.7 microwatts per square centimeter.

As for the two height-finder radars at the North Truro station, they are the FPS-26A and the FPS-6. I was able to acquire detailed information only on the FPS-6, which is manufactured by General Electric. This radar can rotate in any direction and to any azimuth. It operates at a peak power of five megawatts. It works by nodding up and down twenty times a minute, starting below the horizon at minus 2 degrees, in order to detect low-flying aircraft, and moving upward to 32 degrees. (The FPS-6 at the North Truro station is directed over the land mass of Cape Cod at least forty percent of the time; during the rest of the time, it is aimed out over the Atlantic.) This radar has a frequency of 2.7 to 2.9 gigahertz. It has a duty cycle of .0006; a pulse width of 2 microseconds at 330 pulses per second; a horizontal beam width of 3.2 degrees; and a vertical beam width of .85 degrees.

From these data, it is possible to estimate that at a distance of one mile the peak pulse power density of the FPS-6 beam is approximately 170 milliwatts per square centimeter. The average power density is about 100 microwatts per square centimeter, which is a hundred times greater than the exposure level permitted for the general population in the Soviet Union. As for the power density out to eight hundred feet—the circumference of the so-called danger zone around the radomes—Captain Downer had good reason to fear that it might injure someone gliding slowly through it. At eight hundred feet, the peak power density of the pulsed microwave beam from the FPS-6 is about 7,400 milliwatts per square centimeter. The average power density is approximately 4.5 milliwatts per square centimeter.

In order to translate these figures into some analogy that will be familiar to readers of this book, let us return to the confidential briefing paper on the Moscow Signal, which was put out by the State Department in the spring of 1976. Page one of that document informed embassy personnel that the frequency range of the radiation being directed into the embassy building was between .5 and 9.0 gigahertz. (This range includes the frequencies of the FPS–107, FPS-6, and FPS-26A radars at the North Truro Air Force station.) Page 4 of the briefing paper said that "between October 1975 and January 1976 the typical maximum levels measured were up to 13 microwatts per square centimeter," and that the highest level was 18 microwatts. Page 11 of the briefing paper declared that the maximum levels after January dropped to between one and three microwatts, and that "the present screens reduce the current microwave signals to a point well below one microwatt per square centimeter but not to a 'zero level.' "

What this means is that the FPS-6 is irradiating people who live within a radius of one mile of the North Truro radar station with a power level about a hundred times greater than the power level for which the State Department told its Moscow employees it was installing aluminum window screens for their protection. (To know when one is being irradiated by the FPS-6, one merely has to turn on a microwave detection device when an airplane is flying overhead, and listen for the signal that will occur twenty times a minute as the radar nods up and down.) It also means that within ten miles of the station—for example, as far away as Provincetown and Wellfleet—radiation levels from the FPS-6 *alone* may exceed the levels that are in effect for the general population of the Soviet Union. In addition, it may well mean that beachgoers in the vicinity of the station are being exposed to radiation from sidelobes, which are incidental to the main beams of all radars.

As if this were not alarming enough, the State Department was deceiving its employees when it told them that ordinary window screens could reduce microwave radiation in the .5 to 9.0 gigahertz frequency range by a factor of ten. The fact is that microwave radiation in that range (and thus radiation from the three radars at the North Truro station) readily passes through ordinary window screening. It passes through wood. It passes through concrete. It can be deflected only by a sheet of metal. Needless to say, it goes easily through the human skull and the human brain.

Should not the residents of Truro and North Truro insist that the Air Force operate its radars in a way to avoid irradiating the land mass around the station? (Their elementary school lies a mile or so southwest of the radar station.) Should not the citizens of Provincetown and Wellfleet join them, and all of these people be supported by officials of the National Seashore, who encourage tens of thousands of tourists to visit the area each year? They, in turn, should be joined by the thousands of Cape Cod residents who will be exposed to low levels of radiation emanating from the enormously powerful PAVE PAWS radar now being installed at Otis Air Force Base. And, finally, these thousands of people should be joined by millions of Americans who live and work in the vicinity of radar stations, radio transmitters, and television transmitters all across the nation. Only in this way can the hazards described in this book be addressed, and the zapping of America, which now proceeds unabated, be brought under control.

REFERENCES

Many of the references in this book have been cited in the text. The following chapter-by-chapter listings give additional information about some of these references, and include other major sources.

CHAPTER ONE

1. George C. Southworth, *Forty Years of Radio Research* (New York: Gordon and Breach, 1962).
2. Jeremy Bernstein, *Physicist*—Part II (I. I. Rabi), *The New Yorker,* October 20, 1975.
3. John J. O'Neil, *Prodigal Genius: The Life of Nikola Tesla,* (New York: I. Washburn, 1944).
4. A. S. Presman, *Electromagnetic Fields and Life,* (New York: Plenum Press, 1970).

CHAPTER TWO

1. Joel Griffith, Richard Ballantine, *Silent Slaughter,* (Chicago: Henry Regnery, 1972).
2. Ben Patrusky, *The Laser,* (New York: Dodd Mead, 1966).
3. Joseph William Shereschewsky, *Radiology,* 20:246, 1933.
4. William Bierman, Myron M. Schwarzschild, *The Medical Applications of the Short Wave Current,* (Baltimore: Williams & Wilkins, 1942).
5. I. Matelsky, "The Non-ionizing Radiations," *Industrial Hygiene Highlights,* 1: 140–78, 1968.
6. Bernard I. Lidman, Clarence Cohn, *Air Surgeons Bulletin,* Vol. 2, December 1945, pp. 448–49.
7. L. E. Daily, "A Clinical Study of the Results of Exposure of Laboratory Personnel to Radar and High Frequency Radio," U.S. Naval Medical Bulletin, Vol. 41, July 1943, pp. 1052–56.
8. Charles I. Barron, A. A. Love, A. Baraff, "Physical Evaluation of Personnel Exposed to Microwave Emanation," *Journal of Aviation Medicine,* Vol. 26,

December 1955, pp. 442–52.

9. S. I. Brody, "Military Aspects of Biological Effect of Microwave Radiation," *IRE Transactions on Medical Electronics,* Vol. ME-3, February 1956, pp. 8–9.

10. W. W. Mumford, "Some Technical Aspects of Microwave Radiation Hazards," *Proceedings of IRE,* Vol. 49, February 1961, pp. 427–47.

11. Frederic G. Hirsch, "Microwave Cataracts—A Case Report Reevaluated," *Electronic Product Radiation and the Health Physicist,* Proceedings of the 4th Annual Symposium of the Health Physics Society, Louisville, Kentucky, January 28–30, 1970, HEW publication BRH/DEP 70–26.

12. H. Kalant, "Microwave Radiation Hazards," *Canadian Medical Association Journal,* Vol. 81, October 1, 1959, pp. 575–82.

CHAPTER THREE

1. Evan G. Pattishall, ed., *Proceedings of Tri-Service Conference on Biological Hazards of Microwave Radiation.* July 15–16, 1957, The George Washington University.

2. Evan G. Pattishall, Frank W. Banghart, eds., *Proceedings of the Second Tri-Service Conference on Biological Effects of Microwave Energy,* July 8–10, University of Virginia.

3. Charles Susskind, ed., *Proceedings of the Third Annual Tri-Service Conference on Biological Effects of Microwave Radiating Equipments,* August 25–27, 1959, University of California.

4. Mary Fouse Peyton, ed., *Proceedings of the Fourth Annual Tri-Service Conference on the Biological Effects of Microwave Radiation,* August 16–18, 1960 (New York: Plenum Press, 1961).

CHAPTER FOUR

1. Richard D. Grundy, Samuel S. Epstein, eds., *Consumers Health and Product Hazards,* Vol. I (Cambridge: MIT Press, 1974), pp. 173–257.

2. Hearings before the Committee on Commerce, United States Senate, Ninetieth Congress, May 6, 8, 9, 13, and 15, 1968, Serial No. 90–49, U.S. Government Printing Office, Washington, D.C., 1968.

3. S. Prausnitz, C. Susskind, "Effects of Chronic Microwave Irradiation on Mice," *IRE Transactions on Bio-Medical Electronics,* Vol. BME-9, No. 2, April 1962.

4. Stephen F. Cleary, ed., *Proceedings of the Symposium on the Biological Effects and Health Implications of Microwave Radiation,* Richmond, Virginia, September 17–19, 1969, U.S. Dept of HEW, BRH/DBE 70–2, June 1970.

5. Karel Marha, Jan Musil, Hana Tuha, *Electromagnetic Fields and the Life Environment,* (San Francisco: San Francisco Press, 1971).

6. Allan H. Frey, "Human Auditory System Response to Modulated Electromagnetic Energy," *Journal of Applied Physiology,* Vol. 17, No. 4, July 1962, pp. 689–92.

7. Allan H. Frey, "Auditory System Response to Radio Frequency Energy," *Aerospace Medicine,* Vol. 32, December 1961, pp. 1140–42.

CHAPTER FIVE

1. M. Zaret, et al., *Progress Report*, "Occurrence of Lenticular Imperfections in the Eyes of Microwave Workers and Their Association with Environmental Factors," Rome Air Development Center TN–61–226, 1961.
2. M. Zaret, et al., *Final Report*, "A Study of Lenticular Imperfections in the Eyes of a Sample of Microwave Workers and a Control Population, "RADC–TDR–63–125, 1963.
3. M. Zaret, "An Experimental Study of the Cataractogenic Effects of Microwave Radiation," RADC Technical Documentary Report, N. 64–273, October 1964.
4. B. Appleton, "Microwave Cataracts," *Journal of the American Medical Association*, Vol. 229, No. 4, July 22, 1974, pp. 407–8.
5. B. Appleton, "Results of Clinical Surveys for Microwave Ocular Effects," Selected Papers from the Division of Biological Effects Lecture Series, Bureau of Radiological Health, February 1973, DHEW Publication No. (FDA) 73–8031, BRH/DBE 73–3.
6. B. Appleton, et al., "Microwave Lens Effects and Humans," *Archives of Ophthalmology*, Vol. 93, April 1975, pp. 257–58.
7. *1969 Annual Report to the Congress on the Administration of the Radiation Control for Health and Safety Act of 1968*, Bureau of Radiological Health, BRH/OBD 70–3, April 1, 1970, p. 10.

CHAPTER SIX

1. *Radiation Control for Health and Safety*, Hearings before the Committee on Commerce, United States Senate, Ninety-third Congress, March 8, 9, 12, 1973, Serial No. 93–24, U.S. Government Printing Office, Washington, D.C., 1973.
2. T. P. Asanova, A. I. Ravok, "The State of Health of Persons Working in the Electric Field of Outdoor 400 and 500 KV Switchyards," translated by G. Guy Knickerbocker, Electrical Safety and Life Sciences Subcommittee, Power Engineering Society, Institute of Electrical and Electronic Engineers, Inc.
3. Ormond Aebi, Harry Aebi, *The Art & Adventure of Beekeeping*, (Santa Cruz: Unity Press, 1975).
4. P. Czerski, M. L. Shore, et al., eds., *Biologic Effects and Health Hazards of Microwave Radiation*, Proceedings of an International Symposium at Warsaw, Poland, October 15–18, 1973 (Warsaw: Polish Medical Publishers, 1974).
5. M. Zaret, "Electronic Smog as a Potentiating Factor in Cardiovascular Disease," *Medical Research Engineering*, Vol. 12, No. 3.
6. Paul E. Tyler, ed., *Biologic Effects of Nonionizing Radiation*, Conference held by the New York Academy of Sciences, New York City, February 12–15, 1974, Annals of the New York Academy of Sciences, Vol. 247, February 28, 1975.
7. Stephen F. Cleary, ed., *Proceedings of the Symposium on the Biological Effects and Health Implications of Microwave Radiation*, Richmond, Virginia, September 17–19, 1969, U.S. Dept of HEW, BRH/DBE 70–2, June 1970, pp. 116–21.
8. Arnold T. Sigler, Abraham M. Lilienfeld, Bernice H. Cohen, Jeanette E. Westlake, "Radiation Exposure in Parents of Children with Mongolism (Down's Syndrome)", *Bulletin of the John Hopkins Hospital*, Vol. 117, 1965, pp. 374–99.

CHAPTER SEVEN

1. Don R. Justesen, "Microwaves and Behavior," *American Psychologist,* Vol. 30, No. 3, March 1975.

CHAPTER EIGHT

1. S. Barańska, P. Czerski, *Biological Effects of Microwaves,* (Stroudsburg, Pa.: Dowden, Hutchinson & Ross, 1976) pp. 135–36, 168–69.
2. John T. McLaughlin, "Tissue Destruction and Death from Microwave Radiation (Radar)," *California Medicine,* Vol. 86, No. 5, May 1957, pp. 336–39.
3. John T. McLaughlin, "Health Hazards from Microwave Radiation," *Western Medicine,* Vol. 3, April 1962, pp. 126–32.
4. Karel Marha, Jan Musil, Hana Tuha, *Electromagnetic Fields and the Life Environment,* (San Francisco: San Francisco Press, 1971).

CHAPTER NINE

1. Stephen Leary, ed., *Proceedings of the Symposium on the Biological Effects and Health Implications of Microwave Radiation,* Richmond, Virginia, September 17–19, 1969, U.S. Dept of HEW, BRH/DBE 70–2, June 1970, pp. 191–96.

CHAPTER TEN

1. S. Prausnitz, C. Susskind, "Effects of Chronic Microwave Irradiation on Mice," *IRE Transactions on Bio-Medical Electronics,* Vol. BME-9, No. 2, April 1962.
2. P. Czerski, M. L. Shore, et al., eds., *Biologic Effects and Health Hazards of Microwave Radiation,* Proceedings of an International Symposium at Warsaw, Poland, October 15–18, 1973 (Warsaw: Polish Medical Publishers, 1974), pp. 67–74, 189–95.

CHAPTER ELEVEN

1. A. S. Presman, *Electromagnetic Fields and Life,* (New York: Plenum Press, 1970), pp. 141–55.
2. S. Barańska, P. Czerski, *Biological Effects of Microwaves,* (Stroudsburg, Pa.: Dowden, Hutchinson & Ross, 1976), pp. 132–35.

CHAPTER TWELVE

1. Frederick G. Hirsch, A. Bruner, "Proceedings of the Technical Coordination Conference on EMP Biological Effects," sponsored by the Lovelace Foundation for Medical Education and Research, Albuquerque, New Mexico, July 1970.

CHAPTER THIRTEEN

1. Karel Marha, Jan Musil, Hana Tuha, *Electromagnetic Fields and the Life Environment,* (San Francisco: San Francisco Press, 1971), pp. 38–58.

CHAPTER FOURTEEN

1. M. Zaret, "Cataracts and Avionic Radiations," *British Journal of Ophthalmology*, Vol. 161, June 1977.
2. M. Zaret, "Cataracts in Aviation Environments," Letter to *The Lancet*, February 26, 1977.

CHAPTER FIFTEEN

1. John T. McLaughlin, "Tissue Destruction and Death from Microwave Radiation (Radar)," *California Medicine*, Vol. 86, No. 5, May 1957, pp. 336–39.
2. John T. McLaughlin, "Health Hazards from Microwave Radiation," *Western Medicine*, Vol. 3, April 1962, pp. 126–32.

CHAPTER SIXTEEN

1. David S. Rosenthal, Steven C. Beering, "Hypergonadism after Microwave Radiation," *Journal of the American Medical Association*, Vol. 205, No. 4, July 22, 1968, pp. 105–8.
2. Vernon E. Rose, Gerald A. Gellin, Charles H. Powell, H. G. Bourne, "Evaluation and Control of Exposures in Repairing Microwave Ovens," *American Industrial Hygiene Association Journal*, Vol. 30, March–April 1969, pp. 137–42.
3. M. Zaret, "Blindness, Deafness and Vestibular Dysfunction in a Microwave Worker," *The Eye, Ear, Nose and Throat Monthly*, Vol. 54, July 1975, pp. 49–52.

CHAPTER SEVENTEEN

1. S. Barańska, P. Czerski, *Biological Effects of Microwaves*, (Stroudsburg, Pa.: Dowden, Hutchinson & Ross, 1976), pp. 15–16, 117–22.
2. Karel Marha, Jan Musil, Hana Tuha, *Electromagnetic Fields and the Life Environment*, (San Francisco: San Francisco Press, 1971), pp. 59–112.

CHAPTER EIGHTEEN

1. J. D. Dumanskij, M. G. Sandala, "The Biologic and Hygienic Significance of Electromagnetic Fields of Superhigh and Ultrahigh Frequencies in Densely Populated Areas," *Biologic Effects and Health Hazards of Microwave Radiation*, Proceedings of an International Symposium at Warsaw, Poland, October 15–18, (Warsaw: Polish Medical Publishers, 1974), pp. 289–93.

CHAPTER NINETEEN

1. S. M. Michaelson, "Thermal Effects of Single and Repeated Exposures to Microwaves—a Review," *Biologic Effects and Health Hazards of Microwave Radiation*, Proceedings of an International Symposium at Warsaw, Poland, October 15–18, (Warsaw: Polish Medical Publishers, 1974), pp. 1–14.
2. *Radiation Control for Health and Safety*, Hearings before the Committee on

Commerce, Ninety-third Congress, March 8, 9, 12, 1973, Serial No. 93–24, U.S. Government Printing Office, Washington, D.C., 1973, pp. 113–72.

CHAPTER TWENTY

1. L. W. Ricketts, J. E. Bridges, J. Miletta, *EMP Radiation and Protective Techniques,* (New York: John Wiley & Sons, 1976.)
2. William C. Milroy, ed., "Biomedical Aspects of Nonionizing Radiation," Proceedings of a Symposium held at the Naval Weapons Laboratory, Dahlgren, Virginia, July 10, 1973.

CHAPTER TWENTY-ONE

1. William C. Milroy, ed., "Biomedical Aspects of Nonionizing Radiation," Proceedings of a Symposium held at the Naval Weapons Laboratory, Dahlgren, Virginia, July 10, 1973, pp. 40, 49.

CHAPTER TWENTY-TWO

1. *Radiation Control for Health and Safety,* Hearings before the Committee on Commerce, United States Senate, Ninety-third Congress, March 8, 9, 12, 1973, Serial No. 93–24, U.S. Government Printing Office, Washington, D.C., 1973, pp. 104–6.

CHAPTER TWENTY-THREE

1. S. Prausnitz, C. Susskind, "Effects of Chronic Microwave Irradiation on Mice," *IRE Transactions on Bio-Medical Electronics,* Vol. BME-9, No. 2, April 1962.
2. S. Barańska, P. Czerski, *Biological Effects of Microwaves,* (Stroudsburg, Pa.: Dowden, Hutchinson & Ross, 1976), pp. 137–46.

CHAPTER TWENTY-FOUR

1. Ronald L. Adams, R. A. Williams, "Biological Effects of Electromagnetic Radiation (Radiowaves and Microwaves) Eurasian Communist Countries," Defense Intelligence Agency, U.S. Army Medical Intelligence and Information Agency, Report No. DST–1810S–074–76, March 1976.

CHAPTER TWENTY-FIVE

1. Paul E. Tyler, ed., *Biologic Effects of Nonionizing Radiation,* Conference held by the New York Academy of Sciences, New York City, February 12–15, 1974, Annals of the New York Academy of Sciences, Vol. 247, February 28, 1974, pp. 10–11.
2. Hearings before the Board of Public Utility Commissioners, Newark, New Jersey, Docket No. 754–248, Vol. I and II, May 15, July 10, 1975.

Index

ABM system, 267–68, 271, 273, 289
ABRES (Advanced Ballistic Re-entry System), 239
Adey, Ross, 84
AEGIS, 239
Aerospace Corporation, 248
Aerospace Daily, 242, 269
Aerospace Medicine, 51
AFL-CIO, Industrial Union Department of, 216
agriculture, microwaves in, 9
Air Force, U.S., 8, 31, 32, 86, 144–45, 156, 158–59, 163, 241, 242–47, 270, 289–90
  Aerospace Medical Division of, 69, 198–99
  Aerospace Medicine School of, 242, 246, 260
  Air Defense Command of, 219
  Cape Cod (762nd) Radar Squadron base of, 319–24
  early warning satellites of, 266
  electromagnetic pulse (EMP) project of, 153–54

  "golf ball" (AN/FPS-45) of, 219–27
  Intelligence, 271–72
  Propulsion Laboratory of, 267
  Science Advisory Board of, 272–73
  Space and Missile Systems Organization of (SAMSO), 153–54, 289
  Systems Command of, 243
  Tri-Service Programs of, *see* Tri-Service Programs
  Weapons Laboratory of, 153
Air Line Pilots Association, 186–87
ALCOR, 239
Allen, John L., 274
ALTAIR, 240
Altman, Lawrence K., 82–83
Amana Refrigeration, 308
American Cancer Society, 129
American Foreign Service Association, 99, 100
American Health Foundation, 140, 141–42, 144–45, 146, 147
American Medical Association, Council on

American Medical Association *(continued)*
  Physical Therapy of, 23
American National Standards Institute
  (ANSI), 44, 73, 74, 154–55, 215, 218*n*,
  246, 259, 304
  C-95 Committee on Radio-Frequency
  Hazards of, 263
American Roentgen Ray Society, 21
Anderson, Jack, 69–70, 303–4
AN/FPN-40 Ground Controlled Approach
  Radar, 147–49, 208
AN/FPS-45 radar, *see* "golf ball" radar
  tracking system
AN/FPS-77 Weather Radar, 147–48
AN/FPS-85 radar, 226–27, 241, 242–43
angstroms, defined, 19
AN/TPN-18 radar, 147–49, 208
appendicitis, 115, 197
Appleton, Budd, 63, 79, 87, 256, 302–3
Archives d'Ophtalmologie, 87
Armed Forces Epidemiology Board, 173
Armed Forces Radiobiology Research Insti-
  tute (AFRRI), 230, 251, 255, 261–62
Army, U.S., 8, 31, 37, 55, 63–64, 86, 134, 139,
  145–50, 167, 172, 208, 211, 241, 305
  Adversary Proceedings Division of, 210
  Aeromedical Research Laboratory of, 146,
  147
  Aviation Medicine Research Division of,
  146
  Environmental Hygiene Agency of, 147,
  148, 260
  Medical and Information Agency of, 293
  Medical Research and Development Com-
  mand of (AMRDC), 137, 142–44, 146–47
  Missile Command of (MICOM), 209–10,
  268
  Mobility Research and Development Cen-
  ter of, 255, 296
  Office of the Surgeon General of (OSG),
  139
arthritis, 9, 18, 209
asbestos, 196
ASR-5 radar, 148
Associated Press, 98, 100, 101, 102, 104, 111–12,
  293
Association of Trial Lawyers of America, 304
atomic bomb raids (1945), 21, 129, 251, 282
Austin, Frank H., Jr., 307
Avco Everett Research Laboratory, 268
Aviation Week & Space Technology, 266–67,

268, 272, 278–79
AWACS (Airborne Warning and Control
  System), 240, 241

Baier, Edward J., 161–62, 202
Baillie, H. D., 79
Ballistic Missile Early Warning System
  (BMEWS), 34, 56, 219–20
Barron, Charles I., 29–30, 38, 158
Bartl, Franz, 156, 260
Baum, S. J., 261
Baumgart, Guenther, 307
Beauchamp family, 222–23
Beech, Keyes, 128
Beecher, William, 290–91
Beischer, Dietrich E., 256–57, 265–66
Bell, Herbert E., 161
Bell System, 4–5, 6
Bell Telephone Laboratories, 24, 27, 31, 37,
  156
Bendix Corporation, 181
Berman, Ezra, 134*n*
"Big Boy" study, 119
Binder, David, 269
Biologic Action of Ultrahigh Frequencies, The,
  37
Biological Effects and Health Implications of
  Microwave Radiation symposium
  (1969), 47–50, 52, 121
Biological Effects of Non-Ionizing Radiation
  conference (1974), 303
Biomedical Aspects of Non-Ionizing Radia-
  tion symposium (1973), 256
Birenbaum, Leo, 61, 155–56, 160, 286–87
birth defects, 49, 79, 92, 134–51
Bise, William, 299–300
Blasco, Andrew P., 230, 247, 250
blood abnormalities, 30, 36, 89, 96–97, 103,
  104, 109–15, 119, 127, 128, 132, 190
  see also leukemia
Boeing Company, 154–55, 156, 240, 248, 250,
  251, 259–60, 262–63, 285
Bohlen, Charles, 128–29
Boot and Shoe Workers Union, 214
Boston Globe, 170, 207, 290
Bouchat, Joseph A., 86–87
Bradley International Airport, Conn., 175–
  76, 179–80
bradycardia, 36
brain tumors, 160–62
Braun, Ferdinand, 2

Brezhnev, Leonid I., 96, 202–3
Bridges, J. E., 253
British Journal of Ophthalmology, 183–85
Brodeur, Paul, 107–8
Brooks Air Force Base, Tex., 242, 246
Brown, Frederick Z., 103
Brown, Harold, 283–85
Bruner, Alfred, 158, 160, 256
Brzesinski, Zbigniew, 129, 292
buccal smears, 105, 117
Burdeshaw, John A., 138–40, 146
Bureau of Radiological Health, 46, 47, 67, 73, 76, 78, 79, 130, 140, 141, 144, 145, 146, 147–50, 161, 162, 223, 263, 304, 306, 317
Burlington County Times, 220–21, 223, 224, 225
bursitis, 9, 18

Cadieux, Donald, 175
Caine, Stephen, 263–64
Cairns Army Airfield, Ala., 147–48
Camden Courier-Post, 222, 224–25
Campbell, Douglas, 222
cancer, 23, 115, 128–31, 154, 156, 175–76, 196, 263, 291–92
 in Navy civilian employees, 164–72, 307
 in U.S. Moscow Embassy, 128–31, 292
 X-rays and, 18, 22, 166–67, 170
Cape Cod, Mass., radiation exposure at, 226, 227, 243–44, 246–47, 319–24
cardiac pacemakers, 182, 223–24, 244
cardiovascular problems, 36, 52, 80–84, 163, 209, 213
Carpenter, Russell L., 33, 45, 68–69, 79
Carter, James R., Jr., 128, 129, 240, 276, 283–85, 290, 292
cataracts, 33, 37, 38, 50, 54, 55–60, 63–65, 67–69, 79, 86, 94, 96, 156, 174, 183–85, 238–39, 303–4, 305, 306, 321
 capsular, 56–59, 81
 thermal, 25–26, 59
Census Bureau, U.S., 310
Central Intelligence Agency (CIA), 40, 43, 60, 69, 103, 126, 163, 258, 268, 271–72, 273, 287–88, 290, 297, 298
central nervous system, 33, 35–36, 39–41, 47, 48, 52–53, 77, 80, 84–86, 94, 119–24, 129, 236–38, 297–98, 300, 309
Cesaro, Richard S., 101–2, 120
Chaput, Raymond L., 260
charged particle beam (CPB) weapons,

269–79
 see also directed-energy weapons
childbirth, microwaves used in, 87–88
chromosomal abnormalities, 90, 92, 104–5, 130, 132–33, 234, 260–61
 see also genetic damage
Ciprian, Paul, 181–82
Clayton, W. Graham, Jr., 284
Clemenceau, Georges, 280
Clement, William, 267
Cleveland, Grover, 1
clubfoot, radar and, 134–51
COBRA AMBER radar system, 240
COBRA ANGEL radar system, 240
COBRA BALL radar system, 240
COBRA DANE radar system, 226–27, 240, 241, 243
COBRA JUDY radar system, 240
COBRA MIST radar system, 240
COBRA TALON radar system, 240
Cohn, Victor, 110–11
Colby, William, 273
Coleman, William T., Jr., 180–81
COMPASS COPE, 240
COMPASS COUNTER, 240
COMPASS DART, 240
COMPASS DAWN, 240
COMPASS SAIL, 240
COMPASS TIE, 240
Compton electrons, 252
CONELRAD (Control of Electromagnetic Radiation), 240
Consumers Union, 72–74, 308, 316
CONUS Over-The-Horizon Backscatter (OTH-B) radar, 241–42
Crookes, Sir William, 2
Currie, Malcolm R., 247, 249, 252, 268, 269
Czechoslovakia, microwave investigations in, 48–50, 61, 88–89
Czerski, Przemyslaw, 130, 133, 235–36

Daels, José, 87–88
Dally, Clarence, 18
d'Arsonval, Jacques Arsène, 17
deafness, 203–9
Dean, W., Jr., 262, 264
Defense Communications Agency, 163
Defense Department, U.S., 15, 32, 39–41, 43, 46, 71, 74, 85, 91–92, 133, 152, 157, 163, 165, 230–34, 247–49, 255, 266, 270–71, 277, 280, 289, 299

Defense Department *(continued)*
Advanced Research Projects Agency of (DARPA), 41, 60–61, 69–70, 117–20, 122–23, 133, 249, 252, 255, 267–68, 270, 274, 289, 299
Defense Research and Engineering (DRE) branch of, 43, 230, 247, 274, 307
Electromagnetic Compatibility Analysis Center of (ECAC), 232
Institute for Defense Analysis of, 40, 60, 101, 117, 118–20, 123
Defense Intelligence Agency, 203, 272, 293–97
Defense Nuclear Agency, 8–9, 253, 258
De Forest, Lee, 3, 258
Denver, University of, EMP facility of, 255
Dettor, Charles, 147
diabetes, 56, 59
Diamond, Harry, Laboratory, 253, 255
diathermy, 9, 12, 17, 22–23, 49, 68, 87, 306
directed-energy weapons, 266–78, 281, 289
development of, 255–58
Dirks, Kenneth R., 142
Distant Early Warning (DEW) Line radar station, Oliktok, Alas., 212–13
DIXIE CUP, 240
Dodd, Edwin N., Jr., 230, 247, 250, 256, 263
Donaldson, David D., 66, 68–69, 87
Douglas, John H., 276
Downer, Leland, 321, 322
Down's syndrome (mongolism), 91–92, 104, 133, 185–86
Duke-Elder, Sir Stewart, 79
Duncan, C. W., Jr., 284

Eagleburger, Lawrence S., 100–1, 103
eavesdropping operations, 8, 40, 60, 61, 95, 97–98, 126
Edgerton, Germischausen, and Greer (EG & G) Company, 156, 159
Edison, Thomas Alva, 1, 17–18
Eglin Air Force Base, Fla., 136, 246
"Eighth Card," *see* Kirtland Air Force Base
Einstein, Albert, 18–19
Eisenhower, Dwight D., 248, 249
Ekstrom, Merlin E., 261
Elder, Robert L., 73
electrical current transmission, wireless, 13
electromagnetic pulse (EMP), 8, 154–60, 250–56, 259–64, 265–66, 281, 286–87, 289, 291–92

Air Force project on, 153–54
electronic weapons systems and, 157, 251, 254–56
genetic effects of, 159–60, 260–61, 287
electromagnetic radiation, 16–31
cumulative effects of, 18, 21–22, 47, 49, 77
defined, 2
early experiments in, 16–21
ionizing, 19–22, 43, 48, 194, 317
non-ionizing, 19, 43, 81, 85, 89, 129
electromagnetic radiation (EMR) devices, 2, 3, 8, 89, 231–35, 237–39, 241–42
see also specific devices
Electromagnetic Radiation Management Advisory Council, 14–15, 70, 73–74, 85, 89–90, 92, 101, 130, 132, 133, 174, 228, 256, 260
Electronic Warfare, 226, 266
ELF (extremely-low-frequency radio waves) system, 75, 241, 280–85
Emanuel, Irvin, 185–87
EMP Awareness Course Notes, 253
EMP Radiation and Protective Techniques, 253
endocrine responses to microwaves, 37
Energy Research and Development Administration, 272
Engell, Robert W., 169, 171, 174–78, 179, 180, 182, 197, 199
Environmental Assessment for PAVE PAWS, 243–47
Environmental Hygiene Agency, 210
Environmental Impact Statement (EIS) on radar sites in Maine, 242
Environmental Protection Agency (EPA), 111, 135, 138–40, 141–42, 143, 144, 221, 224, 322
Health Effects Research Division of, 137
Radiation Programs Office of, 309–10
Evans, Captain, 158–59
Evans, Rowland, 98
eye damage, 25–26, 30, 33, 36–38, 45, 54–69, 86–87, 183–85, 200–9, 238–39, 303–4, 305, 306, 321
see also cataracts

Federal Aviation Administration (FAA), 164, 166–67, 169, 173–77, 179–85, 239
Aeromedical Division of, 169, 174, 178
Federal Aviation Science and Technological Association (FASTA), 180

Federal Communications Commission (FCC), 7, 221, 300, 309, 316
Felsing, William A., Jr., 171–72
Finklea, John F., 165, 203, 217
Finland, heart attack rate in, 82–84
Finney, John W., 268–69
Fischer, Bobby, 70
Food and Drug Administration (FDA), 143, 196, 208, 224, 317
Ford, Gerald R., 96, 284, 303
Ford, Wendell H., 307
Fort Dix, N.J., 141
Fort Rucker, Ala., 134–52, 169, 185, 199, 208
Fort Stewart, Ga., 150
Fort Walters, Tex., 150
FPS-6 radar, 322–23, 324
FPS-26A radar, 322–23
FPS-107 radar, 323
Frazier, James W., 260
Freedom of Information Act, 293–94
frequency, defined, 2
Frey, Allan H., 50–53, 84–85, 122, 237, 294–95, 317
Funseth, Robert L., 103, 269

Galvani, Luigi, 16
gamma rays, 19, 90, 129, 182, 195, 252, 253, 254
Gandhi, Ohm, 216–18, 242
Garwin, Richard L., 269–70
Gearhart, Owen, 225
General Dynamics Corporation, 171, 248
General Electric Company, 27, 31, 42, 167, 209, 242, 248, 316–17, 323
  Advanced Electronic Center of, 50
  radar test facility of, 50–51
genetic damage, 14, 19, 21, 47, 70, 90–92, 104–5, 129, 132–52, 159–60, 234, 260–61, 287
Gerber, Naomi, 204–5
Gilliat, Robert L., 299
Ginnold, Richard E., 214–17
Godden, William R., 230, 243, 247, 250, 256
"golf ball" radar tracking system (AN/FPS-45), 219–27
Gordon, Zinaida V., 37, 38, 78–79, 306
Gresinger, Thomas H., 104–5
Grove, H. Mark, 260
Grumman Aerospace, 248, 289
Guy, Arthur W., 305

Hall, Franklin, 321

Hallock, Richard, 287
Hammond, E. Cuyler, 129
hang-gliding, 319–21
Hanscom Air Force Base, Mass., 243
HARM (Hypervelocity Anti-Radiation Missile), 240
Harriman, W. Averell, 40
Harris, Elliot, 203
Harrison, Benjamin, 1
Hartford Courant, 170
Healer, Janet, 172, 256
Health, Education and Welfare Department, U.S., 45–46, 94
heart attacks, 82–84, 163, 209
Heaviside, Oliver, 3
Heilmeier, George H., 249, 267
HEL (high-energy laser) program, 267–68
Heller, John H., 90, 132, 260–61
Helms, Richard M., 287
Hemenway, John D., 100–1
hertz, defined, 19
Hertz, Heinrich Rudolph, 2, 258
High Energy Pulse (HEP) weapons system, 251–52, 266–67
Himmelein, John, 223
Hiroshima, 21, 129, 251
Hirsch, Frederic G., 26–27, 28, 156–58, 159, 160, 259, 303
Hoeffler, D. F., 171
Holloway, J. L., III, 284
Home Appliances Manufacturers Association, 66–67, 76, 236, 305, 307
Hood, O. C., 169–70, 172–74
Horner, Charles E., 204–6
House Armed Services Committee, 284
  Research and Development Subcommittee of, 274
House Defense Appropriations Committee, 248–49
Hughes, Howard, 189
Hughes Aircraft Company, 150, 189, 247, 248, 268, 289
hyperthermia, 28–29

IBEX system, 288–90
infertility, 21, 24, 198–201, 321
infrared radiation, 19, 54, 194
Institute of Electrical and Electronics Engineers, 81, 155, 259, 263, 304
  International Pulsed Power Conference of, 268

Institute of Electrical *(continued)*
  Microwave Theory and Techniques Society of, 316
Institute of Labor Hygiene and Occupational Diseases, USSR, 36, 37, 79–80
Integrated Wide-Band Communications System (IWCS), 162–63
Interdepartment Radio Advisory Committee (IRAC), 262
  Side Effects Working Group Technical Subcommittee of, 262–64
International Congress of Radiology (1925, 1928), 21
International Symposium on the Biologic Effects and Health Hazards of Microwave Radiation, 78, 86
International Telecommunications Union, 300
International Telephone & Telegraph Corporation (ITT), 171, 255
ionosphere, 3, 4, 7, 83
Iran, murder of U.S. technicians in, 252, 287–89, 290

Jacobson, Cecil B., 104–5, 133
Janes, David E., 310–12
Jason Committee, 268, 269
Johns Hopkins University, government contracts of, 248
Johnson, Lyndon B., 42
Johnson, Thomas A., 96, 112–15
Joint Uniform Services Committee on Microwave Ocular Effects, 303
Jones, Herbert, 161
Jutesen, Don R., 121–22

Karches, Gerald J., 155, 260
Karras, Ronald P., 208–10
Katz, Gregory, 321, 322
Kavula, Robert, 220–22, 223, 226
Kay, Arthur, 65
Keegan, George J., 271–73, 275
Kennelly, Arthur Edwin, 3
Kirtland Air Force Base, N.M., 158–59, 255, 270
Kissinger, Henry A., 97, 99, 101, 102, 104, 107, 114
Knauf, George M., 34–35, 167
Kohn, Arnold M., 209–10
Kosikowski, Holly, 319, 321
Koslov, Samuel, 66

Kosygin, Alexei N., 42
Krane, Paul W., 224

Labor Department, U.S., 65, 183, 203, 206, 207, 218, 250–51, 259–60, 264, 303
  Employment Standards Administration of, 204
Labyak, Peter S., 165, 172
Larsen, Lawrence E., 307
lasers, 9, 13, 60, 266–71, 274–76
Leach, William M., 130–31
Lepore, Ralph, Jr., 321
leukemia, 21, 44, 91, 130, 154, 156, 261–63, 291–92
Levitas, A. A., 37, 38
Lilienfeld, Abraham M., 104, 125, 133
Litton Industries, 248, 304
Lockheed Aircraft Corporation, 29–30, 36, 38, 111, 158, 248
Lockheed Missile & Space Company, 248
Lodge, Henry Cabot, 40
Lodge, Sir Oliver Joseph, 2
Los Angeles Times, 95–96
Lovelace Foundation for Medical Education and Research, N.M., 26–27, 156–60, 256, 259, 263
lymphocytosis, 109–10
Lyster Army Hospital, Ala., 135–40, 142, 143, 151

McClellan, John L., 249
McDonnell Douglas Corporation, 248
McIlwain, James T., 120–24
McKinley, William, 1
McLaughlin, John T., 189–97, 198, 202
Magnuson, Warren G., 46
Mahon, George M., 249
Makler, Stephen, 220–21
Malmstrom Air Force Base, Mont., 156
Marconi, Guglielmo, 1–2, 3, 4–5
Marha, Karel, 48–50, 53, 121
Marienthal, George, 165, 171
Marino, Andrew, 75n
Markham, Thomas, 170
Marsol, Claude, 86
Martin-Marietta, EMP facility of, 255
Massachusetts Institute of Technology, government contracts of, 248
Massengill, Earl B., 260
Matthews, Arthur H., 301
Maxwell, James Clerk, 2

Maxwell Air Force Base, Ala., 138

Mayo Clinic, 28, 29, 30, 138

Merriman, George R., Jr., 87

Michaelson, Sol M., 66, 76–78, 79, 87, 236, 237, 256, 260, 283, 305–6

Microray Wireless, 5

microwave detection devices, 322, 324

microwave investigations:
  in Czechoslovakia, 48–50, 61, 88–89
  in Soviet Union, 35–40, 43, 48, 73, 77, 78–81, 88–89, 94, 202, 234, 235, 294–96, 297–98, 307, 318
  in U.S., 29–31, 32–35, 36, 37, 40–41, 43–48, 51–53, 57–65, 72–78, 79, 85–86, 88–94, 103–5, 119–21, 128–29, 133, 135–52, 165–66, 172–74, 210–11, 214–18, 236, 238, 281–82, 296, 305

microwave ovens:
  development of, 9
  discounting hazards of, 122, 212, 308–9, 316
  hazards of leakages from, 45, 64, 66–67, 69, 70, 72–73, 76, 200–2, 316–17
  industry links with defense system, 66, 236, 303
  as radiation source, 12, 47, 72, 74, 228
  standards for, 46, 66–67, 68, 73, 76, 202, 228, 305, 317

microwaves:
  audible, 50–52, 84, 234, 322
  behavioral and neurological effects of, 33, 35–36, 39–41, 43, 47, 48, 50, 52–53, 60, 61, 77, 80, 84–86, 94, 97, 101–2, 112–14, 118–24, 129, 236–38, 290–91, 293–301, 309
  biological effects of, *see specific disorders*
  in directed-energy weapons, 255–58, 266–78, 281, 289
  early development of, 1–5
  female births among workers exposed to, 33–34, 37, 49, 159
  future uses of, 9–10
  government concealment of dangers in, 38–41, 59–60, 63–66, 69–71, 75, 85–86, 96, 100, 105–6, 108–9, 116–18, 120, 123–24, 125–27, 129, 133, 134, 137, 139–40, 142–52, 153, 160–63, 169–74, 185, 188–97, 230, 232–33, 239, 249
  heating effects of, 9, 17, 22, 26, 39, 57, 64, 79, 88, 189–92, 233, 237, 306
  legislation for controls on, 42, 45–47, 72
  lengths of, 5, 19
  in medical treatments, 9, 10, 12, 17, 22–23,
    49, 68, 87–88
  need for public protest against, 324–25
  permissible levels of exposure to, 29–31, 33–35, 37–39, 43–47, 49–50, 55, 61, 64–65, 66–67, 69, 73–74, 76–77, 80–81, 85, 88–89, 116–22, 154, 194, 211, 232–37, 256–61, 304–5, 306, 311–12, 317, 323
  present uses of, summarized, 7–9, 227–29
  as security classified, 8–9, 41, 101, 116–18, 209–10, 226, 232, 293–94, 296, 321
  short-wave vs. long-wave controversy and, 4–5

Microwave Systems News, 267

Middleton, Drew, 270

Miletta, J., 253

Milliken, William G., 282–84

Mills, William A., 66

mind-control techniques, 39–41, 60–61, 293–301

Minuteman missiles, EMP and, 252, 256, 261

Missile Materiel Readiness Command (MIR-COM), 210

Missile Tracking Radar (MTR), 211

Mitre Corporation, 248

Montgomery, Thomas E., 203–8

Moose, Richard, 128

Moscow Embassy, U.S., irradiation of, 15, 42, 95–134, 197, 290–92, 307–8
  cancer connected with, 128–31, 292
  concealed from State Department employees, 40, 69, 98–99, 100, 104–5, 134
  discovery of, 39–40
  employee suits relating to, 98, 99, 127, 134
  epidemiological studies on, 101, 104, 110, 118–19, 125, 128–31, 133
  genetic damage and, 132–34
  health issue in, 40, 95–96, 97–99, 100, 103, 108–12, 114–15, 127, 128, 132–34, 292
  health problems attributed to causes other than, 111–14, 128
  levels of, 96, 100, 103, 109, 116–20, 122–23, 127, 307, 323
  motive for, 40, 60–61, 69, 70, 97, 252, 291
  official positions taken on, 40, 61, 69, 95–98, 99, 100–2, 103, 104, 105–6, 108, 109–14, 126, 127, 128, 133, 134, 269, 292, 323–24
  Pandora Project and, 40, 61, 70, 117–23, 125, 133–34, 307
  press revelations on, 95–96, 97–98, 99–100, 101, 102–4, 107, 112–13, 128–29
  U.S. vs. Soviet responsibility for, 126

Moscow Embassy *(continued)*
 window-screening protection for, 97, 98,
  99, 100, 307, 324
Mumford, William W., 260

Nader, Ralph, 144
Nagasaki, 21, 129, 251, 282
National Academy of Science, 306–7
 Committee on Biosphere Effects of Ex-
  tremely-Low-Frequency Radiation of,
  77, 282–83, 284, 305
 National Research Council of, 165, 282
 Naval Studies Board of, 289, 303
National Aeronautics and Space Administra-
  tion (NASA), 63, 102, 267, 288–90, 305
National Cancer Institute, 23, 129
National Institute for Occupational Safety
  and Health (NIOSH), 154–55, 161–63,
  165–71, 196, 202, 203, 214–18, 260, 312
National Institutes of Health, 204
National Security Agency, 8, 126, 161–63, 268,
  288
NAVAIR publications, 172
Naval Aerospace Medical Research Labora-
  tory, Fla., 75, 86, 256, 265, 281
Naval Air Systems Command, 258, 260
Naval Arctic Research Laboratory, Alas., 213
Naval Electronics Systems Command, 163,
  165, 167–68, 263
Naval Materiel Command, 167
Naval Medical Research and Development
  Command, 144–45
Naval Medical Research Institute, 27, 33
Naval Ordinance Laboratory, 258
Naval Research Laboratories, 24, 28, 30, 257,
  263, 268, 275, 277, 285
Naval Research Office, 50, 235–36, 289, 294,
  305
Naval Ship Engineering Center, 304
Naval Weapons Laboratory, Va., 255, 256,
  257, 258, 263, 265
Navy, U.S.:
 Air Rework Facilities of, 166, 168–69, 172
 civilian employee cancer cases and, 164–72
 Electromagnetic Pulse Radiation Environ-
  ment Stimulator for Ships of (EM-
  PRESS), 255
 Environmental Health Center of, 65, 166,
  170
 exposure level standards of, 29, 31, 34, 259,
  304–5

medical studies of, 24, 30
 Occupational Health Workshop of (1976),
  65
 Zaret ophthalmological study and, 65–66,
  69, 238, 304, 305
Navy Medicine and Surgery Bureau, 165, 169,
  236, 260
 Radiation Effects Advisory Board of, 168
Nelson, Gaylord, 249
New Jersey, "golf ball" radar in, 219–27
New Jersey Utilities Department, 305–6
New York Academy of Sciences, 84, 133
New Yorker magazine, 107–8, 182
New York Times, 82, 96–97, 103, 110, 111, 112,
  127, 247, 268, 269–70, 275, 298, 300,
  315–17
New York Times Building, 312–15
North Atlantic Treaty Organization
  (NATO), 35, 235, 236, 237, 240
 Advisory Group for Aerospace Develop-
  ment of (AGARD), 236
 Standardization Agreements of (STA-
  NAG), 235
Northrup Corporation, 248, 268
North Truro, Mass., Air Force's 762nd
  Radar Squadron base in, 319–24
Novak, Robert, 98
Nuclear Intelligence Panel, CIA, 273

Oberlin *News-Tribune,* 181–82
Occupational Safety and Health Act (1970),
  154, 162
Occupational Safety and Health Administration (OSHA), 154–55, 169*n*, 176, 179, 214–
  16, 262, 306
Osepchuk, John M., 66, 76–77, 87, 256, 260,
  308–9, 316
Osnos, Peter, 112–15
Otis Air Force Base, Mass., 226, 227, 243,
  246, 324

Pandora Project, 40, 61, 70, 125, 133–34, 174,
  183, 297–98
 classification of, 101–2, 117–18
 conflicting studies in, 117–23
 destruction of files in, 307
 termination of, 123
Pappas, Nancy, 170
Parr, Wordie H., 155, 165, 215–17, 312–15
Patel, Kumar, 270
Patti, Silvio, 262, 264

PAVE PAWS (Precision Acquisition of Vehicle Entry Phased Array Warning System) radar, 226–27, 231, 240, 241, 243–47, 324
PAVE PENNY, 240
PAVE SPIKE, 240
PAVE TACK, 240
Pavlov, Ivan Petrovich, 39
Peacock, Peter B., 135–38, 140–45, 151
Peyronie's disease, 202
Philco-Ford Corporation, 160–63, 203, 240
PHOENIX system, 241
Pickering, William H., 289
Planck, Max, 18
PNUT (Possible Nuclear Underground Test), 272–73
Pollack, Herbert, 101, 102, 110–11, 114, 118–19, 127, 131, 132, 133, 174, 256, 307
Portasik, Lt. Colonel, 158, 159
power density, 25–26, 28
Prausnitz, Susan, 43
President's Office of Telecommunications Policy, 14, 70, 73, 85, 88–90, 111, 131, 133, 165, 171, 228, 256, 262–64, 265, 281, 309
Privacy Act (1974), 144, 172
Public Health Service, 22, 91–92
purpura, 193

quantum theory, 18
Quonset Naval Air Station, R.I., 164–65, 167, 169–70, 174–75, 179, 199, 307

radar, radar systems:
acronyms for, 239–41
as audible, 50–52, 322
birds affected by, 244–46
birth defects and, 91–92, 104, 133, 134–52, 185–86, 199
in California, 226, 227, 231
cancer and, 164–72
on Cape Cod, 226, 227, 231, 243–44, 246–47, 319–24
cataracts and, 33, 55–60, 63–65, 68–69, 86–87, 94, 174, 183–85, 199, 238–39, 303–4, 321
in FAA operations, 164–78, 179–85
"golf ball," local effects of, 219–27
hazards to civilian employees in, 203–11, 212–13
hearing and sight losses ascribed to, 203–8, 209

infertility and, 24, 198–99, 321
investigations lacking on effects of, 306–7
K- and K/2-band, 6
police, 7, 227, 322
S-band, 6, 30, 136
tissue destruction and, 189–95
types and uses of, 7, 8
in World War II, 5–6, 24–25, 199
X-band, 6, 30, 43–44, 136
see also microwaves; specific devices and systems
radar picket planes, 65
Radar Victims Network, 303
radiant-energy spectrum, 19
radiation absorbed dose (rad), 21
Radiation Control for Health and Safety Act (1968), 45–47, 66, 72
radiotelephony, 3, 4–5, 6, 7
radio transmission, 6–7, 10, 309–13
AM, 7
Citizen's Band, 7, 228
development of, 1–5
FM, 7, 310–13
radio waves, 1, 6–7, 19
extremely-low-frequency (ELF), 75, 241, 280–85
as health hazard, 15, 22–24, 75, 310–13
long-length vs. short-length, 4–5, 15
Rand Corporation, 66, 248
Randomline, 50
Raytheon Company, 9, 25, 45, 66, 76, 171, 226, 243, 248, 256, 260, 287, 289, 305, 308–9
RCA, 219, 220–21, 222, 225, 233, 239, 248
Rechen, Henry J. L., 161
remote transmitters (RTR), 176, 180
Reppert, Barton, 99–100, 101–2, 104, 117, 293–94
Rhea, John, 267–68
Ribicoff, Abraham, 143–44
Ricketts, L. W., 253
Riggs, Arthur A., 260
Robinson, Clarence A., Jr., 272–73, 275–76, 278–79
Rockland Electric Company, 305–6
Rockwell International Corporation, 171, 247, 248, 268, 270, 287–90
roentgen, defined, 19
Roentgen, Wilhelm Conrad, 2, 17
Rose, M. F., 257–61, 277–79
Rose, Vernon E., 161, 200–3, 217–18

Rosenthal, Saul W., 61
Ross, Adele, 224
Rumpel-Leede test, 192, 193

saccharine, 196
Sadcikova, Maria N., 79–80
SADRAM (Seek and Destroy Radar Assisted Mission), 240–41
SAFEGUARD PAR, 241
Samuels, Sheldon, 216, 217
Sandia Corporation, 26, 156–57, 303
Sanguine Project, see Seafarer Project
satellites, communications and surveillance, 7, 8, 9–12
Satterwhite, W., 140
SAWS (satellite-attack warning system), 289
Schereschewsky, Joseph Williams, 22–23
Schilling, Martin, 226
Schlesinger, James, 287
Schwan, Herman P., 29, 30, 33, 44–45, 195, 256, 283
Schwartz, Peter, 268
Seafarer Project, 75–76, 77–78, 237, 249, 280–85, 305
Sea-Launched Ballistic Missile Detection and Warning System (SLBM), 220, 226–27, 242–43, 273
Sealomatic, 213–16
Seasaw Project, 273–74
Senate, U.S., microwave safety investigations of, 32, 42–43, 72–74, 76–78, 86
Senate Armed Services Committee, 284
Senate Commerce Committee, 42, 44, 45, 46, 72, 305, 307
Senate Defense Appropriations Committee, 248–49
SEPAK (Suspension of Expendable Penetration Aids by Kite), 241
Shapley, Deborah, 267
Sharp, Joseph C., 102, 120–21, 123, 256, 260, 263, 295n-96n
Sher, Lawrence, 49–50, 121–23
Sherr, Sava I., 155, 263–64
Shore, Moris L., 79, 304
Skidmore, Wesley D., 261
solar radiation, 6, 12, 76, 228
Solidyne, Inc., 213
Sontag, James M., 129
Southern Research Institute, 135, 137, 140, 141, 146
Soviet State Institute of Physiotherapy, 36

Soviet Union:
  "directed-energy weapons gap" and, 266–78
  microwave investigations and regulations in, 35–40, 43, 48, 73, 77, 78–81, 88–89, 94, 96, 103, 202, 234, 294–95, 297–98, 307, 311, 318, 323
  mind-control research and, 39–41, 60–61, 293–301
  U.S. Embassy and, see Moscow Embassy, U.S., irradiation of
Spassky, Boris, 70
Spencer, Percy, 25
Sperry Gyroscope Company, 33–34
Sperry Rand Corporation, 33
sprains, microwave treatment of, 9, 67–68
Stanford Research Institute, Calif., 156
State Department, U.S., 95–134, 269, 292, 308, 323, 324
Stender, John, 215
sterility, 21, 24, 33, 37, 49, 50, 198–201, 321
Stodolsnik-Baranska, Professor, 130, 133
Stoessel, Walter J., Jr., 95–96, 97–98, 101, 102–3, 105, 108, 115, 126
Stossel, Thomas F., 127, 128, 131
Susskind, Charles, 43–44, 130

TACAN (Tactical Airborne Navigation equipment), 164–71, 176, 179–81, 218, 307
Tanaka, Shiro, 160–61
Target Tracking Radar (TTR), 211
Technical Coordination Conference on EMP Biological Effects, Lovelace Foundation (1970), 156–60, 259
Teledyne, Inc., 171
Teledyne Ryan Aeronautical, 171
telegraphy, development of, 1–2, 3, 4
television, 6, 7, 14, 42, 46, 218, 308–13
Tell, Richard A., 310–12
Tempest Project, 160–63, 203
Terpilak, Michael S., 221
Terrill, James G., Jr., 46–47
Tesla, Nikola, 12–13, 17, 258, 300–1
Thompson, Llewellyn, 128–29
Thomsen, Dietrick E., 276
Tompkins, Edie, 137–40
Towne, Joseph H., 303
Trebets, Frank, 182
Trestle Project, 255
Tri-Service Programs, 32–35, 36, 47, 54–59, 60, 61, 167, 195, 226, 230, 237, 241, 243,

247, 250–51, 256, 264
troposphere, 7
TRW Systems, 248, 267, 268, 285, 289
Tunney, John V., 72–73, 74, 77–78
Tyler, Paul E., 144–45, 155, 165–66, 230, 236,
   238, 247, 250, 256, 260, 264, 303–4, 307

ultraviolet radiation, 19, 90, 129, 194
United Nations Security Council, 40
United Technologies Corporation, 248, 268

Van Allen, James A., 76
Vance, Cyrus, 290, 292
Varian Associates, 171
Vernadskii, Vladimir Ivanovich, 15
Veterans Administration, 64–65, 94, 303
video display terminals (VDT), 228, 315–16
Villforth, John C., 73, 78, 161, 162, 263
vinyl chloride, 196
Volta, Alessandro, 16

Wade, Nicholas, 271–72, 276–77
Walter Reed Army Institute of Research
   (WRAIR), 41, 61, 102, 118–20, 123, 174,
   256, 263, 295*n*, 307
Warren, Shields, 65
Washington Post, 104, 110, 112, 276, 283, 287
Washington Star, 276
Washington University Preventive Medicine
   Department, 186
Watson, William M., 127, 128

wavelength, defined, 2
Weinbrenner shoe plant, Wisc., 213–17
Western Electric Company, 203, 209
Westinghouse, 241, 248, 322
Wheeler, Andrew C., 161
white-blood-cell count abnormalities, 30, 36,
   89, 96–97, 109–11, 112, 114, 115, 127, 190
Whitehead, Clay T., 73–74
Whitten, Les, 69–70, 303–4
Wiley, John, Company, 253
Wilkening, George M., 283
Williams, Henry M., 170–71
Williams, Susan, 319, 321
Winer, Jonathan, 170, 207
wireless transmissions, 2–5, 17
Wold, James W., 115
Woodward, Bob, 287–88
Worden, Frank, 203
Workmen's Compensation Court, 156
World Health Organization, 78, 82, 84, 111
WQXR radio station, 315
Wren, Christopher S., 127, 128

X-band radar, 6, 30, 43–44, 136
X-rays, 1, 2, 17–21, 22, 42, 46, 48, 90, 91, 129,
   166–68, 170, 172, 174, 180, 182, 195, 210,
   291, 317

Zaret, Milton M., 54–66, 69, 73, 74–76, 79,
   81–84, 86–87, 117, 120, 145, 183–85, 196,
   206–7, 238, 297–98, 301, 304, 305, 315, 318